Automation and New Technology in the Clinical Laboratory

Sponsored by the International Union of Pure and Applied Chemistry (IUPAC), Clinical Chemistry Division (VII), Under the auspices of the International Federation of Clinical Chemistry (IFCC), Japan Society of Clinical Pathology, Japan Society of Clinical Chemistry, Japan Society of Clinical Laboratory Automation

ORGANIZATION

Honorary Praesidium
Koki Motegi
Toshitsugu Oda
Tadashi Kawai

International Committee
Pierangelo Bonini
Carl A. Burtis
Terence D. Geary
Rainer Haeckel
Kiyoshi Okuda
Teiichi Sasaki
Kihachiro Takahara

Organizing Committee
CHAIRMAN: Kiyoshi Okuda
Shigeaki Baba
Jiro Endo
Michio Fujimaki
Koichiro Fujita
Junici Fukuda
Iwao Fukui
Itaru Furuta
Chozo Hayashi
Taizo Hayashi
Jun Igari
Sachio Ikawa
Chuichi Ito
Sachiko Kamei
Masamitsu Kanai
Takashi Kanno
Seiji Kasuga
Masaka Kawade
Tadashi Kawai
Hiroshi Kiyose
Kinya Kouno
Akira Kousaka
Hajime Kudo
Ichiro Kurokawa
Katsuhiko Kuwa
Kiyoshi Miyai
Wataru Mizuta
Mikio Mori
Takashi Murachi
Hajime Naka
Keiichi Naka
Kazuo Niitani
Shozo Nomoto
Yasuhiro Oba
Hiroaki Okabe
Jiro Okawa
Shozo Omori
Kyoichi Ozawa
Yoshikatsu Sakagishi
Tetsuo Sanochi
Masahide Sasaki
Teiichi Sasaki
Mitsuo Sekiguchi
Nobuo Shimojo
Kozo Shiota
Genji Suganuma
Jutaro Tadano
Kihachiro Takahara
Noriyuki Tatsumi
Kunihiro Ueda
Satoshi Ueda
Shiro Uesugi
Toshiaki Usui
Masao Wakabayashi
Eiko Yabuuchi
Minoru Yakata
Mitsuo Yamada
Yoshinori Yamamoto
Manabu Yamanaka

Scientific Committee
CHAIRMAN: Teiichi Sasaki
Masuo Aizawa
Pierangelo Bonini
Carl A. Burtis
Terence D. Geary
Rainer Haeckel
Takekazu Horio
Tadashi Kawai
Hajime Kudo
Kiyoshi Miyai
Keiichi Naka
Kiyoshi Okuda
Teiichi Sasaki
Noriyuki Tatsumi
Chr. Trendelenburg
Alain Truchaud

Secretariat
Kihachiro Takahara
Keiichi Naka

International Union of Pure and Applied Chemistry

Automation and New Technology in the Clinical Laboratory

Proceedings of the IUPAC 3rd International Congress on Automation and New Technology in the Clinical Laboratory held in Kobe, Japan, 5–8 September 1988

EDITED BY

KIYOSHI OKUDA

Department of Laboratory Medicine,
Osaka City University Medical School,
Japan

Blackwell Scientific Publications

OXFORD LONDON

EDINBURGH BOSTON MELBOURNE

and published for them by
Blackwell Scientific Publications
Editorial offices:
Osney Mead, Oxford OX2 0EL
25 John Street, London WC1N 2BL
23 Ainslie Place, Edinburgh EH3 6AJ
3 Cambridge Center, Suite 208
Cambridge, Massachusetts 02142, USA
107 Barry Street, Carlton
Victoria 3053, Australia

First published 1990

Printed in Great Britain
at the Alden Press, Oxford
and bound at the
Green Street Bindery, Oxford

DISTRIBUTORS

Marston Book Services Ltd
PO Box 87
Oxford OX2 0DT
(*Orders*: Tel: 0865 791155
Fax: 0865 791927
Telex: 837515)

USA
Publishers' Business Services
PO Box 447
Brookline Village
Massachusetts 02147
(*Orders*: Tel: (617) 524-7678)

Canada
Oxford University Press
70 Wynford Drive
Don Mills
Ontario M3C 1J9
(*Orders*: Tel: (416) 441-2941)

Australia
Blackwell Scientific Publications
(Australia) Pty Ltd
107 Barry Street
Carlton, Victoria 3053
(*Orders*: Tel: (03) 347-0300)

British Library
Cataloguing in Publication Data

IUPAC International Congress on Automation
and New Technology in the Clinical
Laboratory (3rd: 1988: Kobe, Japan)
Automation and new technology in
the clinical laboratory.
1. Pathology laboratories. Applications
of computer systems.
I. Title II. Okuda, Kiyoshi
616.07'028'5

ISBN 0-632-02819-X

Library of Congress
Cataloguing in Publication Data

IUPAC International Congress on Automation and New Technology in the Clinical Laboratory (3rd: 1988: Kōbe-shi, Japan)—Automation and new technology in the clinical laboratory: proceedings of the IUPAC 3rd International Congress on Automation and New Technology in the Clinical Laboratory held in Kobe, Japan, 5–8 September 1988/edited by Kiyoshi Okuda.
p. cm.
At head of title: International Union of Pure and Applied Chemistry.
ISBN 063202819 X
1. Diagnosis, Laboratory—Automation—Congresses. 2. Diagnosis, Laboratory—Technological innovations—Congresses. I. Okuda, Kiyoshi, 1927– . II. International Union of Pure and Applied Chemistry. III. Title.
RB38.I86 1988 616.07'5—dc20

Contents

Preface

Much of the recent progress in medical science and medical care can be attributed to developments in laboratory medicine. Usually, an advance in methodology leads to developments in the field of science; past innovations in laboratory medicine have always been supported by improvements in methodology achieved through the active introduction, understanding, and application of technology from chemistry, physics, biology, and related fields. For the future development of laboratory medicine, continued close interaction with the new technologies of these related fields is essential.

The 3rd International Congress on Automation and New Technology in the Clinical Laboratory took place at the International Congress Center in Kobe, Japan, on 3–8 September 1988, and was a great success in promoting such interaction. The editor takes great pleasure in thanking all those whose efforts have made possible the publication of these proceedings. I thank, in particular, Drs C. Burtis, P. Bonini, R. Haeckel and T. Geary as members of the International Committee, and also Drs K. Naka and N. Shimojo for their supervision of the Secretariat.

At this meeting, many researchers from Japan and overseas gathered to speak about their research and to exchange opinions on automation in the clinical laboratory, including the theory and practical applications of the latest technologies. I firmly believe that the conference greatly contributed to further developments in clinical laboratory medicine.

Kiyoshi Okuda
Editor
Chairman of the Organizing Committee

Recent technological developments and their impact on laboratory automation

Carl A. Burtis

Chemical Technology and Health Divisions, Oak Ridge National Laboratory,*
Oak Ridge, Tennessee 37831

INTRODUCTION

Several technological developments have occurred during the past 15 years and have resulted in a new generation of analytical systems in which all the instrumental, methodological, and reagent components are integrated into a single self-contained unit (1). Such systems (termed "closed") are highly automated, and many of the analytical operations that once required human intervention or labor are now performed by the system. The availability of these new systems that minimize the need for human involvement in the analytical process will have a significant impact on how the clinical laboratory of the future is staffed, equipped, organized, and operated.

TECHNOLOGIES

The analytical systems currently available to the clinical laboratory are the end products resulting from the combination and integration of several technologies into a single functional unit. These include microchips, chemometrics, robotics, sensors, immunodiagnostics, and prepackaged reagents (2).

Microchips

It is appropriate to begin this section with a discussion on microchips since this technology has produced the modern digital computer, which is considered by many to be the most significant development of the twentieth century. Originally, the first digital computers were built using vacuum tubes (3). However, these computers were physically large (i.e., weighed 30 tons), relatively slow, and required numerous specialists to operate them. As a result of the development of the microchips, computers are now available that range from the powerful mainframes to the small, compact micro and personal units. Computers are constantly being improved, with each new generation being smaller, faster, more powerful, and less expensive than their predecessors (4).

The key to this continuing evolution of powerful computers was the invention of the transistor (5) and its subsequent integration onto microchips of silicon (4). Additional developments made in the areas of microlithography and microfabrication also played major roles, as engineers have been able to approximately double every year the number of electronic components contained on a chip, while at the same time dramatically decreasing the size and unit costs. For example, relatively inexpensive microchips that contain a million components on a 5-mm square of silicon are now available.

One of the most important products of this technology is the microprocessor, which is essentially the central processing unit of a digital computer and is contained on a single microchip. The advent of this device, along with the personal and microcomputers which it spawned, has resulted in a new breed of computerized instruments that incorporates them as core components. These instruments have become known as "smart," "expert," or "intelligent" since they possess memory and logic capabilities, and they have brought a high degree of sophistication to laboratory analyses. The microprocessor serves several functions in analytical instruments. First, it provides for automatic data acquisition, management, reduction, and display; and, with the availability of tremendous memory capacity at a relatively low cost, very sophisticated algorithms can now be routinely implemented. Its second function is process control, which allows the various operating parameters of an instrument to be monitored and, if necessary, automatically adjusted. This type of feedback control ensures optimal operation and, in fact, allows for real-time automation in the laboratory. (An automatic system is defined as a system having a self-acting or self-

*Operated by Martin Marietta Energy Systems, Inc., under contract DE-AC05-84OR21400 with the U.S. Department of Energy.

regulating mechanism; prior to the advent of microprocessors, most analytical instruments in the clinical laboratory were simply mechanized, not automated.) An additional benefit from process control by microprocessors is that real-time monitoring of the performance of various components of a system is useful diagnostically. If a component fails, or is beginning to fail, the microprocessor can alert the operator to take corrective action. This greatly facilitates the maintenance and repair of instruments and ensures their availability on a routine basis.

Another function of the microprocessor is its role in the integration of a hierarchy of computers into a single network. In order to provide a data management system for all the computers found in a clinical laboratory and its hospital environment, all of the computer systems need to be linked into a single integrated network. Difficulties have been encountered in interfacing the myriad types of instruments found in the laboratory into a centralized computer network, since each instrument has unique requirements for interfacing its analog outputs to a digital device. With the advent of microprocessor instruments, such interfacing can be done internally for each instrument. The digital outputs from each instrument can then be transmitted to, and accepted by, the next computer in the network. Computer networking allows the information generated for every patient to be automatically acquired and stored into a unified data base where it can be recalled, processed, and managed. With the linking of terminals and/or intelligent workstations (6-8) to this network of computers, the information generated is immediately available and can be disseminated in real time.

The availability of microprocessors has also revolutionized the basic concepts of instrument design. For example, now many operation functions are controlled either by "software" or by "firmware" [i.e., read-only memory (ROM) chips that have been programmed by the manufacturer]. As a consequence, changes in the operation and capabilities of instruments can now be implemented through changes in software (via a disk), a memory board, or a microchip on a board. Additional testing functions can thus be included, and instrument capabilities can be upgraded very easily. Instrument repair is also made simpler and faster, since malfunction due to a faulty component can often be remedied via replacement of a memory board, either by a service representative or (sometimes) a user. With modern, overnight delivery of replacement parts, instrument repair is usually facilitated and downtime is minimized.

Chemometrics

Chemometrics is defined as the application of mathematical and statistical methods to chemical measurements (9). The key to the evolution of chemometrics as a definable discipline has been the advent of computer technology. The advances in computer capabilities and the software developed for chemometrics have resulted in systems that are able to acquire, store, process, and manage large data sets in real time using a wide variety of sophisticated algorithms.

Since the clinical laboratory has always applied mathematical and statistical methods to produce analytical data, it is not surprising that many of the techniques resulting from advances in chemometrics are now being utilized. These include advanced statistics (10), modeling and parameter estimation (11), resolution (12), imaging (13), pattern recognition (14-16), optimization and control (17-22), artificial intelligence (23-24), and computer-assisted interpretation (25-28).

Robotics

Humans have long been fascinated by the idea of robots that can perform and relieve them of various mundane, strenuous, or dangerous tasks. Recent advances in computer technology, chemometrics, artificial intelligence, and sensor technology have now made it possible for robots to perform such tasks in factories, in space, beneath the sea, and, more recently, in laboratories (29-34).

Currently, the robots that are available for laboratory applications are either pickup and delivery vehicles (35) or sampling and reagent processing units (36). The commercially produced processing robots consist of robotic arms, gripper devices (i.e., hands, sensors), and microcomputers. Joints are added to give the robot three-dimensional mobility. As a result, the robotic arms can move to specified spatial coordinates and can thus perform many of the human arm and finger-pair operations.

Robotic devices have several advantages over the dedicated instruments or manual operations that they replace. The most significant is that they can be easily reprogrammed for a variety of tasks. Consequently, the use of robots offers the laboratory a cost-effective means of achieving complete automation, with the flexibility to perform numerous types of analyses.

Sensors

A sensor is a device that responds to a physical stimulus and generates a resulting impulse. In clinical instrumentation, electrochemical and optical sensors are used for both measurement and monitoring purposes. In addition, bar-code readers are becoming widely employed for identification purposes.

Electrochemical sensors. Over the past decade, important advances in the disciplines of electrochemistry, solid-state chemistry, and membrane technology have led to the commercial production of a wide variety of ion-specific electrodes (ISEs). Many clinical laboratories now routinely use ISEs for measuring blood gases, electrolytes, metabolites, and some amino acids (37-40).

Microsensors called chemically sensitive field-effect transistors (CHEMFETS) and ion-sensitive, field-effect transistors (ISFETS) have been developed (41-44) in an attempt to decrease the size and volume requirements of ISEs. These sensors are solid-state chemical devices that are made by joining ISE membrane material to the sensitive gate area of a field-effect transistor. The microfabrication and microlithographic techniques employed to produce integrated circuit chips can be used to obtain an active element that is only 2 mm^2.

Because of their small size, several microsensors can be manufactured on a single chip to yield a device having multiple-analyte capabilities. To demonstrate the feasibility of this concept, an electrode was fabricated having two ISFET sensors — for independent H^+ and K^+ monitoring (45). Using various ionophores, enzymes, antibodies, and plenty of imagination, it seems conceivable that a single microdetector produced on a single chip could be used to measure a wide range of clinically significant analytes. Such devices could be incorporated into "dip and read" instruments or strategically placed in instruments that utilize flowing streams. Such instruments would not require chemical reagents and would be much less complex than existing clinical analyzers, since all the detector and ancillary electronics could be combined into a single compact unit.

Optical sensors. Spectrophotometric and fluorophotometric methods continue to be the most widely used analytical techniques in the clinical laboratory. Sensors used for these measurements traditionally consisted of a light source, a photomultiplier tube, and some type of monochromator to obtain monochromatic light. However, recent developments in solid-state electronics and manufacturing techniques have made available sensors that utilize small, intense light sources or light-emitting diodes, solid-state detectors, and high quality interference filters. As a result, the optics of modern instrumentation are simpler and more compact, reliable, and versatile than those in the older units. In addition, it was not uncommon for earlier clinical instruments to have several optical monitors contained in a single unit. However, with the availability of fiber optics, modern instruments now only need a single optical unit with multiple paths of light transmitted via individual light pipes. The use of light pipes also eliminates the need for the optical system to be situated in close proximity to the measuring cuvettes; thus, it can now be placed in a location which affords easy access for maintenance and repair.

In addition to these general improvements in the overall optical systems, specific technical developments have been made in both detectors and light sources. For example, linear diode array detectors are now available, and various lasers are being more widely used in clinical instrumentation.

Since both the quality and the quantity of the information gained from a spectrophotometric measurement are directly proportional to the wavelength range monitored, analytical and clinical chemists have long desired instrumentation with multiwavelength measuring capabilities. For research applications, multiwavelength measurements can be obtained with a high-performance scanning spectrophotometer; however, this has not been a time- or cost-effective approach for routine clinical analyses. Consequently, laboratory instruments have used single-wavelength monitors connected in parallel, or in sequence, or a single polychromatic system in which multiple wavelengths are obtained by varying the light source or via mechanical manipulation of the filters, grating, or prism.

Photodiode array and vidicon tube detectors that permit rapid and simultaneous measurements at multiple wavelengths are now commercially available (46). When interfaced with a microcomputer, these detectors permit the rapid collection of intensity data at hundreds of wavelengths, as well as data processing with a variety of sophisticated algorithms.

Until recently, linear diode array technology was available to the clinical laboratory only as a stand-alone spectrophotometer or as a detector for use in a liquid chromatograph. However, the new analytical systems appearing in the clinical marketplace feature linear diode array detectors as integral components (47). Their multiwavelength monitoring capabilities offer the analyst new ways of obtaining, processing, and interpreting data. The results are higher-quality clinical information and an increased ability to explore new analytical approaches. For example, since a complete and updated spectrum is always available, multiple analytes can be simultaneously monitored and the possibility of interferences assessed. In addition, sample and reagent blanking can be performed optically, rather than chemically, and both first- and second-derivative spectrometric techniques can be implemented (which also eliminates background contributions from the chemical reaction in question). Another advantage of significance to clinical laboratories is the fact that linear array detectors have no moving parts; thus, they are more reliable than conventional detectors.

Since a laser is a very powerful light source, it will continue to be used in optical systems where enhanced sensitivity and selectivity are required (48). Already, lasers have been employed in chromatographic detectors (49,50) and in flow cytometers, devices which, in conjunction with monoclonal antibodies, have revolutionized both the quantitative and qualitative aspects of cell counting (51). When used to induce fluorescence, argon-ion lasers have decreased the detection limits for analytically useful dyes to the attogram level (52) and have allowed measurement of very low cytochrome enzyme activities (53). In addition, lasers have been used as ionization sources in atomic absorption spectrometers (54,55) and in mass spectrometers (56). Consequently, trace-metal analysis has been improved, and biological compounds having higher molecular weights can now be quantitated by mass spectrometry.

Bar-code readers. Bar-code labels and readers are being used as a means of identifying patients throughout their stay in a health care facility (57,58). This technology is also being incorporated into analytical systems, not only to identify patients and their specimens but also to identify reagents, lot numbers, and even to enter calibration factors into the systems. This integrated use of bar-code technology throughout the analytical process facilitates the tracking of the information generated for each patient, ensures correct identification, and removes the possibility of human transcription and translation errors. The resulting effect of combining programmable robotic arms with a means of identifying both reagents and specimens via a machine-readable bar-code device allows an analytical system to analyze any specimen for any analyte in any sequence. Thus, the system has selective access capability, a feature desired by clinical chemists.

Immunodiagnostics

In 1959, Berson and Yalow (59) reported the development of a revolutionary new type of assay which combined the specificity inherent in the antibody/antigen interaction and the excellent sensitivity obtainable from radioisotope measurements. Since that time, immunoassays have become one of the most important and widely used of all bioanalytical techniques.

The antibody, or the antiserum in which it is contained, is the key reagent of an immunoassay. Initially, antibodies were obtained by first injecting animals with a quantity of purified or semipurified immunogen, and then processing the blood taken from the immunized animals. Because antibodies are biological compounds, their variability, stability, and availability have been of concern, and a great deal of effort has been expended on ensuring and documenting the essential properties and characteristics of antibody reagents (e.g., affinity, avidity, specificity, stability).

In 1975, Kohler and Milstein (60) reported the development of a cell fusion technique that has revolutionized the immunodiagnostic industry. In this new technology two different types of cells are fused to create a new type, called a hybridoma, which exhibits characteristics derived from both parents. For example, fusing fast-growing myeloma tumor cells with spleen cells derived from an animal that has been immunized with a specific antigen yields hybridomas that secrete antibodies against this antigen. Subsequent selection from the population of fused cells can isolate hybridomas that secrete a monoclonal antibody, having a unique set of biochemical characteristics and properties. In addition to antibody-producing capabilities, the hybridomas acquire the growth characteristics of the myeloma parent and can be propagated by cell culture or other techniques to provide continuous quantities of the monoclonal antibody.

As immunochemical reagents, monoclonal antibodies have two significant advantages over conventional antibody reagents: (1) they have a unique and narrow antigenic specificity, and (2) they can be used to produce large quantities of essentially identical antibodies. Thus, it is possible to prepare large quantities of monoclonal antibodies while maintaining both consistent yields and lot-to-lot quality.

Initially, radioisotopes were used as labels in immunoassays since the capability then existed for measuring very low levels of radioactivity. However, numerous problems associated with radioactivity (i.e., isotope decay, health and safety considerations, waste disposal) led to efforts to utilize other labels. In 1972, Rubenstein, Schneider, and Ullman (61) reported a new type of immunoassay in which the radioactive label was replaced by an enzyme. Since that time, numerous immunoassays have been developed using enzyme, fluorescence, chemiluminescent, or electrochemical tags as signal molecules. These procedures, termed nonisotopic immunoassays, have significant advantages over radioimmunoassays: (1) they provide equivalent sensitivity; (2) their reagents are stable; (3) they pose no safety, health, or disposal problems; and (4) they are amenable to automation with instruments commonly used in the laboratory for routine analysis. Thus, the utility of analytical systems is enhanced as their repertoire of available methods is greatly increased. For example, analytical systems now include methods not only for routine chemistries but also immunomethods for isoenzymes, drugs, hormones, coagulation factors, and tumor markers. In addition, immunoassays are now becoming available for identifying many infectious bacterial and viral organisms — a capability which further enhances the utility of the analytical systems that are now available to the laboratory.

Prepackaged reagents

Recent advances in photographic, coating, plastic, and materials technologies have resulted in prepackaged reagents that are available as packets (62), thin films (63), strips (64,65), or tablets (66). Use of the reagents in a dry form with subsequent reconstitution performed internally within and by the instrument, or upon application of a liquid sample, has several advantages. These include: (1) elimination of the need to manually reconstitute reagents into a liquid form, which is a time-consuming, labor-intensive, and error-prone process; (2) minimization of reagent waste; (3) reduced reagent storage needs; (4) prolonged shelf life; and (5) operational simplicity since multistep procedures are reduced to a single step, which is initiated upon introduction or application of the sample. As a result of these advantages, less technical skill is needed and reagents can be managed in an efficient and cost-effective manner.

System integration

The technologies discussed here have individually influenced the practice of clinical laboratory science. Collectively, their greatest impact has resulted from their integration into the advanced analytical systems that are now available to the laboratory. With these systems, analytical processes such as calibration, monitoring, and computation can be performed automatically with little or no operator intervention. In addition, artificial intelligence is rapidly being incorporated into these systems, and they now have the capability of judging whether they are operating properly, deciding whether they will accept data, and automatically transferring the accepted data through a network of computers to make results immediately accessible to medical practitioners through terminals or work stations. Although these sophisticated systems incorporate the most complex state-of-the-art technology, they have a very simple external appearance and are easy to operate.

These new systems incorporate stable, solid-state electronics, have a minimum of moving parts, and, with use of advanced computer-assisted design and fabrication techniques, are more rugged and reliable than earlier laboratory instruments. They are also capable of self-regulation and self-diagnosis, and most repairs involve only simple changes of a circuit board or module by laboratory personnel. They are becoming increasingly very versatile and have selective-access capability. Only those specific tests ordered are performed; and, as new tests are developed by the manufacturer, they will be quickly implemented in the field by the addition of prepackaged reagents and a new chip, board, or floppy disk.

In addition, the new analytical systems have the capability for automating the entire analytical process, which results in decreased labor costs and, consequently, increased cost effectiveness. Prior to 1957, all the individual steps of an analytical process were performed manually. With the advent of the AutoAnalyzer in 1957 (67), many of these steps were mechanized. When digital electronics appeared in the late 1960s and microprocessors in the 1970s, many of the procedures became automated. The introduction of robotics in the 1980s made it possible to completely automate the analytical process, including sample processing.

SUMMARY

The analytical capabilities of the clinical laboratory have continued to expand and improve as a result of technical developments and advancements made in a wide spectrum of allied disciplines. As a consequence, the clinical laboratory has evolved from the small, manual operations of yesterday to the large, central organizations of today. Technology continues to impact the laboratory, especially with the advent of the fully automated analytical systems that are having such a profound effect on how the laboratory is staffed, equipped, organized, and operated. With the accelerating rate at which new developments are occurring, it is safe to assume that dramatic changes will continue to occur in this area. Consequently, it will become increasingly important for clinical laboratorians to be aware of these new developments, to understand them, and to anticipate how they will be assimilated and integrated into the overall health care system. To quote from a recent Bell Atlantic advertisement, "The genius of the future lies not in technology alone, but in the ability to manage it."

REFERENCES

1. C.A. Burtis, Clin. Chem. 33, 352-357 (1987).
2. C.A. Burtis, The Clinical Laboratory in the New Era, E. Bermes, Ed., pp. 247-287, AACC Press, Washington, D.C. (1985).
3. E.A. Feigenbaum and P. McCorduck, The Fifth Generation, New American Library, New York (1984).
4. A.A. Boraiko, National Geographic 162, 421-458 (1982).
5. J. Bardeen, Science 84, 143-148 (November 1984).
6. R.E. Dessy, Anal. Chem. 57, 77-94A (1985).
7. R.E. Dessy, Anal. Chem. 57, 310-331A (1985).
8. R.E. Dessy, Anal. Chem. 58, 678-689A (1986).

9. B.R. Kowalski, J. Chem. Inf. Comput. Sci. 15, 201-203 (1975).
10. S.N. Deming, Clin. Chem. 32, 1702-1706 (1986).
11. I.E. Frank and B.R. Kowalski, Anal. Chem. 54, 232-243R (1982).
12. M.F. Delaney, Anal. Chem. 56, 261-277R (1984).
13. N.L. Anderson and N.G. Anderson, Clin. Chem. 30, 1898-1905 (1984).
14. R.T.P. Jansen, F.W. Pijpers, and G.A.J.M. DeValk, Anal. Chim. Acta 133, 1-18 (1981).
15. J.P. Bretaudiere, G. Dumont, R. Rej, and M. Bailly, Clin. Chem. 27, 798-805 (1981).
16. B.R. Kowalski, Anal. Chem. 52, 112-122R (1980).
17. R.D. Krause and J.A. Lott, Clin. Chem. 20, 775-782 (1974).
18. S.N. Deming and S.L. Morgan, Anal. Chim. Acta 150, 183-198 (1983).
19. G.S. Rautela, R.D. Snee, and W.K. Miller, Clin. Chem. 24, 1954-1964 (1979).
20. C.A. Burtis, W.D. Bostick, J.B. Overton, and J.E. Mrochek, Anal. Chem. 53, 1154-1159 (1981).
21. N.W. Tietz, C.A. Burtis, P. Duncan et al., Clin. Chem. 29, 751-761 (1983).
22. J.G. Vollenbrock and B.G.M. Vandeginste, Anal. Chem. 133, 85-97 (1981).
23. P.G. King, Intelligent Instruments and Computers, 4 (January 1983).
24. M.M. Waldrop, Science 85, 38-45 (March 1985).
25. J.R. Beck, Clin. Chem. 32, 1707-1713 (1986).
26. J.D. Meyers, Clin. Chem. 32, 1714-1718 (1986).
27. F. Van Lente, W. Castellani, D. Chou, R.N. Matzen, and R.S. Galen, Clin. Chem. 32, 1719-1725 (1986).
28. J.C. Boyd, Clin. Chem. 32, 1726-1733 (1986).
29. E. Fredkin, Res. Dev., 242-249 (June 1984).
30. R. Dessy, Anal. Chem. 55, 1100-1114A (1983).
31. R. Dessy, Anal. Chem. 55, 1232-1242A (1983).
32. P. Albertson, Res. Dev., 76-78 (December 1984).
33. G.L. Hawk, Clin. Chem. 30, 937 (1984).
34. Advances in Laboratory Automation — Robotics, G.L. Hawk and J. Strimaitis, Eds., Vol. I (1983), Vol. II (1984), Zymark Corporation, Hopkinton, Massachusetts.
35. D. Seligson, Clin. Chem. 29, 1154 (1983).
36. B.J. McGrattan and D.J. Macero, Am. Lab., 16-24 (September 1984).
37. M.A. Arnold and M.E. Meyerhoff, Anal. Chem. 56, 20-48R (1984).
38. G.A. Rechnitz, Anal. Chem. 54, 1194-1200A (1982).
39. J.D. Czaban, Anal. Chem. 57, 345-356A (1985).
40. M.A. Arnold and R.L. Solsky, Anal. Chem. 58, 84-101R (1986).
41. J. Janata and R.J. Huber, Ion-Selective Electrodes in Analytical Chemistry, H. Freiser, Ed., Vol. 2, pp. 107-174, Plenum Press, New York (1980).
42. H. Wohltjen, Anal. Chem. 56, 87-103A (1984).
43. S.D. Caras, J. Janata, D. Saupe, and K. Schmitt, Anal. Chem. 57, 1917-1920 (1985).
44. S.D. Caras, D. Petelenz, and J. Janata, Anal. Chem. 57, 1920-1923 (1985).
45. B.A. McKinley, B.A. Houtchens, and J. Janata, Ion-Selective Elect. Rev. 6, 173-185 (1984).
46. W.E. Weiser and H.L. Pardue, Clin. Chem. 29, 1673-1677 (1983).
47. S.G. Schultz, J.T. Holen, J.P. Donohue, and T.A. Francoer, Clin. Chem. 31, 1457-1463 (1985).
48. T.D. Harris, Anal. Chem. 54, 741-750A (1982).
49. R.B. Green, Anal. Chem. 55, 20-32A (1983).
50. M.P. Maskarinec, M.J. Sepaniak, A.T. Balchunus, and J.D. Vargo, Clin. Chem. 30, 1473-1476 (1984).
51. R.A. Hoffman, Biotech. Lab. 2, 38-50 (1984).
52. N.J. Dovichi, M.D. Martin, J.H. Jett, M. Trkula, and R.A. Keller, Anal. Chem. 56, 348-354 (1984).
53. B.Z. Egan, N.E. Lee, C.A. Burtis, J.Y. Kao, and J.M. Holland, Clin. Chem. 29, 1616-1619 (1983).
54. J.C. Travis, G.C. Turk, and R.B. Green, Anal. Chem. 54, 1006-1016A (1982).
55. J.C. Travis, G.C. Turk, and J.R. DeVoe, Clin. Chem. 29, 1683-1686 (1983).
56. R.J. Cotter, Anal. Chem. 56, 485-504A (1984).
57. A. Rappoport, Healthy Industry Lines, 7-8 (March/April 1986).
58. E. Maclin and D.S. Young, Clinical Chemistry, N.W. Tietz, Ed., pp. 238-240, W.B. Saunders, Philadelphia, Pennsylvania (1986).
59. S.A. Berson and R.S. Yalow, J. Clin. Invest. 38, 1996-2006 (1959).
60. G. Kohler and C. Milstein, Nature 256, 495-497 (1975).
61. K.E. Rubenstein, R.S. Schneider, and E.F. Ullman, Biochem. Biophys. Res. Commun. 47, 846-851 (1972).
62. D.S. Young, Fundamentals of Clinical Chemistry, 2nd ed., N.W. Tietz, Ed., pp. 197-199, W.B. Saunders, Philadelphia, Pennsylvania (1976).
63. H.G. Curme, R.L. Columbus, G.M. Dappen et al., Clin. Chem. 24, 1335-1342 (1978).
64. B. Walter, Anal. Chem. 55, 498-514A (1983).
65. B. Chernow, B.A. Diaz, and D. Cruess, Crit. Care Med. 10, 463-465 (1982).
66. R.C. Driscoll, R.B. Edwards, M.D. Liston et al., Clin. Chem. 29, 1609-1615 (1983).
67. L.T. Skeggs, Jr., Am. J. Clin. Pathol. 28, 311-322 (1957).

Portions of this manuscript previously appeared in Clinical Chemistry 33, 352-357, 1987, and are reproduced here with permission.

Developments in dry chemistry, and the situation in Japan

Kiyoshi Okuda

Department of Laboratory Medicine, Osaka City University Medical School, Osaka 545, Japan

Abstract – On the way of development of modern clinical laboratory methods, the dry chemistry has been innovating the process of determination of various constituents in urine and blood at clinics and hospitals, as well as emancipated the laboratory examinations to openfields or every one's home. Preprogrammed laboratory analytic procedures are condenced in a thin and small piece of paper, without any skills you can find many informations anytime and anywhere. These single tests is free from heavy instrumentations and complicated equipments operations. I have been strongly interested in this technology during this decade, and reported several inventions by myself. Here I will review what my colleagues in Japan has been contributing in this field, at 1950's there was the first milestone, 60's we found the next milestone, 70's saw the third milestone and what is happenning today.

INTRODUCTION

During the last three decades, we have seen great advances in the technology of clinical chemistry in which dry reagents are used. As you know, many countries have made great contributions to this field. The United States has consistently led the way, and the innovations from Europian countries in particular, have been of much importance. Japan has perhaps been number 2 after the U. S. in the numbers of developments made. There have been three milestones in dry chemistry during the development of its technology.

On the way of development of modern clinicla1 laboratory methods, the creation of the Clinitest® in 1945 was the first introduction of dry chemistry to this field. It was a dry tablet, not a strip which later became most common. In 1956, two still more convenient test systems were introduced by independent two groups. One was called the Clinistix®, which was developed by Dr. Free, and the other was the Glukotest® by Dr. Comer. Dr. Free popularized the concept of 'dip-and-read' testing in urinalysis, and this is still widely applied throughout the world.

The second milestone was the instrumentation of dry chemistry. In 1967, I introduced the use of reflectance measurements to read strips (ref. 1). Reflectance had previously been used by house painters to standardize or compare the colors of painted walls. Reagent strips and a instrument system for the reading of reflectance emerged for use in the quantitative analysis of both urine and blood constituents.

The next milestone was the application of multiple-layer film techniques. This was first developed by the Kodak company, which reported one method in 1978 at the International Congress on Clinical Chemistry in Mexico City. With this technology, some of the factors that can be controlled include the matrix thickness, fiber density, solvent absorbence, molecular sieving effect, and lamination of different materials. These factors can be combined in new ways to generate more sophisticated dry chemistry systems.

HISTORICAL BACKGROUND

Paper impregnated with litmus was probably the first invention involving dry chemistry in this field, and it appeared in the 19th century. In 1930, Mr. Goro Oikawa introduced a commercially available pH indicator paper at the Japanese Exhibitsion for Chemical Industries. This invention is a little-known milestone even in this field in the development of semi-quantitative estimation using color scales. I am mentioning it today because Japanese have often reported important inventions and innovations in the Japanese language only, so they are not accessible to workers from other countries. As you know, we depend strongly on such pH indicator paper in clinical situations to estimate the pH of body fluids or reagent solutions very instant.

In 1935, Feigl reported a modern dry chemistry technique that combined the reagent and the sample on filter paper. This work suggested many ideas to a number of clinical chemists about possible further applications. A enzymatic method using the glucose oxidase reaction specific for glucose was developed by Keilin and Hartree in 1945. These two inventions helped give rise to the dry chemistry strip in 1956 for the estimation of glucose in urine. As Dr. Free writes in one of his

articles, 'this convenient approach was the basis for subsequent analytical chemical systems for all types of urine tests' (ref. 2).
After the appearance of urine reagent strips for the testing of urinary glucose, we had to wait for eight years for the appearance of the Dextrostix®, used for the semi-quantitative analysis of blood sugar. It had the same basic configuration as urine reagent strips.
In the 1950s, test strips for urinalysis were impregnated fibers on a plastic supporting strip. With this system, control of the propagation of the reaction was difficult, calling for the development of dry-format chemistry with compounds immobilized in a fiber matrix for the testing of constituents. The reaction was somewhat dependent on sample volume. Also, another difficulty the system had arose when one wanted to use the reagent strip with impregnated fibers for the estimation of blood glucose concentration. Blood contains the blood cells in half of the volume, as well as red blood cell includes color materials in it, strongly these disturb the measurement with the reagent strips for urine. Before the application of the blood sample onto the strip, it *must* be necessary to separate out the serum for use as the sample.
The Dextrostix® was introduced in 1964. It had the interesting characteristic of a semipermeable membrane that covered the reagent area. When a drop of whole blood is placed on the strip, soluble glucose passes through the semipermeable membrane. It reacts with glucose oxidase, and the reaction is followed by the catalytic oxidation of a chromogen by peroxidase, producing a blue color. The blood cells are washed off after processed these reaction, therefor no interference come arise from the color materials in blood.
During this period I was particularly interested in dry chemistry. I developed a test strip method for serum bilirubin measurement. This was the first landmark along the path of research that I have been following since then. At that time, I had the idea that it might be possible to measure serum constituents by a dry chemistry method quantitatively. This was accomplished by an adaptation of reflectance meters originally used by workers with dye and paint to compare the reflectances of various colors. I bought one reflectance meter and changed some of its fittings to adapt it to the measurement of reflections from a matte surface. This work was reported at a Japanese conference. I collaborated with the Kyoto-Daiichi Kagaku Company to produce a commercial reflectometer for clinical use of the dry chemistry.
A historical landmark in the development of the clinical reflectance meter was distributed throughout the world by the introduction by Miles Laboratories of such a meter produced by Kyoto Daiichi Kagaku Co. and named the Dextrometer or Eyetone. The introduction of instumentation refined the dry chemistry system, and the era of quantitative analysis for blood constituents with reagent strips began. Unfortunately, I only reported my work on the reflectometer in a minor journal in Japanese, so you will not find my name on this landmark.
Before the introduction of instrumentation, the dry chemistry method did not entirely satisfy clinical chemists and physicians, because of the problem of observer errors. Poor performance with the test strip methods, such as underestimation of blood glucose when it was high and overestimation when it was relatively low, caused by mainly observer errors when the color developed in test strips was evaluated with native eyes under unsufficient illumination.
I quote that the Dextrostix-Eyetone method represented a quick and reliable alternative to conventional laboratory methods for blood sugar estimation. This was five years after the development of the prototype of reflectance meter by us.
In the late 1970s, Kodak developed a technology based on quantitative chemistry done in discrete films that are arranged in multiple layers. With adaptations of this technology, more sophisticated dry chemistry emerged by which a variety of quantitative analyses of blood constituents could be done. Microprocessor-assisted instrumentation was also involved.
Recently, there have been increased numbers of developments in the technology of dry chemistry, and there has also been an extention of applications to such fields as immunochemistry, the study of hormones, drug monitoring, specific gravity, and microbiology (ref. 3).

STRUCTURE OF THE DRY CHEMISTRY STRIPS

Most dry chemistry carriers are one of two types: one uses a paper or a synthetic fiber matrix, and the other uses of film-molding techniques. I often call the former a 'single-layer technique' and the latter a 'multiple-layer technique', but this nomenclature is not exactly correct.

a. Single-layer dry chemistry (with impregnated fibers)

The paper matrices commonly employed consist of α-cellulose with uniform fiber density and a defined thickness. It is usually important that all of the reagents needed for the specific reaction with the component of interest can be dissolved in the same solvent. A suitable second solvent for the later addition of reagents is generally difficult to find, because reagents already laid down in the matrix are easy to redissolve. The reagents are absorbed on the cellulose carrier by saturation of the matrix with a reagent solution, which is then allowed to dry.

The quantity of the reagents and the kinetics of the reaction during an assay are controlled by the reagent concentration in the impregnating solution . Other controlling factors are the volume of the matrix, its fiber density, the amount of solution that can be absorbed by the fibers, the solubility of the reagents in the sample solvent, and the reaction temperature and humidity.

A porous membrane layer is affixed to the top of the paper matrix by the use of various lamination techniques. This helps to separate the serum from the whole blood. This type of test strip for the measurement of serum bilirubin, serum urea nitrogen, and blood glucose were commercialized with the instrument called the Eyetone Mark II (Kyoto Daiichi Kagaku Co.).

b. Multiple-layer dry chemistry
In 1978, my coworkers and I reported on a dry chemistry system for the estimation of blood ammonium. The basic components of the dry chemistry carrier were multiple layers kept together with the use of lamination techniques.

Cross Section of AMITEST®

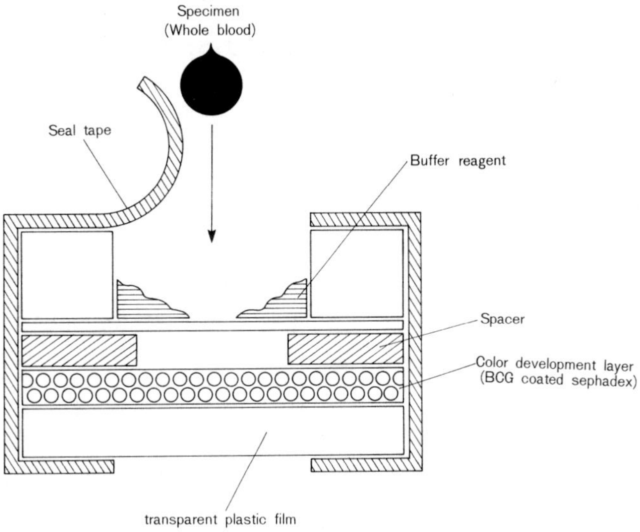

The section of the test element used for blood ammonium is shown in the figure 1. The first matrix layer contains an alkaline buffer at pH 10.3. In these alkaline surroundings, ammonium dissolved in the blood is released and gaseous ammonium first permeates the porous membrane, then to penetrate into the next matrix. The second matrix contains a weak buffer reagent and the pH indicator, which is BCG (blomocresol green). The ammonium that reaches this layer changes the pH of the matrix. We can recognize this by the development of color or by the measurement of reflectance from the colored matrix. The ammonium dry chemistry element was the first that we made that involved multiple layer dry chemistry.
At the same year, 1978, there was a major development in film technology from the Kodak company. The technology was developed originally from color photography, and is based on quantitative chemistry done in films arranged in multiple layers. The layers are constructed by the molding of a porous film that contains the necessary reaction components. Separation membranes and trapping layers can be added as necessary between reagent layers. The thickness of such a carrier may be less than 100 μm.
The reaction during analysis is controlled by the reagent concentration in the molding medium, the thickness of the molded film, the reagent solubility in the sample solvent, and the reaction temperature. Film matrices usually consist of such polymers as cross-linked gelatin, agarose, polyvinyl alcohol, or cellulose acetate. The porosity of the film depends on such factors as the molecular weight of the polymer, the degree of cross-linking, and the concentration of the polymer in the molding medium.
Two of Japanese companies has been rivals since 1980 in this field, the Fuji Film company and the Konica company. The features of Japanese dry chemistry are similar to those of the leader in this race Kodak. They do meet one of the early requirements for dry chemistry, which is simple operation. Thus, whole blood is used as the sample for this dry chemistry. In 1982, Ohkubo reported the fruit of a search for a glucose assay done in whole blood in collaboration with the Fuji Film company (ref. 4). They made an ingenious contrivance at the top of the film, which they called the spreading layer. The spreading layer was constructed with a finely woven thin web having an active surface over which blood spreads quickly and uniformly. Blood cells are filtered off through the cross-linking of this layer. However, plasma diffuses down through to the next layer. They claimed that the results were affected only slightly by the hematocrit of the sample.
c. Electrolyte elements
In 1979, Kodak developed disposable ion-selective electrodes that use film technology (ref. 5).
An ion-selective membrane, consisting of the ionophore valinomycin in a hydrophobic medium, is used to construct a potassium-specific electrode. The electrode consists of a supporting base and a silver plus silver chloride layer that serves as the reference electrode. The salt bridge consists of KCl deposited in a film. The dry reagent carrier consists of two such electrodes joined

by a bridge. The sample is referenced directly to a standard solution that is added at the same time as the deposition of the sample. The potassium concentration is calculated from the potentiometric difference measured between the two electrodes by an electrolyte measuring device.
Similar kinds of dry-reagent electrochemistry have been developed for sodium, chloride and bicarbonate ions.
Fuji Film has developed a sodium-potassium-chloride combined electrolyte element for the combinetion of sodium potassium, and chloride based on the same idea.

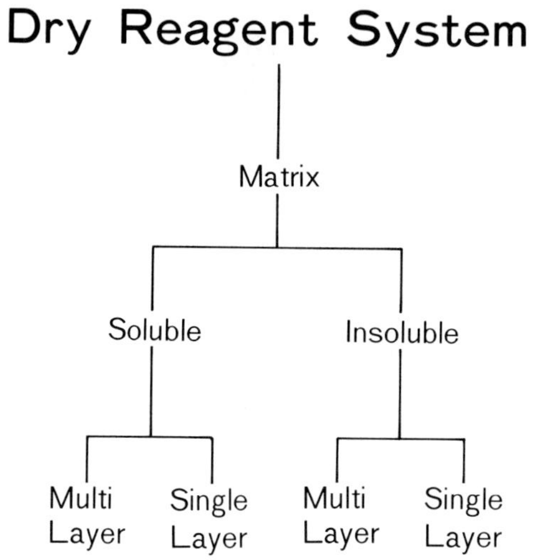

INSTRUMENTATION

A familiar example of reflection is the shining of the moon, which reflects some of the sun's rays that reach it. You will perhaps find that it looks smaller than the image in your memory when it is at the zenith, to the contrary it looks biggen when the full moon is rising at dusk. How about the color? Is it yellow or white? In the old days, Japanese imagined that they could see two rabbits on the surface of the moon, facing each other and pounding rice cakes. I want to mention that the different results as obtained when different people look at the moon can also arise when the color that has developed on a dry reagent strip is being evaluaded. You may see the color as yellowish green, and your colleague may see it as greenish yellow. Many factors affect the results of observation and comparison of test strips, such as differences in the source of the light, the color of the surroundings, and the clearness of the reference color lines. Even one's mental condition can have an effect.
Thus, people hesitate to interpret the color of test strips for use in clinical diagnosis. Also, each company gives an independent interpretation. One sample may gives a result of (+) when assayed with the test strip from company A, but it gives a plus/minus by the test strip from company B. Interpretation has never been standardized.
Variation depending on the different observers or different interpretations can be ignored with the use of reflectometry. As I have mentioned earlier, I reported on the usefulness of the reflectometry in 1967. In early studies in this field, I did not use the theory of optics much, but relied more on experimental data. Many later improvements have been made in the instrumentation of measurement with dry chemistry carriers, but current optical units are basically the same as the one in earlier days.
The Ulbricht sphere contains a light-emitting diode that illuminates the surface of the test strip. The detector detects the reflected light, which is mainly diffuse reflection. Diffuse reflectance is not a true surface phenomenon, but the result of light interacting with various chemical and physical factors in the carrier. These factors include absorption, transmission, and scattering properties of the illuminated materials.
Reflectance measurements are comparable to transmittance measurements in absorption spectrophotometry. The intensity of light reflected by the reaction carrier is measured by comparison to a known reflectance standard. The commonly used percent reflection, or %R, can be expressed by the formula ;

$$\%R = \frac{Is}{Ir} \cdot Rr$$

Is : Reflected light from the reagent carrier
Ir : Reflected light from the reference
Rr : Percent reflectivity of the reference

To make the measurement useful and simple, several theoretical approaches have been tried. The theoretical model for the function of reflectance versus color that develops or the concentration of the analyte was studied by Kubelka & Munk in 1931 (ref. 6). The correlation was later linearized theoretically through the use of a function developed by Williams & Clapper in 1953. The aid of a microprocessor allows the user to store calibration curves and read results directly for the concentration of the analyte.

SYSTEMS AVAILABLE IN JAPAN TODAY

Fuji Film company has been most closely following after the Kodak company. They release their products not only in the Japanese market but also in the world market, including Fuji Dry-Chem 5000 and 2000 for clinical chemistry items. Type 100-N, for ammonium assays, and Type 100-G for glucose assays from Fuji Film company.

The Konica company has recently introduced a product named the Konica Drylab System. At the moment, the system can be used for assays including hemoglobin, urea nitrogen, glucose, total cholesterol, aspartate aminotransferase, alanine aminotransferase, uric acid, triglycerides, total protein, and albumin. The system has the capacity to do 80 tests per hour. It weighs only 18 kgs, being a very compact desk-top analyzer.

Very recently, Kyoto Daiichi Kagaku has developed an automated dry chemistry system named the SPOTCHEM. This system has a built-in microprocessor, which controls the sampler, dispenser, reflectancephotometer, and fully automated after you put a centrifuged sample blood in tube on the sample container : The sampler automatically pipettes an aliquot of serum from the sample container, the platinum nozzle has a liquid sensor. The sample-receiving layer of the dry reagent strip is made of an artificial-fiber net. Its function is to spread the sample uniformly into the reagent layer. The reagent layer is made of a water-soluble polymer that contains the reagents required for the reaction. The water contained in the specimen dissolves the reagent layer and then diffuses back into the upper sample-receiving layer together with the dissolved reagents. In this way, the sample-receiving layer is brought into contact with the contents of the reagent layer. As the results, these two layers compose the detection layer. Then the color that has been developed in the reaction zone is measured by reflectometry. We have evaluated the system, and found the performance of the system is very precise.

Eiken company introduced recentry a dry chemistry strip for chlorides assay in urine or in food even without instrumentation. This has easy dip-and-read concept by the reaction which chloride ion develops a color with the agent of dichlorofluorescein. The general hypothesis that excessive sodium intake plays a role in the genesis of hypertension has been actively debated in recent years. Successful reduction of sodium intake by the success in modifying dietary habits has an effect on blood pressure of hypertensive individuals. However, they say it is ineffective if the patient is not well-motivated or the poorly organized program is run in log term trial. The one of the most difficult problem in such programs is probably they have no easy and good monitoring system of urinary or dietary sodium concentrations for a free-living population. It seems the indirect estimation of sodium concentration by this method may be work using this dry chemistry strip for chlorides. Such unique dry chemistry strips which may be of particular use at laboratories of small hospitals, physicians' offices, and emergency units, have been tried to develop so many in Japan, for exmple you will find a dry chemistry for saliva as an example in this Proceedings issue.

To change the subject, in the management of diabetes, the medical contribution of to self-testing of blood glucose is very great. The Joslin Clinic was the prime advocate for self-testing for glucose in the urine. However, self-testing of urine for glucose was impractical before the development of the Dextrostix® and its reflectometer. The numbers of patients doing self-testing of blood glucose has grown in the hospitalized patients.

In several other ways, dry-chemistry systems are of great usefulness. For example, recent trends in changes in the population of Japan shows that Japan is becoming a country of elderly people at a very fast pace. The population aged over 65 and over has been estimated to reach 20% in the next 30 years. In such society, convenient systems are very much needed both in and out of the hospital for keeping their healthy conditions or for monitorring medical cares.

At the end, the dry chemistry can be call 'the one useful and agreeable'.

REFERENCES

1. K. Okuda, Biochemishe Analytik 2, 55–59 (1978).
2. A. H. Free and H. M. Free, Clin. Chem. 30, 829–838 (1984).
3. J. L. Giegel, M. M. Brotherton, P. Cronin, M. D'Aquino, S. Evans, Z. H. Heller, W. S. Knight, K. Krishnan and M. Sheiman, Clin. Chem. 28, 1894–1898 (1982).
4. A. Ohkubo, S. Kamei, M. Yamanaka, F. Arai, M. Kitajima and A. Kondo, Clin. Chem. 27, 1287–1290 (1981).
5. P. Costello, N. P. Kubasik, B. B. Brody., H. E. Sine, J. A. Bertsch and J. P. D'Souza, Clin. Chem. 29, 129–132 (1983).
6. V. P. Kubelka and F. Munk, Z. Tech. Phys. 12, 593–601 (1931).

also see following review ;

- J. C. Libeer, J. Clin. Chem. Biochem. 23, 645–655 (1985).

Expert systems in clinical chemistry

Christian Trendelenburg

Institut für Laboratoriumsmedizin, Klinikum der Stadt Frankfurt,
D-6230 Frankfurt 80, FRG

Abstract - Appropriate tools for developing expert systems for clinical chemistry purposes and appropriate application domains are essential if daily routine use is intended really. The domains should deal with laboratory data with great influence on the resultant diagnoses. Four expert systems developed for clinical chemistry purposes can be taken as examples. WILFUL (Frick et al.) uses Turbo-Prolog and fuzzy logik for interpreting results of blood coagulation tests. BABAR (Besset et al.) using the expert system shell K.1 is able to create both medically oriented mechanisms for plausibility checks and indications for diagnosis for 50 most common analyses. PROSE (Ahmad and Wells) is written in Prolog and has been tried for areas as diagnosis of hypoglycaemia or comments on digoxin measurements.

PRO.M.D. (Prolog system supporting medical diagnostics), our own expert system, has been written in Prolog-2 professional plus (Expert Systems International, Oxford) as implementation language with all the benefits of Prolog for developing expert systems (easy implementation of symbolic notation, operator concept allowing a sentence like knowledge representation). In addition to the usual production rules the system can deal with concepts like sensitivity, specifity, prevalence and likelihood quotients in an easily usable manner because of the integration of probabilistic reasoning in a rule-based concept. For disorders of lipoprotein metabolism, for thyroid tests and for serology tests of hepatitis we have developed together with domain experts PRO.M.D.-knowledge-bases for daily routine use giving elaborate and very instructive reports for the clinician.

INTRODUCTION

The development of expert systems was influenced mainly by medical oriented projects. Today's increasing availability of professional and scientific expert systems for a variety of industrial and scientific purposes leads to the conclusion that expert systems will come back to medicine for daily routine use. In the following we investigate structure and function of the expert system PRO.M.D. (PROLOG System Supporting Medical Diagnostics), which we developed for applications in Clinical Chemistry and Laboratory Medicine (1), as well as the choice of PROLOG as implementation language. Four other expert systems for Clinical Chemistry question complexes will be discussed. Finally several routine applications with different PRO.M.D. knowledge bases will be shown.

PROLOG AS IMPLEMENTATION LANGUAGE

The experiences with our main tool, PROLOG are very good. One property of PROLOG of itself seeking the method for fulfilling logical declarations, if necessary even by backtracking and new ramifications in the case of several possibilities, is one of the main characteristics of PROLOG distinguishing it from conventional program languages. Further essential characteristics depend on a built-in dynamic database, an efficient implementation of recursive notation as well as the ability to process lists and structures in almost any conceivable form. It is also possible to employ for representing knowledge relationships the so-called operator concept which permits the compilation of interpretable simple sentences and statements and which will be explained in detail later on. All these properties are exceedingly helpful for the so-called symbolic programming. Symbols are defined according to Waterman (2) as character chains for identification of concepts and material behaviour of reality. Such symbols can be combined to set forth the logical relationships between the symbols to form a knowledge based systems which contributes to the common context, which is the main base of an effective exchange of information. In the development of our knowledge-based system PROLOG-2 from Expert Systems International, Oxford has proved exceedingly suitable (3). Many extensions of this special PROLOG-implementation and the declarative symbolic notation do indeed extremely simplify the implementation of ideas and concepts during the development and the improvement of the system compared with conventional programming.

IMPLEMENTATION OF AN INFERENCE ENGINE SUPPORTING MEDICAL DIAGNOSTICS IN THE FIELD OF LABORATORY MEDICINE AND CLINICAL CHEMISTRY

As regards the quality of inference engines, experience shows that generalized inference engines suitable for many question complexes often tend to give moderate results when applied to specific domains. This makes it clear why so far no standardized generally accepted implementation form has been found for inference engines. For this reason an attempt was made to develop an inference engine particularly suitable fo laboratory medicine.

Our main goals in developing our knowledge based system are as follows:

1. Suitability for microcomputers
2. Combination of numerical and non numerical information
3. A first approach to the representation of temporal relations
4. Incorporation of probabilistic reasoning
5. Suitability for different knowledge bases
6. Storing of individual patient files
7. Possibility for reconsultation of individual patient files
8. Facilities for explanation
9. A first approach to knowledge notation in simple sentences
10. A coherent user interface with suggestions of allowed answers to avoid tedious typing in of answers.

During this process we learned, that in contrast to program development using conventional languages, in which as comprehensive as possible a primary concept is important, the methods of gradual refinement are expedient. During the development phase by creating and testing small exemplary knowledge bases for the particular current version of the system pronounced interactions between the system properties and the question complex being represented are generated. In this process in particular the aim must be to continuously improve the inference engine with the objective of enabling area-typical relationships, strategies and other peculiarities to be represented in linguistically easily reproducible form in the formulation of the knowledge components.

Fundamentally, the sequence of processing the rules of the knowledge base can be either a data-directed one or a goal-directed one. In the goal directed processing by calling up underlying rules after predefining a hypothesis all information necessary for confirming the hypothesis is interrogated. If a rule is selected whose reply first requires that another rule be called up, then this other rule is called up first, and so on. In data-directed processing the interrogation takes place firstly in the order of the rules but is then greatly influenced in the course of the processing by the individual fact constellation because rules which on the basis of the facts already known are no longer valid are not processed any more. PRO.M.D. has in modified form both properties because firstly the processing is data-directed and in the further course of the consultation may also be goal-directed. This procedure was implemented because in the case of laboratory medicine knowledge domains are usually symptom-dependent and result-dependent selection from amongst several hypotheses is desired. Specific rule formulations then permit exact examination of a hypothesis in accordance with the use of certainty factors implemented in a similar way as in MYCIN by Shortliffe (4).

STRUCTURE OF RULES

We have implemented several types of rules. With the normal conclusion or inference rule the usual non numerical information can be handled. With the computation rule, it is possible to deal with figures of laboratory results like diagnostic quotients.

The question and answers rules determine whether a certain concept can be asked by the user or must result from intermediate conclusions and whether a conclusion should be used only as intermediate or should be given in the final report. All these features (and additional features are under development) have been added to the system in an incremental approach after development of the basic inference mechanism.

The system permits creation and processing of production rules within the form shown below:

> **if PREMISE then CONCLUSION.**
> **premise consists of:**
> **FINDINGS**
> **Finding: consists of CONDITIONS (concept has attribute)**
> **CONCLUSION may itself a FINDING in following rules**

It is of interest here that conclusions can in turn appear as propositions in subsequent rules. This makes it possible to create complex knowledge bases which in interaction with the user specifically request missing information in accordance with the course of the individual consultation.

The following types of formulation can be assigned to the premises (V) and conclusions (F). Particular attention should be paid to the temporal formulations and the formulations influencing the weighting factors (cf). Actually we are expanding the language concept for the incorporation of probabilistic reasoning into production rules. Examples have been selected from a first knowledge base for supporting serological hepatitis diagnostics:

```
(V  )  anti_hav is at_least slightly_elevated
(V  )  hepatitis_a with_more than 0.4 cf
(V  )  anti_hav is positive
(V F)  hbsag was positive 1 - 5 months ago
(V F)  start of disease was acute 3 - 4 months before
          seroconversion with 0.6 cf
(V  )  "and" and "or" links of premises ...
(  F)  only "and" links of conclusions ...
(  F)  question_time_of symptom_x
(  F)  put hepatitis_b to 0.8/0 cf.
```

The entire knowledge base can be created in a first approximation to a simple sentence formulation. PROLOG greatly supports this through the operator concepts by which language elements as

and, or, with, ago, after, days, month, slightly_elevated

can be used in the usual linguistic form based on the correct logical declaration.

The PROLOG operators are used here to prove the comprehensability of the rules in accordance with the following example:

```
premise:                                                conclusion:
   enzyme_x was greater_than 90 units 4 weeks ago          disease_y with 0.3 cf

                                  ---units                                  ----cf
                greater_than--------- --weeks                ----------with-------
                ------------------------------ago
   ---------was---------------------------------
premise:----------------------------------------
  -------------------------------------------------conclusion:-------------
```

By keeping to certain syntactic rules the knowledge notation is thus made directly in PROLOG syntax without this being noticed by the user. Even the full-stop at the end of the sentence, which is very important to PROLOG because it denotes the end of a logical declaration, can be employed in the usual manner for the user in this type of operator concept application. This thus obviates a serious obstruction in the use of program systems configurable in any manner, that is the conversion of the entry to computer-oriented form. As an extension of the language scope of PRO.M.D. the system will permit in the next configuration level an extended form of knowledge notation including the representation of sensitivity and specificity as well as the financial expenditure and the benefit of a given test. Together with optimization features the system will change the data directed approach towards an improved diagnostic strategy.

FURTHER EXPERT SYSTEMS FOR CLINICAL CHEMISTRY QUESTION COMPLEXES

Three systems will be briefly characterized below as representatives of further expert systems for clinical chemistry uses. No claim to completeness is made. The system of Ahmad and Wells (5) is written in Prolog. In the various development stages of the system an attempt is made to unite the declarative statement (a collection of facts with small set of inferencing procedures for its uses). In a fist stage Ahmad and Wells have created a declarative system with notation of the knowledge in rule form an a simple goal-driven, backward-chaining inferencing mechanism. Confidence factors are used to handle inexact reasoning. Use has shown that with this attempt the procedural knowledge elements frequently additionally employed for clinical algorithms and question complexes can only be poorly imaged. For this reason, in a second attempt a more axiomatic approach was chosen in which the procedural information about the next step is stored within the rule itself. This system has been tried for the following knowledge areas: differential diagnosis of hypoglycemia, classification of hyperlipoproteinemias, clinical comments of digoxin measurements, therapeutic monitoring of thephylline infusion. The present development of the system is pursuing the aim of incorporating the concept of normal values and time series, implementing connections to external program actions and employing so-called blackboard techniques with which the inferences of a relatively large number of expert systems which are related to each other can be combined.

An approach has been adopted by Frick, Sator, Kratzer and Knedel (6) which was very successful as regards the representation of uncertain knowledge. As implementation language Turbo-Prolog was chosen and as field of use the diagnosis of blood coagulation disturbances. The concept of normal and pathological ranges, together with the related problems of the exact description of range transitions was solved by employing the so-called fuzzy logic. The system supports in a graphical screen dialog guide the selection of a diagnosis best fitting a current value combination for an assumed diagnosis. In contrast to many other expert systems it is intended and suitable for real-time use within the scope of laboratory medical plausibility checks.

In contrast to the systems described hitherto Besset (7) has used a commercially available system for creating a knowledge base called BABAR for supporting the work sequence and diagnostics in a medical laboratory. BABAR was created using the expert system shells M.1 and K.1 of FRAMENTEC. The objective is to create with a rule-based system both medically oriented mechanisms for plausibility checks and indications for diagnosis for a commercially operating laboratory in which the 50 most common analyses are carried out. From these analyses BABAR can give indications of 95 diseases which give specific result constellations, possibly to be further checked, or for example make a further analysis in blood coagulation necessary.

APPLICATIONS OF PRO.M.D.

The first application for daily routine use we selected was the interpretation of quantitative lipoprotein electrophoretic tests (precipitation method) in combination with values of serum cholesterol and triglycerides (8,9). The large knowledge base is described elsewhere in this issue.

Selecting other domains for knowledge based system one should keep in mind, that the domain should deal with laboratory data which influence patient care really and which can not be foreseen by the physician by other ways easily. This seems to be the case not with liver enzyme constellations, but with lipoprotein values, with some hormone constellations (e.g. thyroid), with the serological diagnosis of hepatitis and with more complex metabolic evaluations as the interpretation of a variety of laboratory data related with calcium metabolism. For these domains and others (e.g. alkaline phospatase isoenzymes, tumor associated antigens, toxicological screening, cerebrospinal fluid proteins) we have developed or we are developing together with real experts knowledge bases for daily routine use.

References:

1. Trendelenburg, Chr. and Pohl, B.: Pro.M.D. - Medizinische Diagnostik mit Expertensystemen: Eine Einführung mit Disketten für die Expertensystemschale Pro.M.D. (Stuttgart, New York: Thieme-Verlag 1988, ISBN 3-13-730301-X)

2. Waterman, D. A.: Expert Systems 3/1, 16-19, 1986

3. Trendelenburg, Chr.: Proc. 1.st Int. Exp. Syst. Conf, Learned Information Systems, Oxfors, 153-162, 1986

4. Shortliffe, E.H.: Mycin, American Elsevier, New York, 1976

5. Ahmad, K. and Wells, J. G.: In: Computing in Clinical Laboratories (ed. Chr. Trendelenburg), pp. 135-136, Kohl, Brackenheim, 1985

6. Frick, H. G., Sator, H., Kratzer, M. A. A. and Knedel, M.: In: Artificial Intelligence and Advanced Computer Technology Conference (AI-Europa) Proceedings, TCM Exposition Publisher, Liphook, 1986

7. Besset, D.: In: Artificial Intelligence and Advanced Computer Technology Conference (AI-Europa) Proceedings, TCM Exposition Publisher, Liphook, 1986

8. Wieland, H: Mitt. Dt. Ges. Klin. Chem. 16/2, 48-57,1985

9. Trendelenburg, Chr.: Biochimica Clinica 10,928-929,1986

Expert system for the evaluation of disturbances of lipid metabolism and assessment of risk for coronary heart disease

Heinrich Wieland and Christian Trendelenburg

Zentrallabor der Universitaetsklinik Freiburg (F.R.G.)

Abstract - Based on two case-control studies in northern and southern Germany, performed on patients selected for coronary angiography in order to assess the association of lipoprotein parameters with coronary artery disease (CAD) an expert system was developed. It relies on quantitation of lipoproteins after electrophoretical separation and precipitation in the agarose gel by polyanions.
This method is ideally suited to determine the ratio of LDL to HDL (risk index, RI) and also for lipoprotein typing (I-V) and to detect most abnormalities of lipid metabolism.
The clinical significance of a given cholesterol value is estimated by considering the RI and the concentration of LDL. Accordingly therapeutic measures are suggested involving change of lifestyle, dietary recommendations and, if necessary, guidelines for drug treatment. The system considers also other major risk factors for CAD .

Cholesterol and triglycerides are transported by different individual lipoproteins. The biological importance of the different lipoproteins may be opposite. Therefore without the knowledge of actual lipoprotein concentrations the lipid metabolism of an individual cannot be evaluated. Because of the close connection between high concenrations of LDL und low concentrations of HDL with premature atherosclerosis this evaluation should be done on any individual at least once before the age of 30 und repeated at intervals of five years (ref. 1). Clinically safe cholesterol concentrations can be assumed at values below 200 mg/dl. This cut-off point, however, it exceeded by roughly 80 % of the West German adult population. Therefore, there is a a large demand for lipoprotein quantification. The same difficulty as in judging serum cholesterol- und triglyceride-values, however, also exists for evaluation of lipoprotein concentrations. Precise quantitation of LDL and VLDL is lacking in most prospective studies concerning lipoproteins and coronary heart disease. This also holds true for the information regarding the atherogenecity of serum triglyceride values since individuals have been beeen seldom investigated in the fasting state of a duration of at least 12 hours. In additon a variety of different methods have been used and clinical recommendations have to take the methods of analysis in account.

In addition the clinical significance of a certain lipoprotein concentration is largely dependent on other variables regarding the individual patient. These are: age, sex, concomitant lipoprotein concentrations, risk factors such as: hypertension, diabetes and cigarette smoking, body weight and medication. Therefore a considerable uncertainty how to interpret lipoprotein concentrations in a given patient is a common problem. This led us to the development of a knowledge base for the investigation of lipid metabolism.

The method of lipoprotein quantification has been developed 13 years ago (ref. 2). In the meantime two large studies have been conducted, one a case-control-study on patients having undergone coronary angiography (ref. 3); secondly a prospective study on factory workers (ref.4). The results of these two studies are the preliminary basis of our expert system.

The method involved is quantitative lipoprotein electrophoresis which has several advantages over the common quantification of plasma lipoproteins by determining of HDL-cholesterol und calculating LDL-cholesterol by the Friedewald Formula.

These are:

1. Direct determination of beta-lipoproteins (LDL).

2. Differentiation between chylomicrons and prä-beta-lipoproteins (VLDL).
3. Very precise determination of lipoprotein ratios.
4. Recognition of abnormal lipoproteins.

Even the ultracentrifugation procedure recommended by the WHO determins LDL-cholesterol by calculation of the difference of the cholesterol contents of HDL and serum freed of VLDL by ultracentrifugation. Quantitative agarose gel lipoprotein electrophoresis using precipitation of lipoproteins in the gel for staining, allows a direct measurement of the beta-lipoprotein band.

Since chylomicrons do not penetrate agarose gel, their presence can be demonstrated by the discrepancy between the amount of VLDL (pre-beta-lipoproteins) and their presumable contribution to the triglyceride concentration on one side and the whole serum trigylceride concentration on the other side. The possible differentiation between chylomicrons and pre-beta-lipoproteins was the major reason for the clinical usefulness of lipoprotein electrophoresis for typification of hyperlipoproteinemias. The differentiation achieved herewith allows an easy typification and accurate estimate of VLDL-cholesterol and therefore opens the possibility for evaluation of the clinical significance of VLDL-cholesterol in prospective studies. Ultracentrifugation performed as recommended by the WHO is not able to differentiate between VLDL und chylomicrons.

The concentration of macromolecules in the blood depends on the intravasal water concentration. This can be considerably altered by postural changes and venous congestion by a turnicate before venopuncture. Ratios of the different lipoproteins to each other are unaffected by the intravasal water content. In addition no quantitative pipetting-step is necessary to determine ratios. The precision of lipoproteinratios determined by ultracentrifugation is far inferior to that obtained by lipoprotein electrophorsis.
Clinically significant familial dys-beta-lipoproteinemia is as common as familial hypercholesterolemia. It can be diagnosed by lipoprotein electrophoresis in combination with Clofibrat therapy. The usual diagnostic procedures are not able to detect this condition. Since it can be treated very effectively and implicates a high risk for vascular disease this is a considerable advantage of lipoprotein electrophoresis.

In cholestatic liver disease an abnormal lipoprotein (lipoprotein-X) with beta-mobility accummulates in the plasma. This condition is often associated with low HDL-cholesterol values. The abnormal lipoprotein leads to a broad beta-band in electrophoresis and can by this be diagnosed. Lipoprotein (a) is also an atherogenic lipoprotein with pre-beta mobility. Since it is triglyceride-poor a discrepancy between pre-beta concentration and whole serum triglyceride concentration my indicate the presence of this atherogenic lipoprotein which should then be quantified by immunological means. Last not least a normal densitogram of the specimen proves, that all analytical steps were in order and is therefore confirming the validity of the results of lipoprotein quantification. This reassurance can hardly be achieved by the usual purely chemical techniques. A densitogram also is a characteristic of the patient and the lipoproteinprofile and may be remembered much more easily than cholesterol- and lipoprotein-cholesterol-values.
Low dose heparin therapy activates lipoprotein lipase and leads to an alteration of the lipoproteinsystem. These alterations also influence precipitation techniques. Post Heparin Lipolytic Activity yields a characteristical pattern in lipoprotein electrophoresis.

The Expert System first considers the shape of the densitogram by asking certain questions. If it comes to the conclusion that the densitogram is in order the evaluation is started.

The most imporant parameter is beta-lipoprotein cholesterol (LDL-cholesterol), since a hypercholesterolemia it is only clinically significant if it is due to an increase of the LDL concentration. Furthermore, this paramter is a target for the therapy and it has to be used for monitoring. VLDL- (pre-beta) cholesterol is considered as clinically significant if it exceeds 35 mg/dl. If, however, LDL-cholesterol exceeds by far VLDL-cholesterol, the latter is being neglected. Alpha-lipoprotein-cholesterol values (HDL-cholesterol) are considered for risk-evaluation predominantly at beta-lipoprotein-cholesterol values between 140 and 186 mg/dl. Within this range the ratio of beta-Lipoproteins to alpha-Lipoproteins should not exceed 1.5. The lipoprotein measurements are condensed in one number, the so called 'risk-point' in the following way:
risk-point = (beta/cholesterin plus prä-beta-cholesterin) x beta-lipoprotein/alpha-lipoprotein ratio.
This risk-point is used to judge the course of the situation. The risk-point is multiplied by the factor 1.1, if an additional risk factor such as hypertension, cigarette-smoking, coronary heart disease

in the family etc. is present. Each risk factor leads to a multiplication. Above the age of 60 the risk point is multiplied by the factor 0.9.

The risk point is an indicator of the gravity of the disease and accordingly dietary instructions und suggestions for drug therapy are graded. These suggestions differ according to prevalence of hypercholesterolemia or hypertriglyceridemia. In cases of severe hypertriglyceridemia which often makes lipoprotein electrophoresis impossible the danger of pancreatitis is highlighted and drug therapy is suggested.

Because of the widespread use of the typing system of Frederickson, the corresponding types are also mentioned. This is basically unnessary but since a certain type implicated therapy and prognosis, it might be useful for some physcians familiar with lipid metabolism. Apart from risk evaluation alpha-cholesterol (HDL-cholesterol) is used for differentiation between liver disease and familial dyslipoproteinemia and also for explanation of hypercholesterolemias due to oestrogens, alcohol etc..

The concomitant concentration of VLDL-cholesterol leads to questions regarding body-weight und glucose-tolerance and also modifies suggestions for diet and drugs.

Considerable attention is devoted to secondary dyslipoproteinemias due to liver disease, hypothyroiddism or renal disease. Rare abnormalities are also considered (LCAT-deficiancy, Tangier disease, abeta-lipoproteinemia and the heterozygous form of familia dyslipoproteinemia). The system contains many more clinical features. These to describe would use the remaining space.

Expert systems are used either in the laboratory or at the desk of the physician. Our system should be used in the physicians practice since it requires information regarding the patient. In addition lipoprotein quantification is a preventive measure and preventive medicine is not the major goal of large hospitals. Since the recommended measures are useful for the general population, the physician can easily take up the responsibility for the results of the system.
The demand for lipoprotein quantification has considerably increased after introduction of the system two years ago. In the meantime, we were constantly modifying and improving the system considering criticism from the clinic and from outside. The need to update the system is dependent on the scientific progress and new developments in treatment. Presumably a yearly update is sufficient.

This is the first expert system which is used in Germany in several places. It is useful because of the high degree of uncertainty which still exists about the meaning of plasma lipid concentrations. Its constant use may considerably improve the knoweldge of physicians.

Experience has shown that the construction of a useful knowledge base is a matter of extremely good cooperation between the expert und the programmer. The easiest way to achieve this is a programme which enables the expert to construct the base completely by himself using common sense and his knowledge. In addition, it forces the expert to structure the knowledge and deal in more depth with the decision criteria. Construction of a knowledge base is an entertaining and exciting endeavour.

REFERENCES

1. Study Group, European Atherosclerosis Society
The recognition and management of hyperlipidaemia in adults : A policy statement of the European Atherosclerosis Society.
European Heart Journal 9, 571-600 (1988)

2. D. Seidel, H. Wieland, C. Ruppert,
Improved techniques for assessment of plasmalipoprotein patterns. I. Precipitation in gels after electrophoresis with polyanionic compounds.
Clin. Chem. 19, 737-739 (1973)

3. H. Wieland, D. Seidel, V. Wiegand, H. Kreuzer,
Serum lipoproteins and coronary artery disease (CAD)
Comparision of the lipoprotein profile with the results of coronary angiography.
Atherosclerosis 36, 427-439 (1980)

4. P. Cremer, H. Wieland , D. Seidel,
Göttinger Risiko-, Inzidenz- und Prävalenzstudie (GRIPS). Aufbau und bisherige Ergebnisse (Stand Juni 1987)
Münch. med. Wschr. 130, 268-274 (1988)

Dry chemistry on whole blood

S. Kamei

Department of Laboratory Medicine, Faculty of Medicine,
University of Tokyo. Hongo 7-3-1, Bunkyo-ku, Tokyo 113, Japan.

Abstract - An increasing number of clinical test systems based on the dry chemistry have been developed for practical use.The dry chemistry is a technology,in which all the reagents necessary for analysis are kept in a dried state. Typically,they are coated on a paper or film. Water required as a solvent for chemical reactions is supplied from a specimen. Accordingly, the reactions are initiated by the addition of a small amount of specimen. Usual analytical methods in clinical laboratory, including several dry chemistry systems, utilize serum or plasma as a sample. In these cases, separation of serum or plasma is required prior to analysis. It is obvious that the procedure becomes more simple and rapid, if whole blood can be applied as the sample. It is further desirable to utilize the dry chemistry which is one of the most simple analytical methods, for direct analysis of whole blood. Many systems along this line have been developed for the determination of the blood sugar levels. Systems for the determination of various test items in whole blood have also been developed such as DRI-CHEM system by Fuji Photo Film and REFLOTRON system by Boehringer Mannheim. In this paper I will make an introduction to the analytical principles of the dry chemistry systems together with some of their characteristics, and analytical performances and will discuss about advantages as well as disadvantages of these systems and prospects of their practical use.

INTRODUCTION

Recently, analytical methods based on dry chemistry are becoming more and more popular in the field of clinical diagnosis. Dry chemistry can be defined as a technology in which dry reagents are impregnated in a dry matrix. Upon the addition of a sample liquid, the reagents dissolve and react with a specific analyte in the sample liquid to give a detectable signal.

Qualitative or semiquantitative test papers, such as pH-papers and teststrips for urine tests are examples of dry chemistry. They have been widely used in clinical laboratories. Dry chemistry has been improved as a method to be used for quantitative analysis. Various technologies have been developed to meet a variety of needs in laboratories. Examples of these methods are summarized in Table 1. Dry chemistry developed for whole blood analysis is described in this paper.

TABLE 1. Examples of dry chemistry

1. **Qualitative Dry Chemistry** : pH test, Test sticks for urine
2. **Quantitative Dry Chemistry**
    1) **Determination of blood sugar level** :
       GLUCOSTAR, REFLOLUX II, GLUCOSCOT and many others.
    2) **Determination of various test items**
       Multilayer film method : EKTACHEM, DRI-CHEM, DRY LABO
       Test paper method : SERALYZER, REFLOTRON
       Other method : SPOTCHEM

ADVANTAGES AND DISADVANTAGES OF DRY CHEMISTRY

Dry chesmitry methods, in general, have many advantages over conventional wet chemistry as summarized in Table 2. Among these, the dry chemistry method for whole blood is most advantageous for some circumstances, because this method eliminates time and the labor-consuming centrifuge process. It is especially useful when real-time diagnosis is required, since the results are obtained on the spot a few minutes after the blood collection.

TABLE 2. Characteristic features of dry chemistry

Advantages	1. No preparation of reagents or buffers required. 2. No plumbing required. Only electric power source. 3. No technical training for operation required. 4. Small sample volume. 5. Compact instrument with small space. 6. Easy to operate. 7. Easy maintenance of instrument. 8. No centrifuge required for sample preparation.
Disadvantages	1. Test menu is not large enough (about 10 tests). 2. Relatively high cost for consumables.

DRY CHEMISTRY SYSTEMS FOR WHOLE BLOOD ANALYSIS

Dry chemistry systems for whole blood analysis are summarized in Table 3. There are several portable systems for self-monitoring blood sugar by the use of dry chemistry technology. Some of them are quite compact and weigh only about 150 grams. On the other hand, the DRI-CHEM system of Fuji Photo Film and the REFLOTRON system of Boeringer Mannheim currently cover more than 10 tests and are being expanded to a larger system.

TABLE 3. Dry chemistry systems for whole blood analysis

Manufacturer	Reagent	Test Menu ( ):under development	Reagent Matrix	Analyzer
Fuji Photo Film	DRI-CHEM Slide	GLU Na K Cl NH_3 CRE BUN Hb UA TG CHO ···	Multilayer Film	FDC Analyzer Series multi/single auto/manual
Boehringer-Mannheim	REFLOQUANT Teststrip	GLU BUN GGT CHO TG Hb AST ALT UA BIL AMY(CRE LDH CK ···)	Paper	REFLOTRON multi manual
Miles Laboratories		GLU	Paper	GLUCOSTAR
Kyoto DIC		GLU	Film	GLUCOSCOT
Boehringer-Mannheim		GLU	Paper	REFLOLUX II
many others		GLU		

FUJI DRI-CHEM SLIDE

Fuji Photo Film developed the DRI-CHEM system based on multi-coating film technology like that which Eastman Kodak applied to its EKTACHEM system (ref. 1). However, Fuji succeeded in developing a method for whole blood analysis (ref. 2).

Figure 1 shows the structure and the analytical principle of the DRI-CHEM creatinine slide for whole blood (ref. 3). Six functional layers are laminated on a polyester film. The uppermost is a spreading layer consisting of woven cloth specifically treated to optimize the spreading of whole blood. Under the spreading layer is an ammonium-scavenging layer containing glutamate dehydrogenase, and NADP to eliminate endogenous ammonium in the blood. The next layer contains pH-buffer that stops ammonium from leaking out of the slide. The fourth layer is a creatinine-reacting layer containing creatinine iminohydrolase that hydrolyses the creatinine to give ammonium. Under that layer is a porous membrane which passes gaseous ammonium. The gaseous ammonium reaches the indicator layer which contains a pH-indicator. It reacts with the concentration of creatinine in the blood sample. Optical reflection density is measured through transparent support.

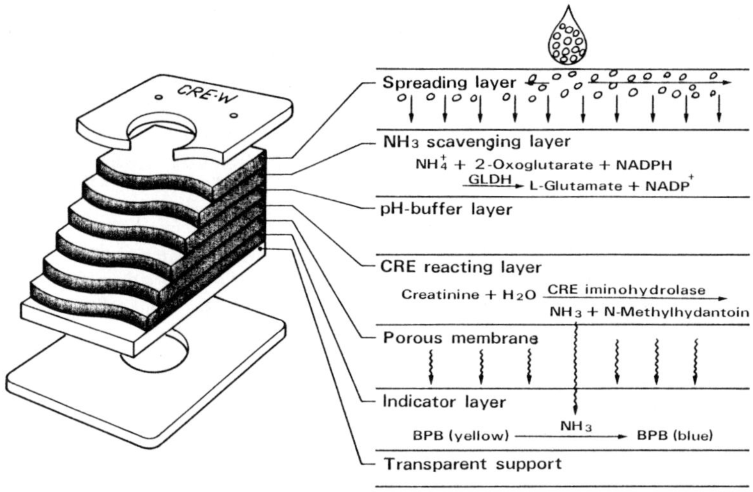

Fig. 1. Structure and analytical principle of DRI-CHEM creatinine slide

DRI-CHEM ELECTROLYTE SLIDE

DRI-CHEM has also a potentiometric slide for whole blood analysis (ref. 4). Three electrolytes-sodium, potassium and chloride- are measured simultaneously with one slide. The results are obtained in one minute on a compact portable-sized instrument.

Figure 2 shows the appearance, structure and analytical principle of the slide. Three multilayer, film-type, ion selective electrodes are incorporated into one slide. Each film electrode is separated electrically into two part-one, for the sample and one for the reference solution. When drops of sample and reference solution are simultaneously applied to the slide, they diffuse through the liquid-distributing elements made of non-woven cloth to reach each of the three ion selective film electrodes. At the same time, a part of the sample and a part of the reference solution diffuse through a piece of thread to form an ionic bridge and construct an electrical circuit. The potential difference between the sample and reference solution is measured by potentiometer.

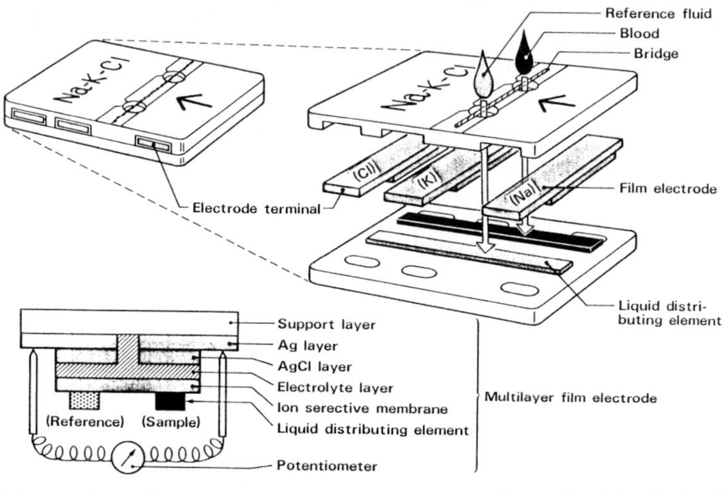

Fig. 2. Appearance, structure and analytical principle of DRI-CHEM Na-K-Cl slide

REFLOTRON TESTSTRIP

Boehringer Mannheim developed the REFLOTRON system. It consists of a compact analyzer, REFLOTRON and teststrips.

Figure 3 shows the configuration and analytical principle of the teststrip. It has two functional parts: one for separation of plasma from blood cells and the other for detection reactions. When a drop of whole blood is applied to the strip, blood cells are filtered out while it diffuses through a separation matereial made of glass wool filter paper. Below the separation material, there is a layer which contains auxilliary reagents, for example, ascorbate oxidase or enzyme activator, to eliminate some interferents. The plasma portion is transferred through the transport layer to the reagent layer where the detection reaction takes place. Optical reflective density of the color developed is measured through a transparent foil (ref. 5).

The construction of the slide or teststrip and the reactions involved are quite complicated, but, they are designed and menufactured so precisely that the analytical performances of the slide or teststrip satisfy the precision and accuracy, generally required in clinical laboratories.

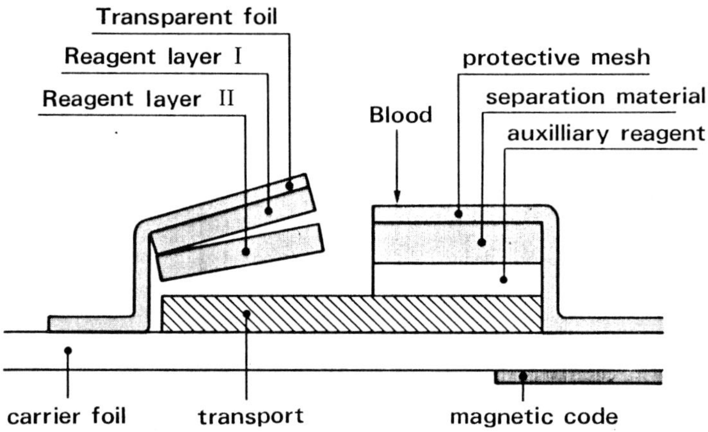

Fig. 3. Structure and analytical principle of REFLOTRON teststrip

HOW TO MAKE STANDARD CURVES

In dry chemistry systems, optical reflection densities of color developed in the film are not linear to the concentrations of analytes in the sample. In addtion, optical reflection density does not give a 100 % reading at zero concentration. These make dry chemistry difficult to treat theoritically, in comparison to conventional wet chemistry systems for which the theoretical basis is well established.

In dry chemistry systems, a standard curve is based on the experimental results. It is prepared by the following steps:
1st. Samples of various concentrations are collected.
2nd. Concentrations of a specific analyte in whole blood samples are measured by the dry chemistry systems to determine the optical density of the samples.
3rd. The plasma obtained from the same whole blood samples are measured with an established method to determine the assigned value of each sample.
4th. The optical density vs concentration relationship is obtained by plotting the results.
5th. The above relationship is simulated and a mathematical expression is stored in computer memory of the instrument (Fig. 4).

Although theoretical expressions of the standard curve are possible after quite a complicated mathematical treatment, experimental procedure is usually used since it is more practical. To have good performance, the reproducibility of the test results for each specific sample is very important.

PERFORMANCES OF DRI-CHEM AND REFLOTRON

Performances of the DRI-CHEM system and the REFLOTRON system are examined and the results are summarized. Table 4 shows the precision data of DRI-CHEM creatinine (ref. 3). Within-run CVs obtained with whole blood samples, as well as between-day CVs obtained with serum samples, are less than 2 % for most tests.

Figure 5 shows the precision data of REFLOTRON glucose and hemoglobin (ref. 5). Day-to-day CVs are about 3 % for most tests. It is expected that between-day precisions are not much different from within-run precisions since it is one of the characteristic features of dry chemistry and is already well established with plasma and sera.

As is seen from these table and figure, both systems gave good, acceptable results over the concentration range important for clinical diagnosis. On the other hand, the precisions at lower and higher concentration ranges are poor in general, because of the non-linearity of the standard curves.

A method comparison between wet chemistry and the DRI-CHEM system using several test items, as well as between wet chemistry and the REFLOTRON system gave good, acceptable resutls.

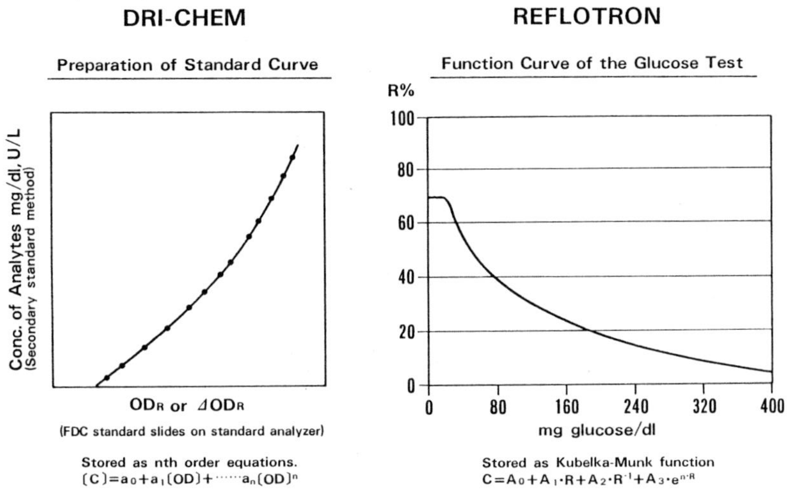

Fig. 4. How to make standard curves

TABLE 4. Precision data of DRI-CHEM

Within-Assay (CRE-W)

n=20	Sample 1	Sample 2	Sample 3	Sample 4
X̄ (mg/dl)	0.80	4.66	8.66	12.28
SD(mg/dl)	0.06	0.08	0.15	0.14
CV(%)	8.11	1.77	1.69	1.11

Day-to-day (CRE-P)

	Sample 1	Sample 2	Sample 3
X̄ (mg/dl)	1.26	6.03	10.52
SD(mg/dl)	0.05	0.04	0.10
CV(%)	4.0	0.7	1.0

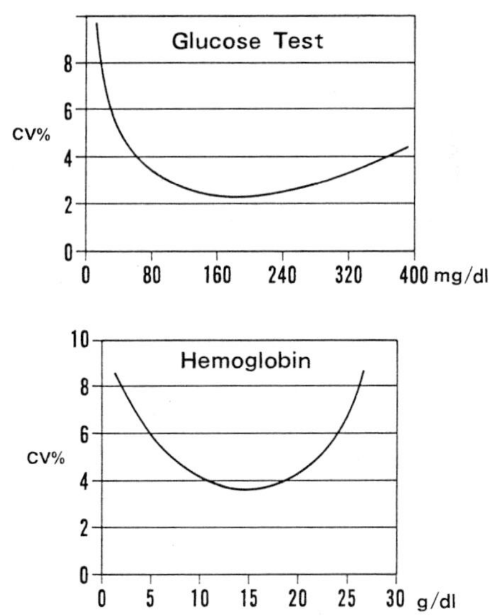

Fig. 5. Precision data of REFLOTRON (CV % day-to-day)

CHARACTERISTICS AND PROBLEMS SPECIFIC TO WHOLE BLOOD ANALYSIS

Some analytical features which are considered to be characteristic of dry chemistry systems:

<u>Turbidity</u>
Since the optical reflection density is measured against a white difusing background, the turbidity of the samples, which is a potential interferent to wet chemistry, has not affect, at all, on the results obtained with dry chemistry.

Hemoglobin and bilirubin
Both hemoglobin and bilirubin have a large molecular size, and the layers in dry chemistry can be designed to function as molecular sieves. These high molecular weight intereferents can be effectively blocked so that the results are free from the optical disturbance caused by them.
Elimination of endogenous substances
Functional layers to eliminate endogenous interferents can be incorporated into the multilayer structure: for example, layers containing ascorbate oxidase to eliminate endogenous ascorbate, or glutamate dehydrogenase to eliminate endogenous ammonium. Buffering layers are also designed to eliminate some intereferents.
Effect of sample volume
About this innovative feature of dry chemistry, the data will be shown later.

Some problems specific to whole blood analysis with dry chemistry:

Effect of sample viscosity
Dry chesmitry systems tend to be more affected than wet chemistry by the variation of protein concentrations. The viscosity of the sample affects its spreading and diffusing directly, because no dilution of the sample takes place in dry chemistry. This viscosity dependency is more serious with whole blood analysis since the hematocrit of whole blood varies over a large range. When hematocrit varies 20 % to 55 %, the viscosity change of the sample is 17 to 40 cps. This problem will be discussed later.
Effect of pH
The effect of the pH of the samples also tends to be more prominent with dry chemistry than with wet chemistry for the same reason.
Avoiding hemolysis
When whole blood is used as a sample, hemolysis completely destroys the results for some tests (such as pottasium, LDH and AST) because their concentration inside of the blood cells is far different from the concentration outside. The materials, as well as the configuration of the analytical elements, must be carefully selected so that no hemolysis takes place during the analytical process.
Quality control
There is no standard solution of natural whole blood which can be used for the purpose of quality control in dry chemistry. An artificial standard solution which gives comparable results to those obtained with whole blood is developed as a control solution or calibrator for the DRI-CHEM system.

EFFECT OF SAMPLE VOLUME

One of the innovative features of dry chemistry is the compensating function of spreading layer or DRI-CHEM or of the separation material of REFLOTRON which improves the precision by minimizing the dependency of the results on the sample volume. This function is especially important for the whole blood analysis since it is difficult to quantitate the small volume precisely. Figure 6 (ref. 6,7) show the performances of the DRI-CHEM uric acid slide and the REFLOTRON triglyceride teststrip respectively. With both systems the effect of sample volume variations on the results is minimized to about one-third.

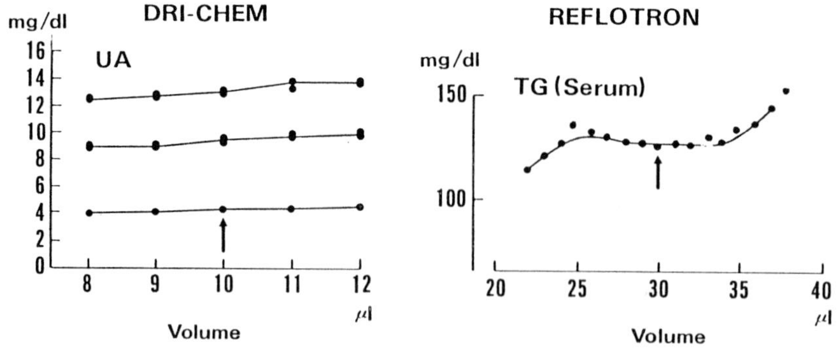

Fig. 6. Effect of sample volume

EFFECT OF HEMATOCRIT

The dependency on hematocrit was examined with both the DRI-CHEM system and the REFLOTRON system (Fig. 7). The upper figures are the results obtained with DRI-CHEM glucose and urea nitrogen (ref. 8,9). Lower figures are the results obtained with REFLOTRON glucose and triglyceride (ref. 10,7). Between 20 % and 55 %, the results are basically independent of hematocrit; but lower or higher than this range, the results obtained are lower than the expected value. The expected value is defined as the results obtained with hematocrit of normal range. Since it is not common to have a sample with hematocrit outside of the 20 % to 60 % range, the problem is not very serious in practice.

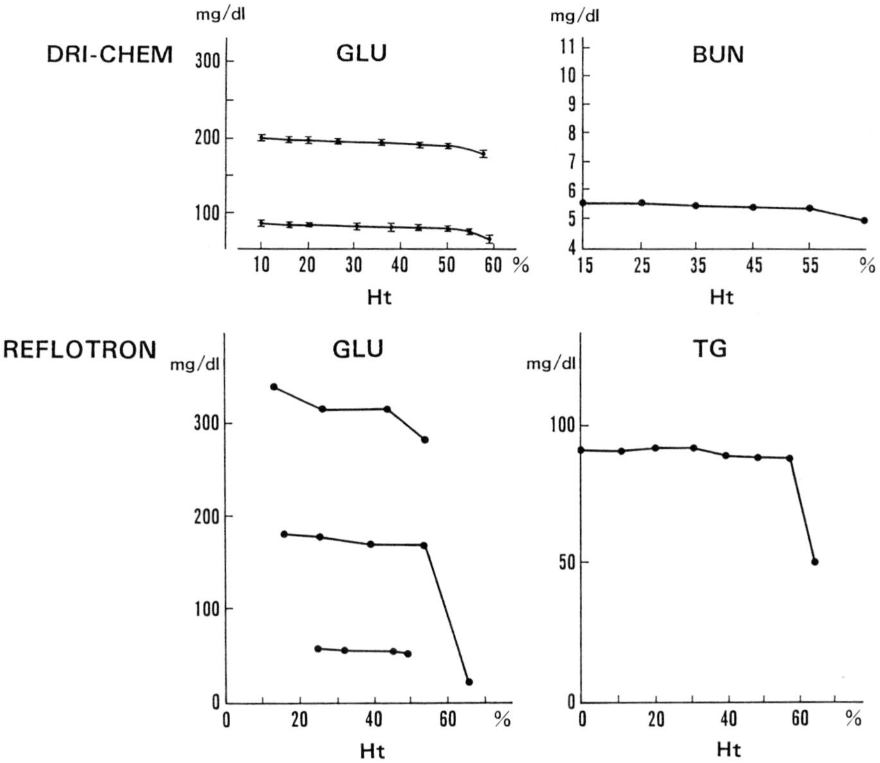

Fig. 7. Effect of hematocrit

OUT PATIENT WARD

In the out-patient ward for diabetics at our hospital, a patient goes to a clinical technologist to get a blood sugar test before going to meet a doctor. The technologist cuts his ear lobe and takes 6 µl of whole blood directly from the ear with a disposable pipette and then, applies the blood sample to a DRI-CHEM glucose slide which is on the DRI-CHEM-1000 analyzer. After 6 minutes, the patient is given his print-out result and goes to see his doctor.

FUJI DRI-CHEM 5000

A FUJI DRI-CHEM 5000 is used in an emergency test room of our hospital. Up to ten slides can be done this instrument at a time; 100 µl of sample, whole blood, plasma or sera is aspirated from a sample cup. Then, the rest of the process preceeds automatically: sample spotting, incubation, optical measurement and printing out the results. The name of each test, as well as the specimen, is differentiated by bar codes. Therefore, at each measurement no in-put operation is neccesary. The throughput of this instrument is about 100 tests per hour depending upon the test menu to be run.

REFLOTRON

30 µl of whole blood sample is applied to a teststrip, and then, the strip is placed in the REFLOTRON analyzer. The results are obtained in 2 to 3 minutes. The name of the test is differentiated by magnetic code on the back of each strip. The magnetic code gives further information, such as the type of the test, preincubation time, wavelength, calculation factor and so on. Thus, in all test items a common teststrip can be used for the test of whole blood, plasma and serum samples.

FUTURE PROSPECT OF DRY CHEMISTRY

Table 5 summerized the future prospect of dry chemistry. Dry chemistry systems, especially those for whole blood analysis, are quite useful for real-time clinical diagnosis at the emergency room, out-patient ward, CCU and ICU. These systems are also useful at satellite laboratories at remote sites in large hospitals or small clinics in isolated locations. Furthermore, I would like to stress that dry chemistry systems for whole blood analysis will be used as powerful tools in improving the medical care conditions in developing countries.

TABLE 5. Future prospect of dry chemistry

1. Real-time Diagnosis
- **Emergency/Urgent Tests**
- **Bed-side Tests**
  - **CCU, ICU, Operation Room, Blood Dialysis ···**
- **Acute Out-patient Ward**
  - **Diabetes Mellitus ···**

2. Decentralized Testing
- **Satellite Clinical Laboratories**
- **Doctor's Offices**
- **Islands or Isolated Locations**

3. Developing Countries

REFERENCES

1. K.C. Kennard, Abstracts of X Internat. Cong. Clin. Chem., Mexico City, p. 13 (1978)
2. A. Ohkubo, S. Kamei, M. Yamanaka, F. Arai, M. Kitajima and A. Kondo, Jap. J. Clin. Pathol., 28 suppl., 67 (1980)
3. S. Ohkubo, H. Hana, H. Yokota, S. Kamei, A. Ohkubo, Y. Sekikawa, N. Yanaginuma, T. Arai and H. Katsuyama, Jap. J. Clin. Pathol., 35 suppl., 76 (1987)
4. A. Ohkubo, S. Kamei, M. Yamanaka, O. Sekimoto, K. Miura, Y. Saito, M. Terashima, Y. Iwata and M. Kitajima, J. Clin. Lab. Inst. Reag., 9, 315-320 (1986)
5. Boehringer Mannheim internal information.
6. H. Yokota, S. Ohkubo, S. Kamei, A. Ohkubo, M. Yamanaka, F. Arai, H. Katsuyama and K. Miura, J. Clin. Lab. Inst. Reag., 10, 65-69 (1987)
7. N. Takagi, N. Yazawa, M. Hirasawa, H. Tomoyasu, R. Uzawa, K. Gomi and H. Ishii, J. Clin. Lab. Inst. Reag., 9, 43-47 (1986)
8. A. Ohkubo, S. Kamei, M. Yamanaka, F. Arai, M. Kitajima and A. Kondo, Clin. Chem., 27, 1287-190 (1981)
9. Fuji Photo Film internal information.
10. C. Takeuchi, T. Iizuka and Y. Hayashi, J. Clin. Lab. Inst. Reag., 9, 35-42 (1986)

Systems using whole blood separation by centrifugal force

A. Truchaud. (Hôpital de Meaux, 77104 France),
C. Burtis (Oak Ridge Tennessee 37831 USA).

Abstract

Plasma separation from whole blood is possible either by filtration or by centrifugation. Several centrifugal systems have been developed to automatically process aliquots of whole blood into aliquots of plasma : a capillary processor and aliquoter, the Vision system and the Satelit 900. Results and analytical performances of these systems are directly comparable to those of big multiparametric analyzers as long as the same reagents may be used with absorbance measurements in an optical cuvette.

Centrifugation of whole blood to produce serum or plasma is a classical preanalytical step in clinical chemistry. Routinely, tubes containing aliquots of whole blood are centrifuged in batches in large laboratory centrifuges which separate either plasma or serum and then transferred into other containers. This processing step is a key step in processing the morning workload of samples in a central laboratory, and is an important constraint and a source of errors for emergency laboratories and for doctor's office work.

In chemistry, measurements on whole blood samples are limited to direct potentiometry by Ion Selective Electrodes. But some analyzers accept whole blood samples because they process automatically the separation of the plasma by different principles. Here, we present systems using centrifugal force, dry chemistry analyzers being the subject of an other article.

A capillary processor and aliquoter was presented in 1986 by C. BURTIS. (Ref 1).
The Vision system was presented at the Oak Ridge conference in 1985 (ref2) and we presented the Satelit system at the Oak Ridge conference in 1987 (ref 3).

CAPILLARY PROCESSOR AND ALIQUOTER (CPA)

The CPA consists of transfer and sampling disks and a processing rotor. A combination of centrifugal force and capillary action is used whithout any mechanical moving parts. The transfer disk can accommodate up to 16 capillaries inserted in a spoke arrangement. These capillaries are constructed from 2.54-cm lengths of 2.24-mm (i.d.) tubing and, when filled, contain approximately 100 uL of blood each. When the transfer disk is placed in the processing unit, the contents of each capillary will be transferred by centrifugal force into a processing chamber.

The sampling disk also can hold as many as 16 capillaries, which have internal diameters smaller than those of the transfer capillaries, and are constructed from 2.54-cm lenghts of precision-bore tubing. Aliquots of specific volumes can be prepared by using capillaries of different internal diameters. This provides the CPA with multivolume capabilities so that sample volumes can be matched with the volumes required for specific chemical assays.
The central processing rotor is fabricated from a disk of clear acrylic plastic into which has been machined 16 individual chambers, each of which will accept a transfer and sampling capillary.

Queries shoud be sent to A. Truchaud
Laboratoire de Biochimie
Centre Hospitalier de Meaux
77104 MEAUX FRANCE

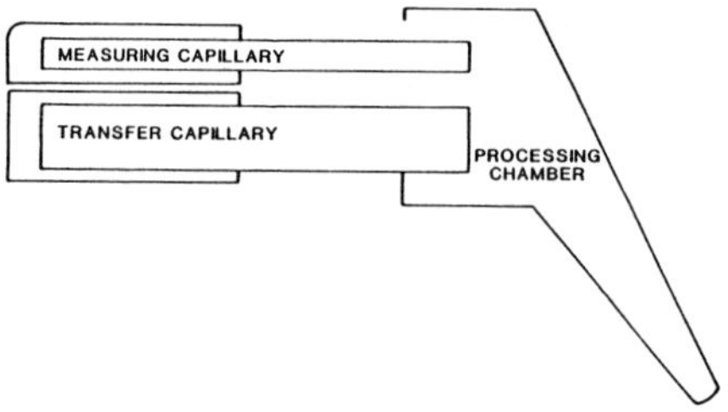

Fig. 1. Side view of one channel of the CPA

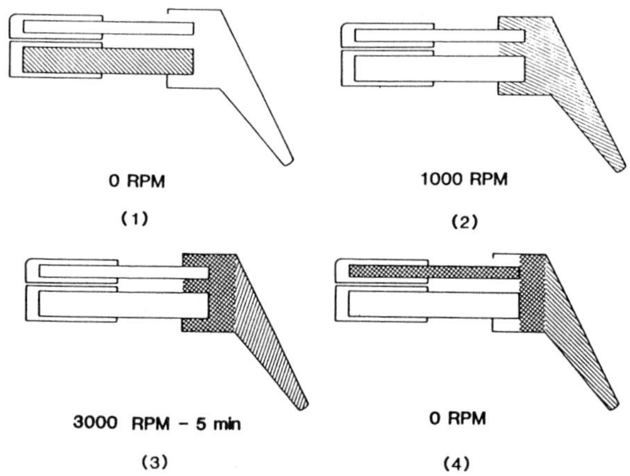

Fig.2. Shematic representation of the process used by the CPA to produce a measured aliquot of plasma from an aliquot of blood.
In View 1 with the rotor at rest, the transfer disk containing capillaries filled with blood is placed into the lower level of the processing unit. The sampling disk is then stacked on top of the transfer disk. When the rotor is accelerated to 1000 rpm (View 2), the contents of the transfer capillaries are propelled into their respective processing chambers. Plasma is then separated from cellular components by increasing the rotor speed to 4000 rpm and maintening it there for 5 min (View 3). When the centrifugal field is removed by decreasing the rotor speed to zero, an aliquot of plasma is withdrawn by capillaries (View 4). The sampling disk is then removed for subsequent analysis. Although not shown in View 4, plasma is also withdrawn into the transfer capillaries. However, because the transfer disk remains in the processing unit, this does not affect the subsequent analytical step.

Table 1. Photometric Evaluation of the Aliquoting and Transfer Capabilities of the CPA, Compared with a Mechanical Pipettor (M).

Volume, Ul	Pipettor	Absorbance[a] Mean	SD	CV, %
1	M	0.0435	0.0014	3.1
	CPA	0.0441	0.0026	6.1
2	M	0.0821	0.0018	2.1
	CPA	0.0866	0.0017	2.0
5	M	0.2018	0.0011	0.5
	CPA	0.2040	0.0046	2.2
10	M	0.3795	0.0018	0.5
	CPA	0.3803	0.0052	1.4

n = 16 observations each. [a]At 400 nm, 0.5-cm pathlength.

Precision and accuracy in the photometric evaluation of the capability of the measuring capillaries for quantitatively delivering their contents into a reaction mixture, the absorbance of the diluted PNP dye volumes indicates the quantity of dye contained in each capillary tube and the effectiveness with which the dye was transferred and delivered. The results, presented in table 1, suggest a linear relationship between capillary volume (x) and absorbance (y) : $y = 0.0912x + 0.0013$ (SEE = 0.0009).
For comparison, similar dilutions were made with a mechanical pipette and obtained comparable absorbances.
So the CPA can process 1 to 10 uL aliquots of plasma with precison and accuracy.

Main uses of the CPA could be :

- the processing of liquids in low gravity conditions like in space,
- a front end sample processor for centrifugal analyzers,
- a sampling unit in two-phase systems i.e. solvent extraction or heterogeneous immunoassays.

THE VISION SYSTEM

The Vision System is a benchtop instrument, using a plastic tespack containing liquid reagents. It was developed by ABBOTT Laboratories (North Chicago, IL. 60064, USA).

Behind an apparent simplicity is hidden a very high technology :

- a mechanical centrifuge that allows a rotation at 1.800 rpm but also, during the course of analysis, the testpack itself is rotated 90° counter-clockwise within 2 seconds, while the main centrifuge till rotates at 1899 rpm.

So, during operation, the test-pack holders rotate back and forth about their normal axes to change the relative g-force vector within the tespack. This action allows fluids to flow between chambers inside the testpack, accomplishing the necessary steps for blood analysis. Furthermore, a self balancing mechanism allows to run from one to 10 tespacks.
A flash lamp and diode array spectrometer provide for optical measurements of 10 testpacks at as many as eight wavelengths simultaneously.
Absorbances are measured during incubation for kinetic analyses (enzymes) and at the end of incubation for equilibrium reactions (general chemistries). The analytical results are calculated and printed, the centrifuge stops, and the testpack is discarded.
To run an assay, introduce 40-80 uL of blood sample into the opening on the testpack cover. Or, place into the testpack end blood acquired by skin puncture and collected into a capillary tube. Position the testpack in the instrument, close the cover, and press the "Run" button. Ten or fewer testpacks, for any combination of available assays, can be placed in the analyzer during a single run. Results are available in less than 10 min and are printed with a 20-column printer. In a separate step, each assay is calibrated by placing two drops of the three calibrator solutions into three separate testpacks, loading the instrument, and pressing the "Calibrate" button. As many as three assays can be calibrated simultaneously.

A large panel of tests are available ; Analytical performances were evaluated in differents ways :

- Jocelyn HICKS made a classical evaluation of the precision which was found excellent and of the correlation with a KODAK EKTACHEM 700. (ref 4).

- Edward SACHS made a correlation study from whole blood versus plasma with the Vision Analyzer which proves the good quality of the separation of the plasma. (ref 5).

THE SATELIT SYSTEM

The Satelit System was developed by Kis company in Grenoble (FRANCE), in cooperation with our team.

The Satelit 900 is a desktop analyser of 15Kg for easy carrying.
The device is based on a disposable testpack with two parts : one is a collector for capillary whole blood, including a part for plasma separation ; the other is a multichambered testpack for measuring and mixing plasma or serum sample with reagents in an optical cuvette with a 5 mm optical lenght. Each part is injection molded and ultrasonically welded.
The Satelit System was developed by Kis company in Grenoble (FRANCE), in cooperation with our team.
The Satelit analyzer is built around a centrifugal rotor with five tespack holders, a self balancing mechanism, a mechanism to rotate the testpacks 180°, then changing the direction of the centrifugal force inside the testpack and an optical system for absorbance measurements.

First, the assay and the reagent lot are checked by a barcode on the testpacks.
During the first centrifugation at 1,800 rpm, reagents are moved into the main chamber including the optical cuvette), mixed, and warmed, and at the end a reagent blank is measured to check reagent integrity ; in the meanwhile, whole blood is being centrifuged in the collector part. After two minutes, the cartridges are rotated at low speed and a new acceleration moves plasma from the collecting part, or any sample from the second chamber, into the sample-measuring chamber, where an aliquot of 10 uL is measured. Sample and reagents are mixed after a second testpack rotation and a new acceleration - stop-run-acceleration. Absorbances are measured after 5 S. to detect eventual reaction interferents in the sample (E.G. hemoglobin, lipids, bilirubin). Then absorbances are measured at any scheduled times from 5 to 240 s. and used to calculate the analytical results. Results are printed for one to five determinations for one to five patients with normal reference intervals and any warning.
So, all the steps of a classical analysis are achieved fully automatically inside the testpack.

We can emphasize some details :
- Usually, systems accepting whole blood require additional parts ; the collecting part of the Satelit avoids any capillary, tips, pipette and gives the assurance to have the right anticoagulant.
- Precision in the metering of the specimen was tested with a concentrated solution of NADH used as a sample, diluted in the testpack by this buffer used as a reagent.
On 20 dilutions, a 1,8 % CV was obtained.
- Plasma sample inlet allows to use only 20 ul of plasma, serum or calibration solution.
- Optical system : in the Satelit system, a tungsten lamp and diode array spectropotometer provide for optical measurements of five testpacks at as many as eight wavelengths simultaneously from : 340 to 690 nanometers. The optical system is linear to 4 A at 340 nm and 2,5 A for other wavelengths.

The lamp is mounted in a preset part for easy replacement. The holographic array is enclosed in a metallic block wich is damp and dust proof. No moving parts in the optics assures for reliability.
So, the flexibility of the optical system is very good, compared to reflectometry systems.
Temperature is controlled at 37° ± 0.1 ; C by an air-heating system ; we tested the delay to warm testpacks from different temperatures to 37°C by using a cresol red solution which absorbance is related to temperature ; whith a testpack warmed 5 minutes at room temperature, the equilibrium is reached 20 s after the beginning of the measurements .i.e. 3 minutes after the beginning of the process.

REAGENTS : it is possible to put a liquid reagent in one or two components into the reagent container : 30 to 100 ul in one chamber, 100 to 1000 ul in the other chamber. It is also possible to put in the mixing chamber a tableted reagent which will be dissolved by a diluent or by orther reagents.
With 10 ul of specimen, this allows dilution ratios for 1/15 to 1/100.

To use the system, the operator collects 60 ul of capillary whole blood, he interlocks the collector with the reagent testpack, he unseals the reagent container by pushing it, he positions the tespack into the analyzer, he identifies the patient through the keyboard and the five assays are displayed, he starts the process ; a few minutes later, results are printed beside normal range.

ANALYTICAL PERFORMANCES

We will report now the first results of the analytical performances of the system from an internal evaluation performed in our laboratory.

Prototypes lots of reagent testpacks were produced in an experimental unit with commercially available reagents from Medical Analysis Systems (Canarillo, California USA).

To check the quality of plasma separation, we compared the results obtained with whole blood and plasma samples for glucose and urea determinations on 40 patients.

Equations of linear regression were :
(Y whole blood ; X plasma)

UREA :	$Y = 1.07\ X - .402$	$r = .986$
GLUCOSE :	$Y = .93\ X + .41$	$r = .990$

Precision was tested on Beckman Decision Control Sera for Glucose, Urea, and Amylase, and on serum pools for Cholesterol Creatine Kinase and bilirubine (Table 1).

Comparison study on 100 patient simples was performed versus Beckman Astra 8 for Urea and Glucose, versus an IL Multistat III with reagents from Biomerieux for cholesterol, amylase bilirubine and creatinine kinase. Results are given on table 1.

TABLE 1

ANALYTE	PRECISION		COMPARISON			LINEAR RANGE
	MEAN	CV %	SLOPE	INTER.	R	
GLUCOSE mmoles/L	2,63 7,06 15,09	3,0 2,1 2,3	.978	+ .03	.996	0,20 – 50 mmoles/l
UREA mmoles/L	2,9 7,1	6,5 6,0	.964	+ .21	.992	1 – 40 mmoles/l
CHOLESTEROL mmoles/L	2,50 4,86	5,1 4,2	1.03	+ .02	.982	0,5 – 15 mmoles/L
CK UI/L	40 207	10,4 4,9	.984	– 5	.999	20 – 1500 UI/L
AMYLASE UI/L	100 200	6,7 6,3	1.05	– 4,4	.997	20 – 1000 UI/L

These preliminary results assess the validity of the concept of the Satelit 900. Performances will certainly be upgraded by final technical improvements decided in the analyzer and the testpack after this internal evaluation.

CONCLUSION

The ability of analytical systems to use whole blood samples reduces manipulations and then the risk of infections contamination.
The integration an automatic process of plasma separation by centrifugal force allows to use classical reagents with multi-wavelenghts absorbance measurements.

A large panel of parametry and furthermore a fast adaptation of new reagents may be provided.

REFERENCES

1. C.A. Burtis , W.F. Johnson, and W.A. Walker, Development of a simple device for processing whole-blood samples into measured aliquots of plasma, Clin. Chem. 32, 1642-47 (1986).
2. S.G. Shultz , J.T. Holen, J.P. Dunohue, and T.A. Francoeur, Two-dimensional centrifugation for desktop Clinical Chemistry. Clin. Chem. 31, 1457 – 63, (1985). (1985).
3. A. Truchaud, Y. Gourmelin, J.P. Simon, G. Jamin, D. Gros, M. Cadoux, D. Seydoux, X. Launois, and J.P. Cloarec. From blood collection to issuing results : a new system that performs all the steps of Clinical Chemistry. Clin. Chem. 33, 1560 (1987).
4. J.M. Hicks, and M. Iosefsuhn., Another physician office analyzer : the Abbott Vision evaluated. Clin. Chem 33, 817-19 (1987).
5. E. Sachs, B. Sachs, and L. Bernstein, Correlation studies for whole blood versus plasma with the "VISION" analyzer. Clin. Chem. 33, 1268 (1987).

Clinical biochemistry of erythrocytes

Bonini P.A, Ceriotti F, Mosca A*, Paleari R.

Istituto Scientifico H.S. Raffaele, Laboratorio Analisi,
* Universita' degli Studi di Milano, Via Olgettina 60, 20132
Milano, Italy

Abstract - The metabolic pathways of human erythrocytes are directed mainly to the production of sustances and energy for the specialized functions of these cells. The analytical approach to the study of such metabolism is usually difficult, because of the relevant interference of the proteic matrix of the cells.
In the last years our research group developed a new potentiometric technology, based on differential measurements of pH, which has been succesfully applied to the study of some peculiar aspects of the erythrocytic metabolism. The main advantages of this techinque, in comparison with the traditional spectrometric analysis, are: a) lack of interference from sample colour and turbidity; b) automatic sample blank subtraction; c) simpler analytical reaction schemes.
In the present report we shall illustrate the application of the differential pH technology to the study of the following clinical-biochemical problems: 1) assay of G6PDH activity, 2) acetylcholinesterase assay in erythrocytes and whole blood, 3) ATP and Magnesium assay.

Why we need a clinical biochemistry of erythrocytes? Which are the analytical problems related to the practical and correct determinations of erythrocytic parameters? The answer is that in many forms of anemia there are important modifications of erythrocyte components and that the monitoring of erythrocytes parameters during storage could be of relevant importance for a safe and effective blood transfusion.
Red blood cells activities are largely concerned with the exchange of oxygen, but there are also some other important metabolic pathways to be usefully investigated.
Glycolysis and the connected pentose shunt pathway are critically important to the red cell, first to provide energy for various functions, and second to modulate hemoglobin function. The glycolysis accomplishes the generation of three important substances: ATP, DPG and the reduction of NAD+ to NADH.
The 2-3DPG has the very important role of affecting the release of oxygen by hemoglobin, but we have no intention to face the complex field connected to hemoglobin and the gaseous exchanges in this paper.
Considering the glycolytic system, for each molecule passing through this pathway to lactic acid, a net syntesis of 2 molecules of ATP occurs. In fact 2 moles of ATP are employed for the phosphorilation of glucose to G-6-P and of F-6-P to F-1,6-P while 4 moles are produced at the phosphoglycerokinase and pyruvate kinase steps (each mole of glucose is splitted in two trioses).
APT plays a number of important roles in the mature red cell: 1) phosphorylation of sugars (mainly glucose), 2) transmembrane transport of K+ and Na+; 3) maintenence of cell shape; 4) syntesis of purine and pyridine nucleotides; 5) regulation of glycolysis by allosteric inhibition of phosphofructokinase. Many of the ATP functions are mediated by the presence of magnesium.
Another important function of the anaerobic glycolysis is the reduction of NAD to NADH, which is accomplished at the glyceraldeide-3-P step. The reduced cofactor is used by the methemoglobin reductase that is responsible for the reduction of methemoglobin. In fact hemoglobin is continously oxydized to methemoglobin, a nonfunctional product with iron in the ferric state.
After a carbohydrate passes through the various steps of glycolysis it ends up as pyruvic acid or lactic acid. These molecules are both freely diffusible through the red cell membrane and the levels are in equilibrium with the plasmatic ones. The equilibrium between pyruvate and lactate is

regulated by LDH and plays an important role in the red cell metabolism. In fact the conversion of pyruvate into lactate produces NAD+ that has a regulatory effect on the glycolysis at glyceraldeide 3-P step.
A collateral cycle in the glycolytic process is the pentose phosphate shunt The two most important functions of this pathway are the reduction of NADP to NADPH and the production of phosphoribosyl-pyrophosphate. The NADPH is used by glutathione reductase to keep almost all glutathione within the red cell in the reduced state. Reduced glutathione is used to protect the cell from oxidant damage. Phosphoribosyl-pyrophosphate is used for the syntesis of adenine nucleotides.
From the brief exposition on erythrocyte metabolism appears clearly the important role played by some analytes like ATP, Mg and G-6PD. We will point out the importance of these metabolites and enzymes in some diseases and the possibility to determine them on whole blood or washed erythrocytes through appropriate technologies. Particularly we will describe the Delta-pH metry which is the technique developed in our institute (1).

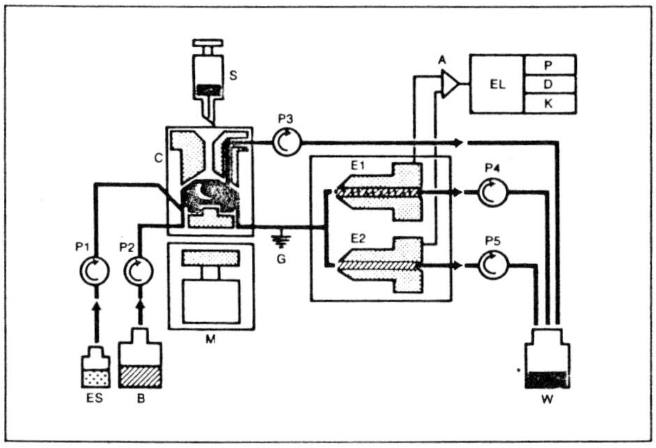

Fig. 1 Schematic representation of a delta-pH apparatus; the explanation of the symbols is in the text.

In Fig. 1 a schematic diagram of a delta-pH apparatus is illustrated. There is a mixing chamber (C) where the reaction takes place that is filled by the peristaltic pump P2 with a buffer from a separate reservoir (B); by means of the peristaltic pump P3, the content of the mixing chamber can be brought to constant volume (typically 800 ul). The content of the mixing chamber can be mixed by means of a magnetic stirrer (M). The two capillary electrodes (E1 and E2) (Ingold AG, Zurich, CH) having an internal volume of about 25 ul, can be filled with the reaction mixture (contained in the mixing chamber) by the action of the peristaltic pumps P4 and P5, respectively.
The measure cycle is started by the operator, when he manually introduces a known amount of the sample . The stirring motor is automatically activated for 2 s to mix the content of the mixing chamber, then about 300 ul of the reaction mixture are aspirated into the electrodes. Pump 1 then injects into the mixing chamber a known quantity of the reaction starter, the stirring motor is activated again for 2 s, and the pump 5 aspirates about 300 ul of this reaction mixture (containing the starter) into electrode 2. After a suitable time, the difference in pH between the reaction mixtures respectively contained in the electrode 1 (sample blank) and 2 (reaction to be measured) is calculated from the difference in potential between the two electrodes. With this technique is possible to follow any kind of reaction in which a pH variation is involved, and the method is completely unaffected by sample colour or turbidity.
The major features of this technique are the following: 1) it does not suffer from any colorimetric interference from hemoglobin, 2) it permits an automatic blank subtraction and in some cases 3)the use of whole blood instead of washed erythrocytes, 4) it uses simpler reaction schemes. For these reasons this technique is particularly suited to study red blood cells where the high hemoglobin content heavily interferes with traditional colorimetry. In this report we present the application of this technique to the study of some critical aspects of erythrocyte biochemistry.

GLUCOSE-6-PHOSPHATE DEHYDROGENASE

The erythrocytic G-6-PD deficiency is a genetically transferred X-linked disease. It is the most prevalent heterogeneous enzyme defect in humans, being responsible for two clinical syndromes: spontaneous chronic congenital nonspherocytic anemia and episodic hemolytic anemia induced by drugs, food (fava beans) and bacterial or viral infections. The accurate quantitative determination of G-6-PD activty is possible only using the WHO recommended method (2) that is time consuming and requires high technical skill.

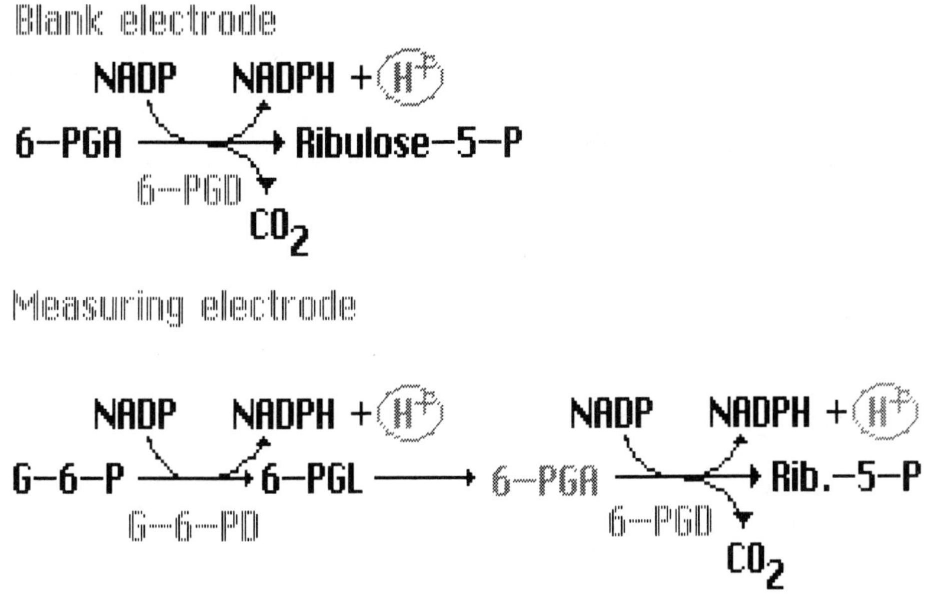

Fig. 2 Reaction scheme of the G6PD determination

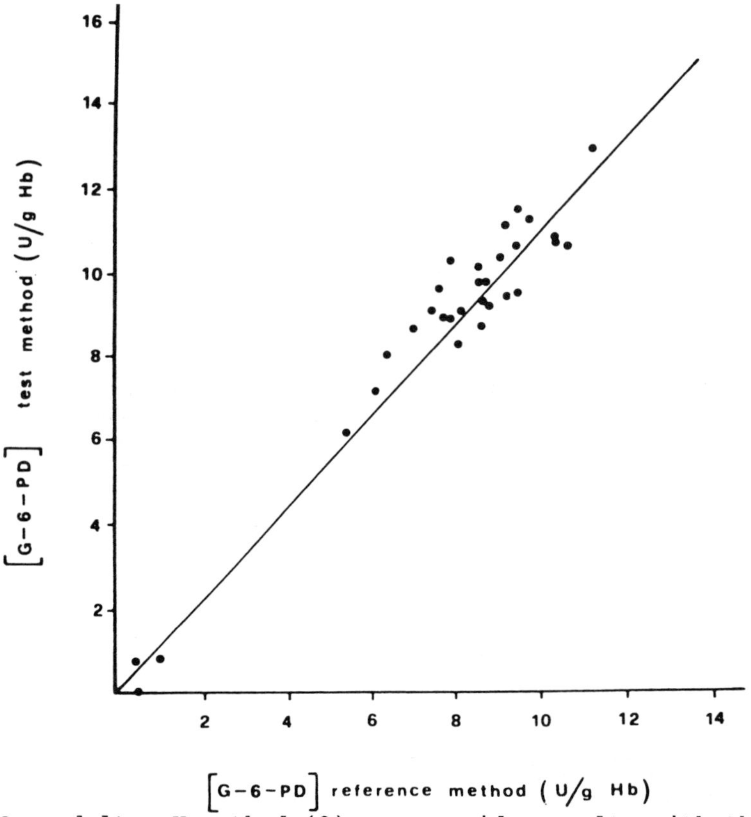

Fig. 3 Correlation between our method (y axis) and the WHO method (x axis).
y= 1.13x + 0.02
r = 0.971

Our delta-pH method (3) can provide results with the same accuracy and with even better precision but in shorter time and without any particular skill. The method is based on the reactions shown in Fig. 2.In the blank electrode only the interfering 6-phosphogluconate-dehydrogenase reaction takes place and is automatically subtracted. After a short lag-phase (10-20 s) a delta pH over a 60 s period is recorded. Fig. 3 illustrates the correlation between our method and the recommended WHO method using washed erythrocytes. It is also possible to use whole blood (volume of sample needed: 10 ul) as a screening procedure, obtaining sligthly higher results (about 10%) caused by the interference due to the G-6-PD content of leucocytes and platelets.

ACETYLCHOLINESTERASE

This enzyme is a component of the red cell membrane, but its function in the erythrocyte metabolism is still unknown. In fact an inherited deficiency or a pharmacological inhibition do not seem to affect the red cell survival or function. Nevertheless the erythrocyte acetycholinesterase determination has a great interest as a marker of environment pollution. Its levels are markedly reduced in intoxications from organophosphate and carbamate pesticides.
The RBC ACHE determination is useful also in the diagnosis of a rare disease: the paroxysmal nocturnal hemoglobinuria, in this disease the ACHE levels are frequently low. The principle of the reaction is shown in Fig. 4.

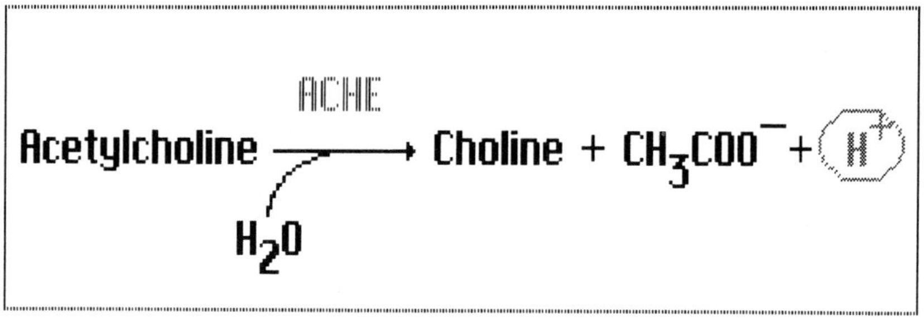

Fig. 4 Reaction scheme of the acetylcholinesterase determination

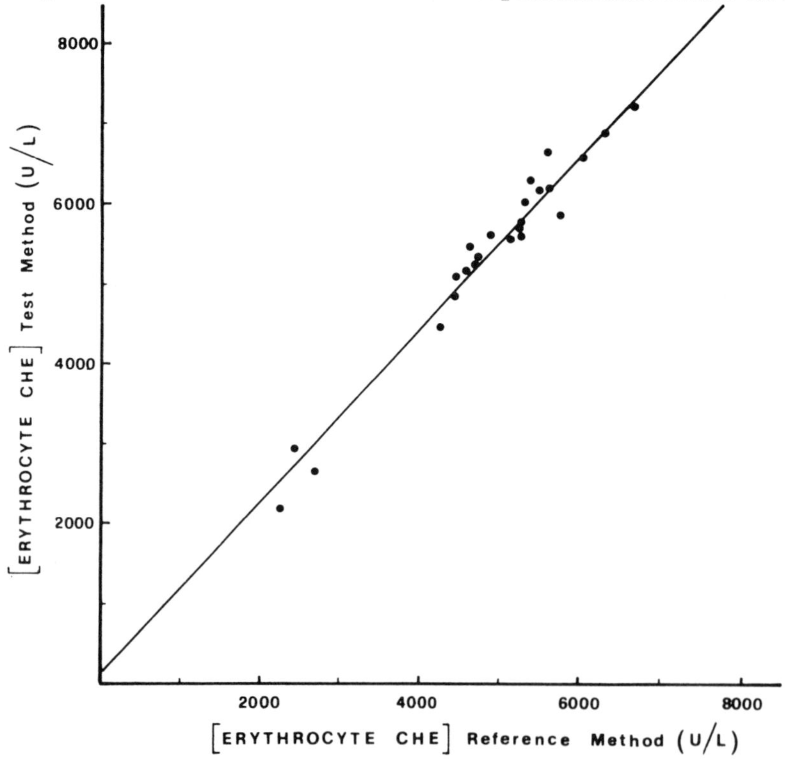

Fig. 5 Correlation between our method (y axis) and the Ellman method (x axis). y=0.938x + 87 r=0.9694

The reaction is performed on whole blood using 10 ul of sample, the interference of plasma pseudocholinesterase is eliminated by the addition of a specific inhibitor (quinidine sulphate).
The correlation with the colorimetric method is shown in Fig. 5.

ATP

As discussed previously, ATP plays a central role in the erythrocyte metabolism. Its levels are a useful parameter to monitor the cell vitality; in fact they are reduced in many pathological conditions, such as some

glycolytic enzyme deficits (pyruvate kinase, hexokinase, G-6-PD), diabetes, chronic renal failure, cardiac and hepatic injuries.
Current methods used to measure the ATP levels usually need the execution of a deproteinization or an extraction step. Our delta-pH based method can be performed on whole blood (50 ul) inactivated with a heat treatment (5 min at 65 C). The principle of the test is illustrated in Fig. 6.

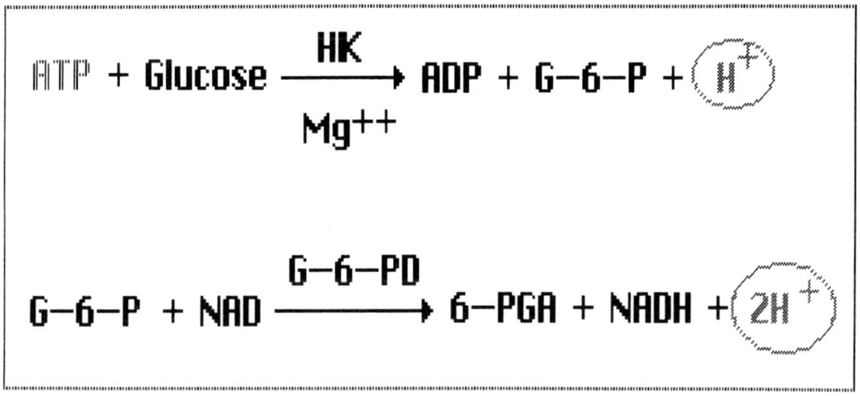

Fig. 6 Reaction scheme for ATP determination

The correlation with a colorimetric method (Sigma)(Fig. 7) shows a significant underestimation of our method. We excluded experimentally the possibility of a distruction of ATP during the heat treatment. We believe that the deproteinization procedure liberates some ATP which is protein bound and that is not analyzed when measuring undeproteinized samples.

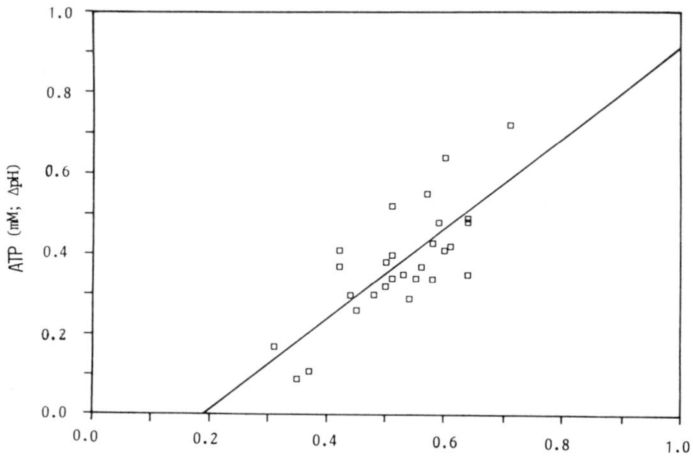

Fig. 7 Correlation between our method (y axis) and the Sigma method (x axis).
y = 1.222x - 0.21
r = 0.779

MAGNESIUM

Magnesium is an essential cofactor of many kinases and has an important role in the glycolytic process, in pentose phosphate shunt, in transmembrane ion transport and cell shape maintenance.
The erythrocytic Mg level seems to be a good indicator of the total body Mg content. With the aging of the red cells there is a reduction of the Mg concentration and a low erythrocytic Mg level seems to reduce the red cell life and to induce ultrastructural membrane defects. Moreover a prolonged increase of RBC Mg level has been recently observed after a miocardial infarction.
The principle of our measurement is illustrated in Fig. 8.
The correlation with a colorimetric enzimatic method is shown in Fig. 9.

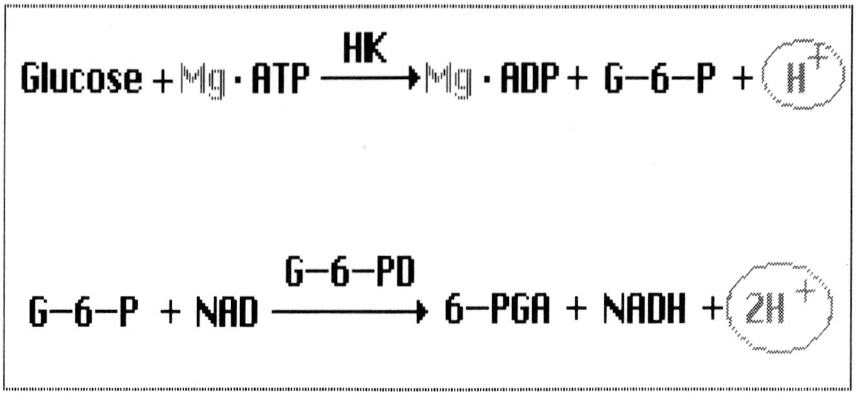

Fig. 8 Reaction scheme of the determination of magnesium

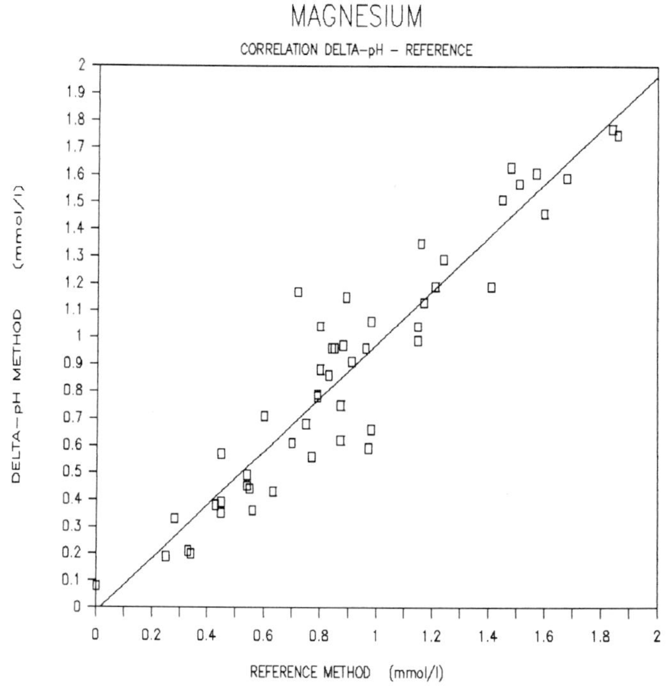

Fig. 9 Correlation between our method (y axis) and a photometric enzymatic method (x axis).
$y = 0.989x - 0.03$
$r = 0.942$

In conclusion, 1st: there is a large evidence of the importance of the avaiability of reliable, routine methods to determine biochemical parameters of erythrocytes, possibly using whole blood , either to diagnose some diseases, or to check the quality of the blood to be transfused ;
2nd: our proposed methodology seems to largely fulfill the requirements of an optimal technique for this purpose. Other parameters will be avaiable in near future and we look for international collaboration to improve our results.

This research has been partially supported by CNR (Consiglio Nazionale delle Ricerche).

REFERENCES

1) Luzzana M, Dossi G, Mosca A, et al. Clin Chem 29,80-85 (1983)
2) Report of a WHO Scientific Group. Standardization of procedures for the study of glucose-6-phosphate dehydrogenase. WHO Tech. Rep. Ser. 1967;366
3) Barenghi L, Ceriotti F, Ripamonti M. Clin Chem 33,579- 582 (1987)
4) Barenghi L, Ceriotti F, Luzzana M, et al. Ann Clin Biochem 23,538-545 (1986)
5) Ellman GL, Courtney KD, Andreas V, Featherstone RM. Biochem Pharmacol 7,88-95 (1961)

Pulsed field gel electrophoretic snapshots of chromosomes

Cassandra L. Smith*, Jose P. Abad#, and Guy Condemine#

Departments of *Microbiology, *Psychiatry, and #Genetics and Development, College of Physicians and Surgeons, Columbia University, N.Y. 10032

Abstract - Pulsed field gel electrophoresis and large DNA technology allow the analysis and manipulation of molecules that range in size up to 10 million base pairs. This means that it is now possible to do molecular studies on whole chromosomes from virtually any organism. These techniques have revolutionized studies on protozoans, fungi, bacteria, and the human genome.

INTRODUCTION

In the past most molecular studies on DNA focused on specific genes or small regions of genomes. The advent of pulsed field gel (PFG) electrophoresis (ref. 1) and large DNA technologies (refs. 2-7) now allows manipulation and characterization of DNA molecules 100 times larger than have previously been worked with. Thus, it is now possible to do molecular studies on whole chromosomes.

PFG electrophoresis was first applied to separating the chromosomes of various yeasts (ref. 8) and parasitic protozoa (ref. 9) because the chromosomal DNAs from these organisms were within the size range first resolved by this technique, i.e. from 0.05 to 1 million base pairs (Mb). Initial studies with *Saccharomyces cerevisiae* (ref. 8) and on the small Trypanosome (ref. 10) chromosomes simply and directly determined, for the first time, numbers and sizes of chromosomal DNAs and allowed the characterization of important chromosomal rearrangements. Some of the identified chromosomal polymorphisms in parasites helped clarify aspects of infectious disease processes and were even used for diagnostic purposes.

EXPANDING THE PFG FRACTIONATION SIZE LIMIT

Subsequent experiments have expanded the size range of DNA molecules amenable to analysis by PFG electrophoresis to at least 10 Mb (refs. 11-12). These DNA molecules are enormous. If they were stretched out they would be 1 mm in length. These new size limits have recently allowed the identification and comparison of chromosomal DNAs from an ever increasing number of organisms, such as *Schizosaccharomyces pombe* (ref. 11), *Neurospora crassa* (ref. 12), *Candida albicans* (refs. 13-14), *Plasmodium falciparum* (refs. 15-16), *Giardia lamblia* (ref. 17, Smith *et al.*, unpublished), and the previously unkown large number of large chromosomal DNAs of Trypanosomes (Smith *et al.*, unpublished). The smallest human chromosome is 50 Mb; this is only 5 times the size of the largest size DNA molecule that has been fractionated bv PFG electrophoresis. At this time, the true size limit for DNA fractionation by PFG electrophoresis is unknown. Also unknown is the size limit of intact DNA molecules that can be isolated, manipulated, or cloned.

PFG ELECTROPHORETIC SIZE STANDARDS

In order to analyze DNA molecules by PFG electrophoresis reliable size standards needed to be developed. The first standards used in this technique were bacteriophage DNAs (lambda, T7, T2, and T4) and the chromosomal DNAs of *S. cerevisiae*. The sizes of the former DNAs were known, but they only extended up to 180 kilobases (kb); while only approximate sizes of the later molecules were known they appeared to extend up to at least 1 Mb. The first accurate DNA length standards that extended to 1 Mb were made by tandemly annealing bacteriophage DNAs at high concentrations (refs. 2, 18). In fact, these size standards extend above 6 Mb, but in practice definite bands can only be resolved to about 1.5 Mb.

Since physical maps have been constructed for the three chromosomes of *S. pombe* (Fan *et al.*, unpublished), their sizes are known (3.5, 4.7, and 5.7 Mb). This means that these chromosomal DNAs can be used for size standards for molecules above 1.5 Mb. Finer size standards in this range have been developed using the partial restriction enzyme digestion products from the *S. pombe* chromosomes (Ringquist *et al.*, unpublished).

PURIFICATION AND MANIPULATION OF INTACT CHROMOSOMES

Large intact DNA molecules cannot be purified using the usual solution procedures because such molecules are exquisitely sensitive to shear damage. Thus, DNA purification procedures were developed in agarose to prevent shear damage (ref. 1). A summary of specific agarose procedures for DNA purification and manipulation from a wide variety of organisms can be found in reference 19. Essentially, live cells from virtually any organism are suspended in agarose, and the suspension is distributed into a mold which forms blocks of agarose called inserts. If the organism has a cell wall, like bacteria and yeast, it is treated *in situ* with reagents that remove the cell wall material. Naked cells from all organisms are lysed *in situ* and treated with various reagents that clean up the DNA and, if necessary, make the DNA amenable to enzymatic manipulation.

Although circular bacterial chromosomes are within the size range amenable to PFG resolution, these molecules will not enter agarose gels unless they are linearized. The simplest way to linearize these molecules is to treat them with a restriction enzyme (refs. 2, 19). Restriction enzymes with large recognition sites facilitate chromosome mapping experiments because they cut the genome at a limited number of places. Now, only two restriction enzymes are known with 8 bp recognition sequences, *Not* I and *Sfi* I (Figure 1A). These enzymes should produce fragments which average 64 kb from an organism with a 50% GC content and random base distribution. Although *E. coli* has such a GC content, genomic *Not* I and *Sfi* I restriction fragments average 200 kb, whereas in the closely related bacterium, *Salmonella typhimurium*, fragments average 64 kb (Figure 1A). Thus, even closely related organisms can be easily distinguished.

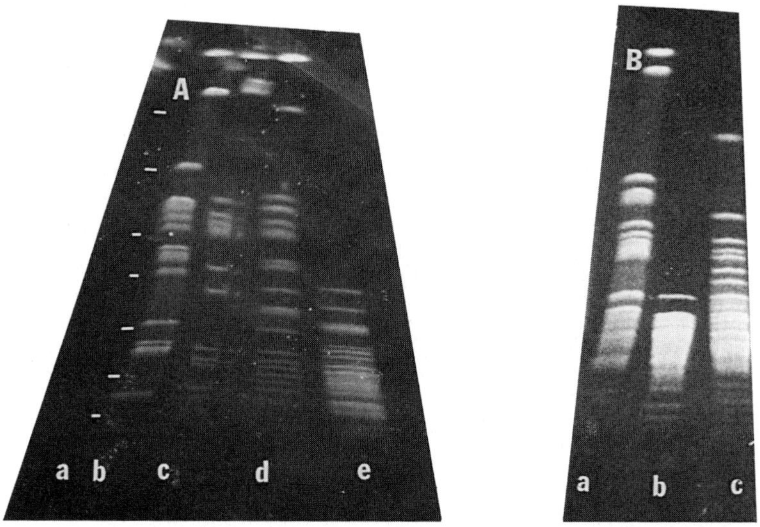

Figure 1. Genomic Restriction Enzyme Digestion. A. *E. coli* and *S. typhimurium* digested with *Not* I. Bacterial chromosomal DNA purified in agarose was digested with various restriction enzymes and fractioned by PFG electrophoresis on a Pharmacia-LKB Pulsaphor apparatus for 40 hrs at 330 V and 15 C using 30 sec pulse times. Lane a - Annealed lambda phage DNA (monomer = 48.5 kb), b - *E. coli* K12, c - *E. coli* B, d - *E. coli* C and e - *S. typhimurium*. B. *E. coli* K12 digested with restriction enzymes with 6 bp recognition sites. Lane a - *Xba* I, b - *Nhe* I and c - *Spe* I.

Preliminary experiments with new organisms should simply test a wide variety of restriction enzymes with 6 bp recognition sites for their ability to generate a small number of large genomic restriction fragments. The restriction enzyme *Dra* I generates large fragments in *Mycobacterium* species because it recognizes the sequence TTTAAA and these organisms have high GC content (Smith, Jacobs, and Bloom, unpublished observations). Surprisingly, very large genomic restriction fragments also are produced from *E. coli* with restriction enzymes having the nonsense codon, TAG, in their recognition sequence (Figure 1B). The restriction enzyme *Avr* II (CCTAGG) produces fragments whose average size is greater than that of *Not* I and *Sfi* I; *Xba* I (TCTAGA) and *Spe* I (ACTAGT) produce fragments that range from 0.02 up to 0.8 Mb, while *Nhe* I (GCTAGC) produces fragments ranging from 0.02 up to only 0.2 Mb. It is not yet clear whether the ability of these enzymes to produce large fragments extends to other organisms. Even the restriction enzyme *Bam* HI has proved useful in comparing different Archaebacteria (ref. 20).

CONSTRUCTION OF GENOMIC RESTRICTION MAPS

Using large DNA technology, complete low resolution physical maps of *E. coli* (ref. 21) and *S. pombe* (Fan *et al.*, unpublished) have been completed along with large regions of various mammalian chromosomes (refs. 22, 23, 24). The existing technology permits such maps to be constructed from virtually any organism. The construction of these maps is particularly eased by the use of linking clones (refs. 2, 3, 4) as probes in hybridization experiments along with partial restriction mapping strategies that are especially well suited to PFG. Linking clones are those clones which contain sequences recognized by infrequently cutting enzyme. A *Not* I linking clone used as a probe in a hybridization experiment to *Not* I digested DNA will identify the two large fragments that lie next to each other. Partial digestion strategies are particularly well suited to PFG because resolution increases as the size of the DNA increases. Thus, hybridization experiments with single copy probes to partially digested genomic DNA fractionated by PFG electrophoresis has scanned 3% of human chromosome 21 in a single experiment.

SCANNING CHROMOSOMES FOR DNA POLYMORPHISMS

The detection of genomic polymorphisms allows one to analyze the relationship between different isolates and to identify unknown organisms. Many organisms such as *S. cerevisiae* and various protozoans have their genomes divided into enough chromosomes so that DNA polymorphism between different isolates are easily detected by PFG electrophoresis by simple chromosome fractionation experiments (see above). However, genomes of other organisms are not divided into many chromosomes. For instance, prokaryotes have single chromosomes. DNA polymorphisms may be detected in these organisms by specifically fragmenting their genomes into a reasonable number of large restriction fragments that can be resolved by PFG electrophoresis.

Large DNA technology can also be applied to obtain snapshots of large regions of more complex eukaryotic genomes. The pattern of large restriction fragments obtained from mammalian genomes thus far appears to be too complex to analyze directly. However, hybridization experiments with multicopy probes or with pools of single copy probes allow large regions of the genome to be scanned in single experiments (Figure 2).

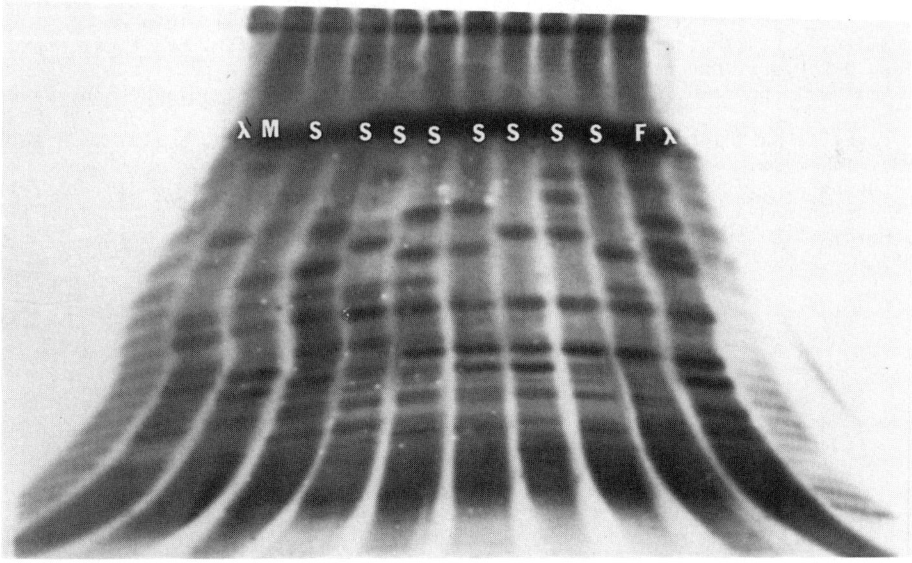

Figure 2. Detection of DNA polymorphism in a family over a large region of the human genome. DNA from human lymphoblastoid cells purified in agarose was digested with the restriction enzyme *Xho* I, fractionated by PFG electrophoresis as described in the legend to Figure 1 using 100 sec pulse time. λ -annealed lambda bacteriophage DNA (monomer = 48.5 kb). M - mother, F - father. and S - siblings. The gel was hybridized with a chromosome X alphoid repeat probe.

The size limits of DNA molecules amenable to analysis and manipulation has drastically changed as have the types of molecular studies now possible on whole chromosomes and genomes. The application of the new large DNA technologies to a variety of biological systems and problems has only just begun. The full impact of these technologies on biology will not be realized until scientists change their thinking to accommodate the new technical possibilities.

ACKNOWLEDGEMENTS

This work was supported by grants from DOE (DG-FG02-87ER-GD825), NIH (GM14825), Pharmacia-LKB and the MacArthur Foundation.

REFERENCES

1. D.C. Schwartz, W. Saffran, J. Welsh, R. Haas, M. Goldenberg, and C.R. Cantor. Cold Spring Harbor Symp. Quant. Biol. 47, 189-195 (1983).
2. C.L. Smith, P. Warburton, A. Gaal and C.R. Cantor. In, Genetic Engineering, eds. J.K. Setlow and A. Hollaender, Plenum, NY, 8, 45-70 (1986).
3. C.L. Smith, S.K. Lawrance, G.A. Gillespie, C.R. Cantor, S.M. Weissman and F.S. Collins. In, Methods in Enzymology, "Molecular Genetics of Mammalian Cells", ed. M. Gottesman, Academic Press, New York, 151, 461-489 (1987).
4. C.L. Smith and C.R. Cantor. In, Methods in Enzymology, "Recombinant DNA", ed. R. Wu, Academic Press, New York, 151, 461-489 (1987).
5. C.L. Smith and C.R. Cantor. TIBS 12, 284-287 (1987).
6. R. Anand. TIG 23, 278-283 (1986).
7. D.P. Barlow and H. Lehrach. TIG 3, 167-171 (1987).
8. D.C. Schwartz and C.R. Cantor. Cell 37, 67-76 (1984).
9. L. Van der Ploeg, D. Schwartz, C.R. Cantor, and P. Borst. Cell 37, 77-86 (1984).
10. S. Holmes-Giannini, M. Schittine, J.S. Keithly, P. Warburton, C.R. Cantor, and L.H.T. Van der Ploeg. Science 232, 761-763 (1986).
11. C.L. Smith, T. Matsumoto, O. Niwa, S. Klco, J.B. Fan, M. Yanagida and C.R. Cantor. Nucl. Acids Res. 15, 4481-4490 (1987).
12. M.J. Orbach, D. Vollrath, R.W. Davis, and C. Yanofsky. Molecular and Cellular Biology 8, 1469-1473 (1988).
13. D. Vollrath and R. Davis. Nucl. Acids Res. 15, 7865-7877 (1987).
14. R.G. Snell, I.F. Hermans, R.J. Wilkins, and B.E. Corner. Nucl. Acids Res. 15, 3625-3630 (1987).
15. T. Wellems, D. Walliker, C.L. Smith, V. Rosario, W. Maloy, R. Howard, R. Carter, and T. McCutchen. Cell 49, 633-642 (1987).
16. L.H.T. Van der Ploeg, M. Smits, T. Ponnudurai, A. Vermeulen, J.H.E.T. Meuwissen, and G. Langsley. Science 299, 658-661 (1985).
17. R.D. Adam, T.E. Nash, and T.E. Wellems. Nucl. Acids Res. 16, 4555-4567 (1988).
18. M.K. Mathew, C.L. Smith, and C.R. Cantor. Biochemistry (1988). In press.
19. C.L. Smith, S.R. Klco, and C.R. Cantor. In, Genome Analysis: A Practical Approach, ed. K. Davies. IRL Press, Oxford, England (1988). In press.
20. C.L. Smith, J. Econome, A. Schutt, S. Klco, and C.R. Cantor. Science 236, 1448-1453. (1987).
21. J.L. Sanz, I. Marin, L. Ramirez, J.P. Abad, C.L. Smith, and R. Amils. Nucl Acids Res. (1988). In press.
22. S.K. Lawrance, C.L. Smith, S.M. Weissman, and C.R. Cantor. Science 235, 1387-1390 (1987).
23. W.R.A. Brown and A.P. Bird. Nature 322, 477-481. (1986).
24. D.A. Hardy, J.I. Bell, E.O. Long, T. Lindsten, and H.O. McDevitt. Nature 323, 453-455 (1986).

Separation of antibody by affinity gel electrophoresis

Kazusuke TAKEO

Department of Biochemistry, Yamaguchi University School of Medicine, Ube 755, Japan

Abstract - We have developed a new types of two-dimensional electrophoresis measuring the difference in charged state of proteins in the first direction and the difference of their biological activity in the second direction. Thus, rabbit anti-DNP antibodies have been separated in the first direction by IEF and in the second direction by affinity electrophoresis. By this method, purified rabbit anti-DNP antibodies have been separated into several hundred IgG spots. Each spot appears to be homogenesou. While at the beginning of the immunization IgG having lower pI and higher dissociation constant were predominant, after one to two weeks of the immunization IgG spots having the higher pI became predominant. Carrier proteins of the hapten appeared to have no effect on their heterogeneity. On the basis of the electrophoretic patterns and the affinity for DNP-hapten, those IgG spots can be grouped into several monoclonal IgG families. Preparative affinity electrophoresis in a scale of one milligram order of IgG samples has also been develped.

INTRODUCTION

Induced antibodies against a single antigenic determinant are heterogeneous. In order to separate those heterogeneous antibodies into individual immunoglobulins, isoelectric focusing (ref. 1, 2) or two-dimensional electrophoresis (ref. 3, 4) have been used. In spite of their high resolving power, satisfactory resoltuion of polyclonal antibodies still has not been attained.

Two-dimensional electrophoresis based on the diversity of charge in the first direction and on the difference of biological activity in the second direction should be feasible for separating heterogeneous protein mixture of equal molecular weight, such as induced antibodies. Under these considerations, we have developed a new type of two-dimensional electrophoresis carring in the first direction by isoelectric focusing (IEF) and in the second direction by affinity electrophoresis(AEP) (ref. 5, 6, 7). Thus, rabbit anti-DNP antibodies have been separated into more than hundred immunoglobulin spots. Each spot appears to be homogenous. On the basis of the unique electrophoresis patterns and the affinity for the hapten, these immunoglobulin spots can be grouped into several IgG families. Each IgG family appears to be monoclonal. This affinity technieque could contribute to elucidation of the mechanism of heterogeneous antibody production from the angle of protein chemistry.

ANALYTICAL TWO-DIMENSIONAL AFFINITY ELECTROPHORESIS

Analytical two-dimensional affinity electrophoreswis (analytical 2D-AEP) is composed of, as the first electrophoresis, IEF on capillary PAG and, as the second electrophoresis, affinity electrophoresis on semimicro scale PAG slab. Table I shows the conditions for the first and the second electrophoresis. At the second electrophoresis, slightly acidic buffer system of Reisfeld (ref. 8) was usually used. In this case, the final pH of the gel becomes to 3.9. Affinity ligand, DNP-PA was added uniform in the separating gel and the gel was polymerized in dark. At the same time, the separating gel, lacking the affinity ligand was prepared as the reference gel. Concentration of DNP-residues of the affinity ligand was calculated from the absorption at 360 nm using DNP-glycine as the standard. Western blot was carried out in the glycine-HCl buffer, pH 2.5, using blotting apparatus having cooling device. Using the double antibody fixation technique, followed by the peroxidase activity staining, 1 - 2 ug of anti-DNP-IgG can be stained clearly separated in two-dimension.

Preparation of anti-DNP antibodies: Rabbits were hyperimmunized with DNP-carrier protein conjugates as antigen (5 mg as an emulsion of an equal volume mixture of the complete Freund's adjuvant). As the carrier protein, human gamma-globulin(HGG), rabbit serum albumin(RSA), chicken serum albumin(CSA), egg white lysozyme(EWL), and concanavalin A(Con A) were utilized. The animals were bled periodically and the anti-DNP antibodies were purified by affinity chromatography using DNP-lysine Sepharose 4B column. The obtained antibody preparations are composed of almost only the IgG class of antibodies.

Fig. 1 shows the 2D-affinity patterns (Picture B and C) of one of the anti-DNP-antibody preparations (1Z-4). For the reference, the capillary IEF pattern (Picture A) obtained from the same antibody using 10 ug antibody and Coomassee staining is also presented. The antibody is separated into a large number of bands in the pH range between 5 and 8. Picture B is the

Fig. 1 Two-dimensional affinity electrophoresis pattern of rabbit anti-DNP antibody (1Z-4)

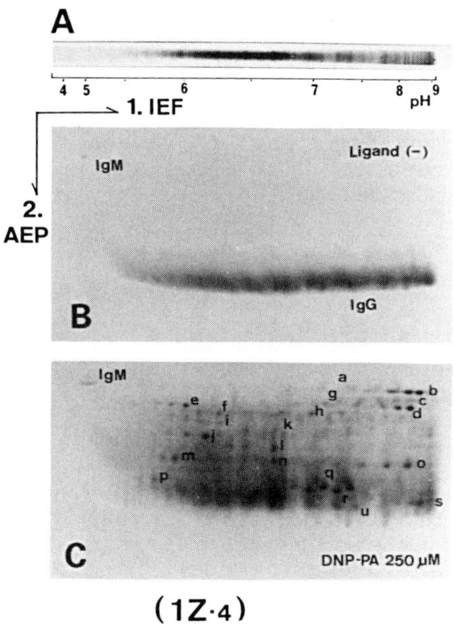

Table I Condition of analytical two-dimensional affinity electrophoresis

The first electrophoresis

Capillary PAG IEF (1.3 x 65 mm)		
Gel composition: T = 5%, C = 3%		
Ampholite	pH 4 - 6.5	0.63%
	pH 6.5 - 9	0.63%
	pH 5 - 8	1.25%
Glycerol		10%
Lysine		1.5 mM
Urea		6M
TEMED		0.1%
Amm. persulf.		0.05%
Electrode solution:		
Cathode		1 N NaOH
Anode		0.04M glutamaic acid

The second electrophoresis

AEP in slab PAG (75 x 75 x 1 mm)
Gel composition: T = 5.1%, C = 2.6%
Buffer system:
Slightly acidic buffer system reported by Reisfeld (ref.8) (the final pH = 3.9)
Affinity ligand:
DNP-PA 0 - 500 uM in slab PAG
(PA; allylamine-acrylamide copolymer)

reference 2D-affinity pattern of the same antibody obtained at the absence of DNP-PA. The antibody migrates as a straight line. A trace of IgM spot is demonstrated at the corner of the pattern. When the second electrophoresis was carried out at the presence of 250 uM DNP-PA, as seen in Picture C, the antibody is separated into several hundred spots. Among them, clearly stained spots can be grouped at least into 21 (a to u) anti-DNP IgG families. Every family is composed of several IgG spots having the identical affinity, but different pI. The higher the affinity, the stronger the decrease of mobility. The apparent dissociation constants of each IgG family can be calculated from the affinity pattern according to the affinity theory (ref. 6, 7). They are amounted to be the values from 10^{-4}M to 10^{-7}M.

Fig. 2 shows 2D-affinity patterns of another preparation of anti-DNP IgG (1S-6) at two different pH in the second electrophoresis. Under the slightly acidic condition of the Reisfeld system (pH 3.9) and at the absence of the affinity ligand (picture A), the IgG preparation migrates as a straight line as in the case of the previous antibody. At the presence of DNP-PA (picture B), the IgG preparation was separated into a large number of spots. The clearly recognized IgG spots can be grouped into 19 families from a to s. Under the slightly alkaline condition of Ornstein-Davis system (pH 9.5)(ref. 9, 10) as the second electrophoresis and at the absence of DNP-PA (picture C), the IgG preparation migrates as a broad line inclining to the cathodic side. At the presence of DNP-PA (picture D), the IgG preparation was separated into a large number of spots, but not so sharp. However, still the separated spots can be grouped

Fig. 2 Two-dimensional affinity electrophoresis patterns of rabbit anti-DNP antibody (1S-6) obtained at two different pH values

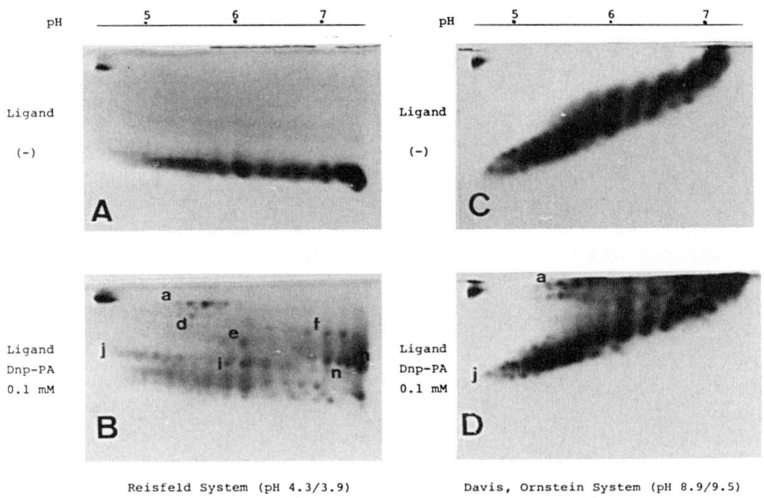

Fig. 3 The time course of antibody production (2F) and 2D-AEP patterns after immunization with DNP-RSA.

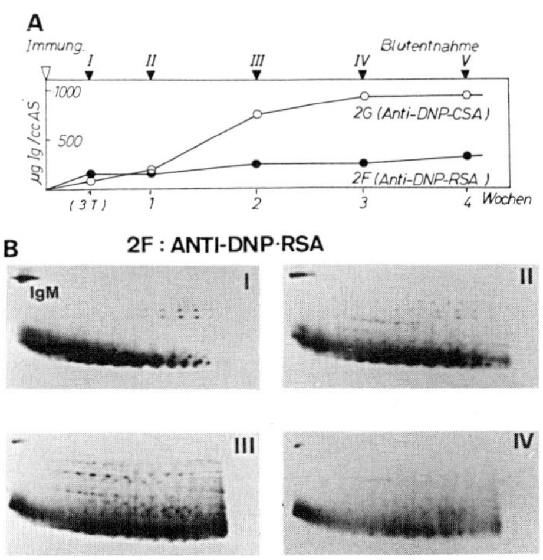

Fig. 4 The time course of antibody production (2G) and 2D-AEP patterns after immunization with DNP-CSA.

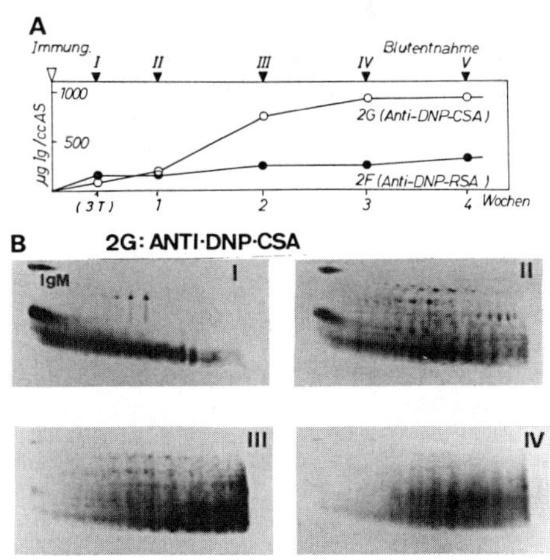

into several families corresponding to those obtained at the slightly acidic condition. This result verifies the assumption, that each IgG family is monoclonal.

From this affinity patterns, the apparent dissociation constants were calculated. For Families a and j, they amounted at pH 3.9 to be 3.7 x 10^{-5}M and 1.9 x 10^{-4}M and at pH 9.5, they are 2.2 x 10^{-5}M and 3.4 x 10^{-4}M, respectively. This results indicate that, Family a has a higher affinity at the alkaline condition, while Family j has a higher affinity at the acidic condition. Because at the slightly acidic condition of the Reisfeld buffer system, much clearer and sharper patterns have been obtained, we have utilize the Reisfeld buffer system as the standard second electrophoresis throughout the experiments.

Picture A of Fig. 3 shows the time course of antibody production after immunization. The abscissa is time in week and the ordinate antibody concentration in antisera. Antibody concentrations were calculted assuming that the yield of the antibody prepared by the affinity chromatography is theoretical. The closed circles(2F) is the antibody concentration obtained from antiserum prepared against DNP-rabbit serum albumin(DNP-RSA) and the open circles(2G) is that prepared against DNP-chicken serum albumin (DNP-CSA) as antigen. Few milliliters of blood was taken 3 days(I), 1(II), 2(III), 3(IV), and 4(V) weeks after the immunizations. While DNP-RSA is weak antigen and antibody concentration was only gradually increased from 157 ug to 320 ug per ml, DNP-CSA is a potent antigen and 3 weeks after the immunization, antibody concentration was increased from 87 ug to 910 ug per ml. Picture B of Fig. 3 shows the 2D-affinity patterns of anti-DNP-RSA antibody in various stages of the immunization. While the patterns of the anti-DNP antibody prepared from bloods taken 1 and 2 weeks after the

Fig. 5 Two-dimensional affinity electrophoresis patterns of anti-DNP antibodies induced against DNP-conjugates with various carrier protein.

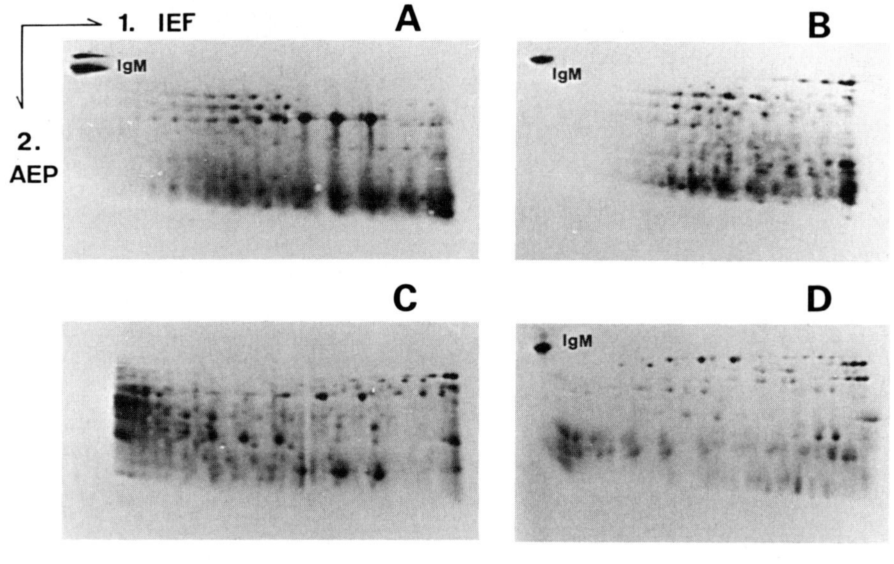

immunization (II and III) show sharp and clear patterns with highly heterogenous distribution, 2D-affinity pattern obtained from blood taken 3 weeks after the immunization (IV) shows diffuse pattern. The dissimilation of antibody appears to start from the second or third week after immunization.

Picture A in Fig. 4 is the identical time course pattern with that presented in Fig. 3. In Picture B in Fig. 4, 2D-affinity patterns of anti-DNP-CSA antibody in various stages of the immunization were presented. While the antibody concentration was much higher than that of anti-DNP-RSA antibody, the sharpness and the degree of heterogeneity of the patterns were almost of the same order. Three weeks after immunization, its 2D-affinity pattern became diffuse as in the case of the anti-DNP-RSA antibody. These results suggested that carrier protein of hapten-antigen affects on the level of antibody production, but does not affect on the degree of antibody heterogeneity.

Fig. 5 shows the 2D-affinity patterns of anti-DNP antibodies induced against DNP-conjugates with various carrier protein. Picture A is that against DNP-rabbit serum albumin, Picture B against DNP-chichen serum albumin, Picture C against DNP-lysozyme, and Picture D against DNP-concanavalin A, respectively. While the serum concentration of each antibody and its electrophoretic patterns are different from each other, they are all equally highly heterogeneous. Those results verify the assumption that the carrier protein of DNP-antigens affects on the level of antibody production, but does not affect on the antibody heterogeneity.

PREPARATIVE TWO-DIMENSIONAL AFFINITY ELECTROPHORESIS

Table II shows the conditions of the preparative 2-D affinity electrophoresis. The first electrophoresis was performed using a larger capillary, 3.5mm in diameter and 14.5 cm in length. To this column 0.5 to 1 mg antibody sample can be applied. The second electrophoresis was carried out with the preparative PAG electrophoresis apparatus (ref. 11), 15 cm in width, 8.5 cm in height, and 3 mm in thickness. Electroblotting was performed in the 50 times diluted phosphate buffered saline containing 2 mM DNP-glycine at pH 7.4. The blotted nitrocellulose membrane was stained by dipping into 0.5% Ponceau Red in 1% acetic acid and washed with 1% acetic acid. The stained NC membranes were stored in cool protecting from drying. Fig. 6 shows one of the preparative 2D-affinity patterns of

Table II Conditions for preparative two dimensional affinity electrophoresis

The first electrophoresis

Column PAG IEF (3.5 x 145 mm)
Gel composition:
As same as for the analytical method (T = 5%, C = 3%, pH 4.0 - 9.0)

The second electrophoresis

AEP in slab PAG (15 cm x 8.5 cm x 3 mm)
Gel composition and buffer system:
As same as for the analytical method (T = 5.1%, C = 2.6%, the final pH = 3.9)
Affinity ligand: 400 uM DNP-PA

Detection and extraction

Western blot:
NC membrane in the presence of 2 mM DNP-glycine, pH 7.4
Staining: 0.5% Ponceau Red 3 R in 1% acetic acid
Extraction: 70% formic acid

Fig. 6 Two dimensional affinity electrophoresis pattern of anti-DNP antibody (1S-6) in preparative scale.

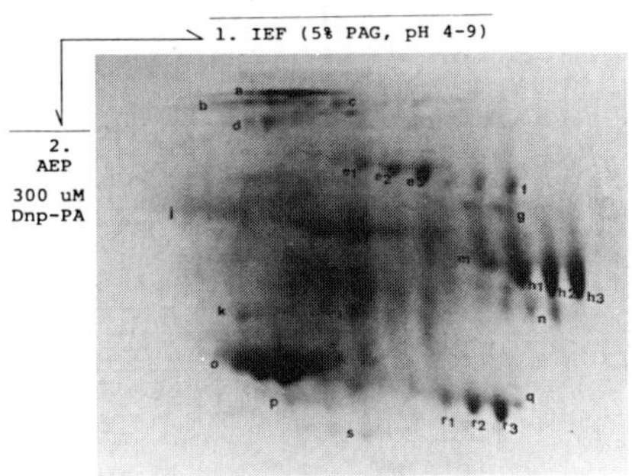

Fig. 7 SDS-PAGE patterns of the anti-DNP IgG samples extracted from the spots on the NC membrane with 70% formic acid

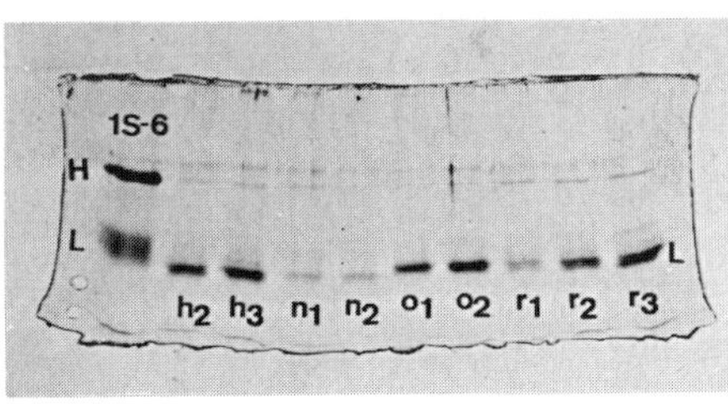

anti-DNP antibody (1S-6). The antibody was separated well as in the case of the analytical AEP. IgG from each spot can be extracted with 70% formic acid.

Fig. 7 shows the SDS-electrophoresis pattern of the IgG samples extracted from spots on the nitrocellulose membrane with 70% formic acid. At the left end of the picture, the pattern of the original IgG sample (1S-6) was also shown as the reference. Its light chain migrated as a broad band. While the yield of extraction of IgG, especially of the heavy chains were very low, generally only 20 to 30%, those electrophoretic patterns were sharp. Nevertheless, electrophoretic patterns of those spots, which were extracted from the same families (for example, h_2 and h_3, or r_1, r_2 and r_3, and so on) showed the identical pattern. Those results verify the assumption that every IgG family is composed of monoclonal IgG. In regard to the applicability of two-dimensional affinity electrophoresis to preparative scale, however, there are many problems to be solved. But its application will give us the useful technical means in the field of immunochemistry.

CONCLUSION

Two-dimensional affinity electrophoresis presented here offers a powerful tool for elucidation of heterogeneity of antibodies and its production mechamism. Its resolving power is the highest one among the similar resolution techniques. Furthermore, one sheet of 2D-affinity pattern gives many important informations on immunoglobulins:

1) It gives not only pI distribution pattern of immunoglobulin, but also
2) its affinity distribution.
3) The apparent dissociation constants for all IgG spots can be calculated from one sheet of 2D-affinity pattern.
4) The technique is appricable to follow the process of the appearance and the disappearance of individual immunoglobulins in serum at physiological and also at pathological conditions.

REFERENCES

1. C. Wood and E. A. Kabat, Arch. Biochem. Biophys., 212, 262-276 (1981).
2. N. Congy and C. Mihaesco, Immunology, 35, 307-315 (1978).
3. N. L. Anderson, S. L. Nance, T. W. Pearson and N. G. Anderson, Electrophoresis, 3, 135-142 (1982).
4. T. Manabe, Y. Takahashi, N. Higuchi and T. Okuyama, Electrophoresis, 6, 462-467 (1985).
5. K. Takeo and S. Nakamura, Arch. Biochem. Biophys., 151, 1-7 (1972).
6. K. Takeo, Electrophoresis, 5, 187-195 (1984).
7. K. Takeo, Advances Electrophoresis, 1, 229-279 (1987).
8. R. A. Reisfeld, U. J. Lewis and D. E. Williams, Nature, Lond., 195, 281-283 (1962).
9. B. J. Davis, Ann. N. Y. Acad. Sci., 121, 404-427 (1964).
10. L. Ornstein, Ann. N. Y. Acad. Sci., 121, 321-349 (1964).
11. K. Takeo, R. Suzuno, M. Fujimoto, A. Kuwahara, H. Ogata and S. Nakamura, Bull. Yamaguchi Med. Sch., 23, 165-183 (1976).

Ionic-floating chromatography of biopolymers

Tomisaburo Kakuno, Bok-Hwan Kim, Jinpei Yamashita and Takekazu Horio

Institute for Protein Research, Osaka University, Suita, Osaka 565, Japan

Abstract - Biopolymers are easily adsorbed to the gel matrix of HPLC packings by nonspecific interaction which causes retardation and broadening of elution peaks and as the results poor yields. On the contrary, ionic repulsion between a biopolymer and a gel matrix shifts the elution time earlier than the expectant value. The repulsion could be applicable to prevent the nonspecific adsorption of biopolymers to the gel matrix. Nucleic acids such as DNA and RNA tend to be adsorbed to the gel matrix owing to their hydrophobicity. When the nucleic acids with negative charge interact with a cation-exchange group (negative charge), they are supposed to be prevented from the adsorption to the gel matrix as if they were floated in the pore of the gel. By the use of the charged molecular-sieve gel in the presence of salts, nucleic acids and proteins were separated better than that by the conventional noncharged molecular-sieve gel. We propose to call it ionic-floating chromatography.

INTRODUCTION

HPLC is widely used in basic sience research and applied research. Various of chromatographies have been developed and many kinds of gel packings are now on the market, however, the nonspecific adsorption of biopolymers to gels arises from ionic and hydrophobic interactions. Sometimes, these seriously affect the performance of the chromatography. The two interactions act in an opposing manner with the addition of salts; an increase in salt concentration reduces the ionic interaction while strengthening the hydrophobic interaction.

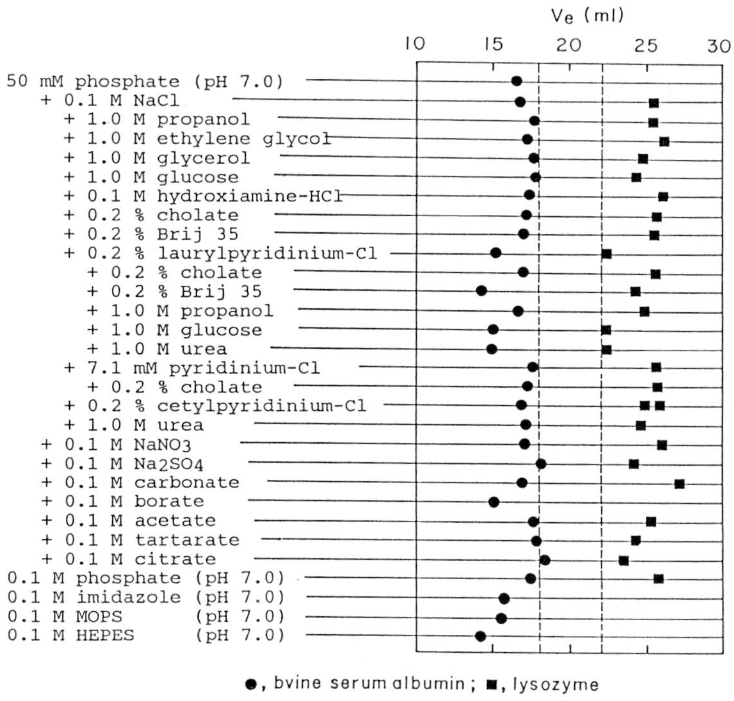

Fig. 1 Effect of various running buffers on Ve of BSA and lysozyme

SILICA-BASED MOLECULAR-SIEVE GEL

Silica-based gels, in which silanol groups are masked with glyceropropyl groups are popular for separating biopolymers such as proteins. However, a major problem is that it is impossible to mask all the silanol groups and avoid the matrix effect. Most proteins are distributed along a calibration line of molecular weight versus elution volume (Ve) with TSK-gel G3000SW, However, lysozyme is retarded from the estimated value of Ve while BSA precedes it. These two proteins are useful samples to examine the secondary interaction between proteins and gel matrix. For improving the above problems, we have tried to find a better running buffer than the standard buffer (50 mM phosphate (pH 7.0) + 0.2 M NaCl). By using 50 mM phosphate at pH 7.0 as the base buffer, the effects of various additives on the elution volume were examined with lysozyme and BSA. The left broken line represents the Ve value estimated from the calibration curve, and the right broken line is of BSA. With the base buffer only, BSA was eluted at an earlier point than the predicted value but the lysozyme was not. With the addition of 0.1 M NaCl, lysozyme was eluted but it was away from the calibration line. When various OH group-containing compounds were added to the buffer, the Ve of the two proteins were closer to the calibration line. Glucose and citrate gave the best results. Other additives had a one-sided effect. Where it was suitable for BSA, it was not for lysozyme and vice versa. Generally speaking, the OH-rich compounds gave relatively good results but we could not identify an ideal buffer for both proteins. There were limitations which prevented the secondary adsorption of proteins on silica-based SW columns even when the running buffer was replaced. Another disadvantage of silica-based gel is its instability under alkaline conditions.

POLYMER-BASED COLUMNS

Polymer gels have been recently developed and widely used in the separation of biopolymers. The resolution of the polymer gel is now comparable to that of silica-based gel. It has the advantage of high stability at alkaline pH values. In general however, polymer gels show a matrix effect in which biopolymers are suddenly adsorbed in the presence of high concentration of salts. Shodex Ionpak KS columns contain polymer gel which consists of stylene-divinylbenzene copolymer with a porous structure and sulfonate group as a cation-exchange ligand. There are six kinds of Ionpak KS columns depending on their exclusion limits (TABLE 1).

TABLE 1. Shodex Ionpak KS-800 series

Material; stylene-divinylbenzene copolymer

Exclusion limit (Shodex STANDARD P-82 Pullulan);

Ionpak KS-801	1×10^3
KS-802	1×10^4
KS-803	1×10^4
KS-804	1×10^5
KS-805	1×10^6
KS-806	1×10^7

Ligand; sulfonic acid group

Column size; diameter 8 mm, length 300 mm

IONIC REPULSION BETWEEN GEL AND BIOPOLYMER

When a gel has a negative charge, it repels a biopolymer with a negative charge. This ionic repulsion could be used in preventing nonspecific adsorption of biopolymers to the gel matrix. Nucleic acids bear negative charges at neutral pH and are thought to be repelled by a cation-exchange ligands. By using Ionpak KS series which are negatively charged molecular-sieve columns, we examined the elution profiles of deoxyadenine pentadecamer in the presence of various concentrations of sodium sulfate. With KS-803, the elution peak of $p(dA)_{15}$ shifted with the addition of salt (Fig. 2). In the presence of 10 mM Tris-acetate buffer only, the oligonucleotide was eluted first where it corresponded to the void volume of the column. However, with the addition of sodium sulfate, the peak was shifted toward a larger volume with increasing concentration, and reached an approximate maximum at higher than 0.25 M of the salt (Fig. 3). These figures show the dependency of salt concentrations on the Ve of $p(dA)_{15}$ with three kinds of Ionpak columns, KS-803, KS-804, and KS-805. In the absence of Na_2SO_4, the Ve corresponded to the Vo with KS-803 and KS-804. In KS-804, the dependency of Ve on salt concentration was remarkable. As the concentration of salt increased, the Ve increased and then reached a plateau. Under these conditions, the so-called repulsion chromatography is observed. In KS-805, the Ve was not equal to the Vo. It is conceivable that the pore size of the gel is so large that the ionic repulsion between the oligonucleotide and the gel surface might be negligible. In the presence of 0.2 M or higher sodium sulfate, every curve was parallel. This means that the repulsion is eliminated though the adsorption is microscopically suppressed by the short-range repulsion and molecular-sieving is occuring. The schematic model shows how DNA and the gel interact with each other in the absence and the presence of the salt (Fig. 4). In the absence of salt, a negatively charged DNA should be repelled by the negatively charged groups on the gel matrix. Thus, it has a difficult time entering the pore. On the other hand, the repulsion will be weakened in the presence of salt and DNA molecules easily penetrate into the depth of the pore. Accordingly, DNA molecules might move around as if they were floating from the surface of gel. We suggest calling this mode ionic-floating chromatography.

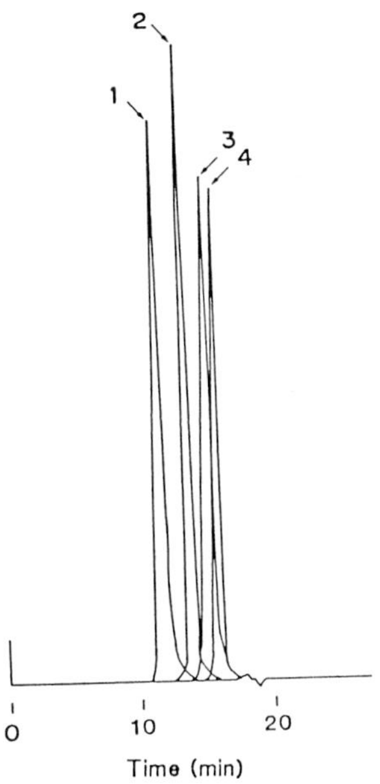

1) 10 mM Tris-acetate + 1 mM EDTA (pH 7.5)

2) TAE buffer + 0.10 M Na_2SO_4

3) TAE buffer + 0.25 M Na_2SO_4

4) TAE buffer + 0.50 M Na_2SO_4

Fig. 2 Effect of salt concentration on elution profile of $p(dA)_{15}$

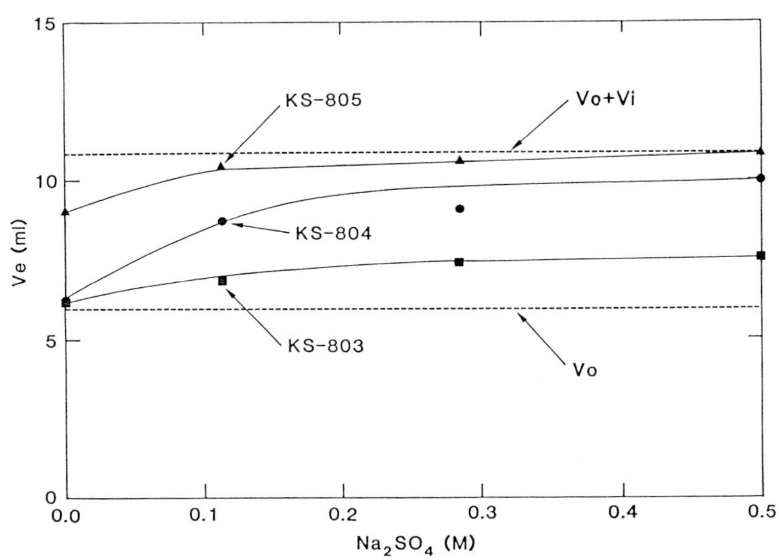

Fig. 3 Effect of salt concentration on Ve of $p(dA)_{15}$

IONIC-FLOATING CHROMATOGRAPHY OF OLIGONUCLEOTIDES

In our study, four kinds of oligodeoxyadenines: pentamer, decamer, pentadecamer, and pentacosamer were separated with adequate resolution and high recovery by ionic-floating molecular-sieve chromatography using KS-802 and KS-803 connected in a series (Fig. 5).

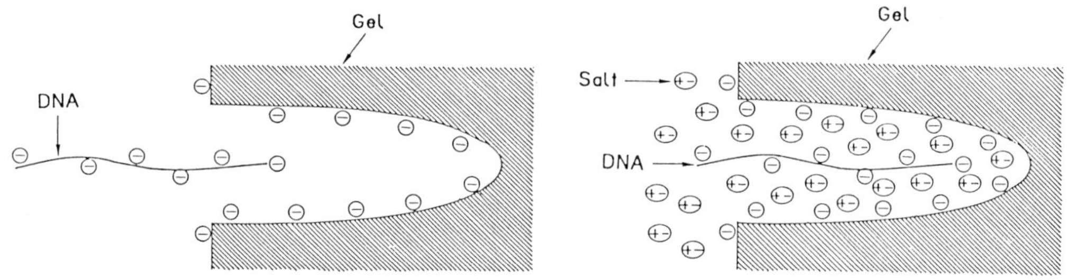

Fig. 4 Schematic model of interaction between DNA and gel.

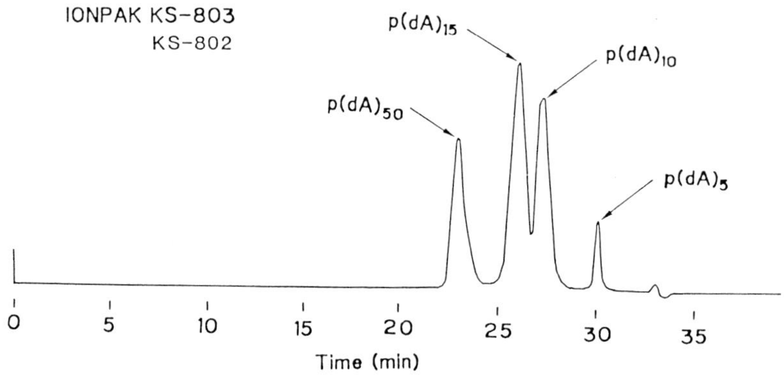

Fig. 5 Separation of oligonucleotides by ionic-floating chromatography

IONIC-FLOATING CHROMATOGRAPHY OF PROTEINS

On the basis of above information, we have applied this technique for separation of proteins. For ionic-floating chromatography, better results occur with samples that do not

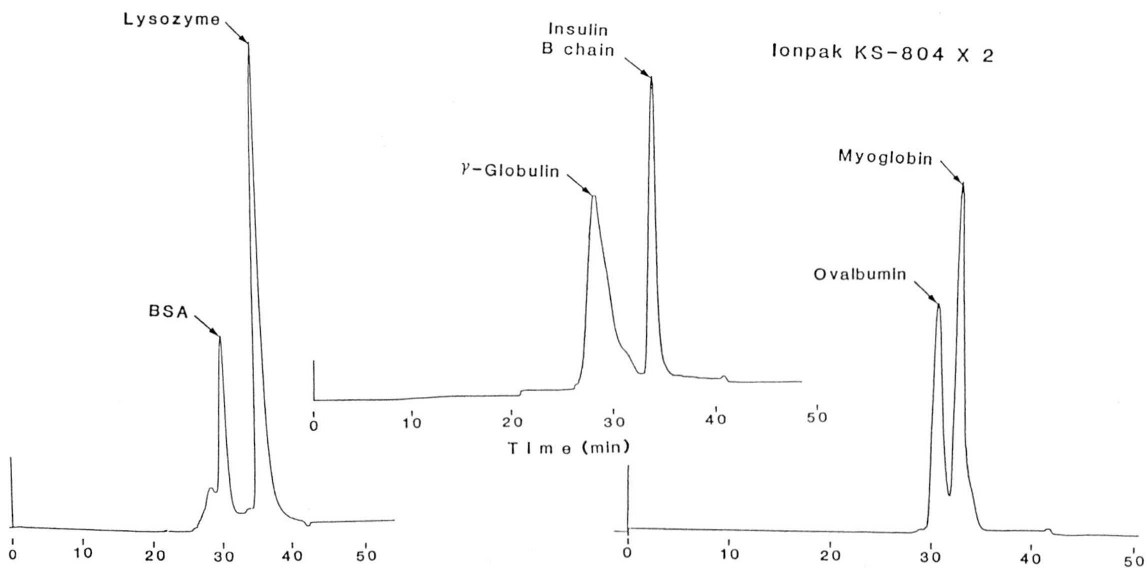

Fig. 6 Separation of proteins by ionic-floating chromatography

contain the opposite polarity to the gels. At pH 12, all the dissociated groups of amino acids possess a negative or zero charge. The running buffer for protein separation contained 20 mM sodium phosphate (pH 12) with 50 mM sodium sulfate and 0.25% SDS. The ionic strength of the buffer was reduced by 1/4 of the oligonucleotide separation buffer to avoid hydrophobic interactions during protein separation. As shown in Fig. 6, the peaks were sharp. The height equivalent to the theoretical plate (HETP) for BSA with KS-804 was 0.13. This was comparable to TSK gel G3000SW. Since most proteins have their isoelectric points in the acidic region and have a negative net charge at a neutral pH, it might be possible to perform the ionic-floating molecular-sieve chromatography also at a neutral pH.

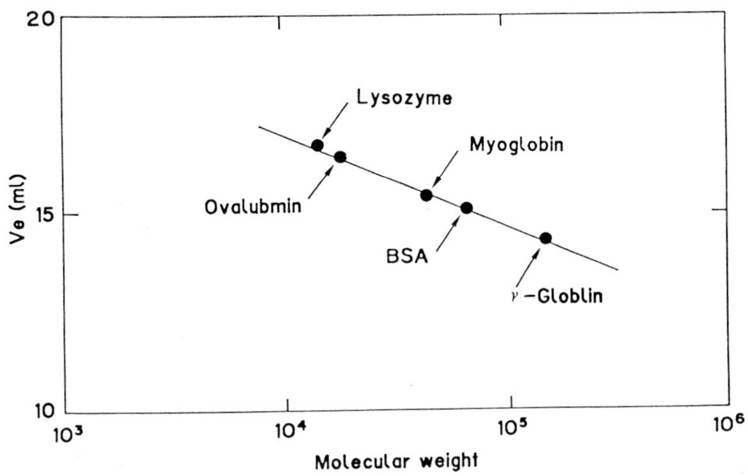

Fig. 7 Relationship between molecular weight and Ve with proteins

A plot of the logarithm of molecular weight versus Ve for proteins is shown in Fig. 7. Five kinds of proteins: lysozyme, ovalbumin, myoglobin, BSA, and γ-globulin were fitted to the calibration curve. In immuno-affinity chromatography, proteins are sometimes hard to elute from an antibody-bound affinity column. The ionic-floating chromatography might be useful for high-yield elution of proteins from such an immuno-affinity column. To prevent a nonspecific adsorption of biopolymers to gel matrix, we have proposed the ionic-floating chromatography. It might also be effective in purifying micro-scale quantities of biopolymers.

Recent trend in progress of immunodiagnostics

Tadashi Kawai

Department of Clinical Pathology, The Jichi Medical School,
Tochigi, 329-04, Japan

Abstract - The development of the versatile and sensitive analytical technique of quantitative radioimmunoassay has revolutionized diagnostic methodology in clinical medicine and has provided a powerful analytical tool in biomedical research. Recently, there has been a growing interest in the use of non-isotopic immunoassays for monitoring the distribution of free and antibody-bound ligands. The following non-isotopic labels have been used in immunoassays: bacteriophages, free radicals, fluorescent groups, chemiluminescent groups, synthetic particles, red blood cells, electron-dense materials, metals, enzymes, and prosthetic groups. There are many reasons of replacing the radioisotopic labels with nonradioactive ones. Enzymes have been most commonly used as well as latex particles and fluorescent materials. These non-isotopic immunoassays have been developed first in reagent kits, and then in partly or fully automated systems.Major advantages of using automated systems include to avoid tedious and complex manual procedures, and to set a strict reactional condition in order to improve their precision significantly. However, their automated systems are usually expensive and far from a compact set-up. There has been no system that could avoid satisfactorily the prozone phenomenon inherent to any antigen-antibody reaction. A recent trend in the development of automated immunoassay systems for clinical use, except for luminescent assays which are covered in the other sections, is reviewed.

One of the major challenges for modern medical science is the translation of basic immunological advances into diagnostic and therapeutic procedures applied clinically. Much of this work has been done in the clinical immunology laboratory, where a great variety of the recent ly developed immunoassay principles are performed on various clinical samples. The clinical laboratory results are then utilized by many clinicians in the diagnosis and treatment of clinical disorders. The wide application of these immunological laboratory tests has led to better understanding of the pathogenesis of clinical disorders. In turn, this better understanding has stimulated further basic scientific research in immunology.

The goals of laboratory medicine are to improve the availability, accuracy, and precision of a group of medically important laboratory tests to assure correct interpretation, to assess the the significance of new tests introduced into clinical medicine. It is particularly important for the industry to supply the immunological reagents or kits which show good performance characteristics. Most of the immunological reagents cannot be made or produced in routine clinical laboratories, and they must be brought into clinical laboratories through various industrial services.

HISTORY OF IMMUNOLOGICAL ASSAYS

In 1896, Herbert E. Durham and Max von Gruber (ref.1) first observed specific agglutination reaction. As early as 1897, Georges F. I. Widal and Arthur Sicard already developed a test for the diagnosis of typhoid fever, namely Widal test on the basis of the Gruber-Durham reaction (ref.2). Since then, many different kinds of in vitro antigen-antibody reactions have been found, including precipitation reaction, complement fixation reaction and others (ref.2). Quantitative study of antigen-antibody reaction was first developed by Michael Heidelberger and Forrest E. Kendall in 1935-36 (ref.3). The series of this study eventually resulted in development of turbidimetric and nephelometric immunoassays. In 1946, Jacques Oudin (ref.4) found a precipitin reaction in gels, and this has made a great impact on further development in the quantitation of many major protein constituents in biological fluids.

Antigen-antibody reaction is highly specific and sensitive, and various laboratory tests based on antigen-antibody reaction could become very simple, once the method has been established. However, antigen-antibody reaction is by no measns absolutely specific and may show cross reactivity, and its major disadvantage is to show the prozone phenomenon due to antigen excess. Nevertheless, in the past more than two decades, immunological laboratory methods have gradually become increasingly more refined and simplified. Because of their inherent specificity and sensitivity, these methods have now achieved a central role in modern clinical laboratory science.

One of the other major factors which have influenced the rapid advances in immunoassay is the significant improvement in the procedures to make the antibody reagents and also improvement in the analytical instruments. Namely, the use of adjuvants and carrier proteins for immunizing experimental animals has made available specific antisera even for small antigenic substances and haptens. Also the introduction of hybridoma technology to make various monoclonal antibodies has made us able to measure even small epitopes which have never isolated by classical immunological research techniques (ref. 5). Furthermore, the development of the versatile and sensitive analytical technique of quantitative radioimmunoassay by R.S. Yalow and S. A. Berson (ref. 6) in 1959 has revolutionized diagnostic methodology in clinical medicine and has provided a powerful analytical tool in biomedical research and clinical practice.

DEVELOPMENT OF NON-ISOTOPIC IMMUNOASSAYS

Recently, the use of non-isotopic labels for monitoring the distribution of free and antibody bound ligands in immunological assays has been drawing much attention in clinical laboratory. The following labels have been used in immunoassays: bacteriophages (ref.7), free radicals (ref.8), fluorescent groups (ref.9), chemiluminescent groups (ref.10), synthetic particles (ref.11), red blood cells (ref.12), electron-dense materials (ref.13), metals (ref.14), enzyme (ref.15-19) and prosthetic groups (ref.20). Major reasons for current interests in replacing the radioisotopic labels with non-isotopic ones are (a) the relatively short half-life of gamma-emitting isotopes which creates logistic problems in the preparation of labeled ligands for immunoassays, (b) the impairment of immunological reactivity and specificity owing to the structural damages caused by the gamma-ray radiation of the isotopes, (c) the use of expensive toxic, flammable liquid scintillants for beta-ray emitting isotopes, and effective disposal of scintillants can be problematic, and (d) the possible health hazards involved in the use of radioisotopes (ref. 18). Among the non-isotopic labels previously described, enzymes have been most commonly used as well as latex particles and fluorescent materials.

DEVELOPMENT OF AUTOMATED IMMUNOASSAY SYSTEMS

Various non-isotopic immunoassays have been developed in reagent kits at first, particularly enzyme immunoassays. However, the enzyme immunoassay procedures are usually tedious and time consuming. Therefore, the increasing needs and wider application of these immunoassays have prompted automation of various immunoassay procedures in the past decade. Conventional chemical automatic analyzers are used for turbidimetric immuno-precipitation and immuno-agglutination methods, and nephelometry, particularly laser nephelometry for immunoprecipitation and passive latex agglutination, fluorometry for fluorescent immunoassays, and luminometry for chemiluminescent immunoassays.

Major advantages of using automated systems include to avoid tedious and complex manual procedures, and to set a strict reactional condition in order to improve their performance signif icantly. In addition, a recent panic in relation to human immunodeficiency virus infection(AIDS) and other infectious diseases prompted to introduce into clinical laboratories closed-system automatic instruments, particularly to prevent all laboratorians from dangerous biohazards. However, their automated systems are usually expensive and far from a compact setup. There has been no system that could avoid satisfactorily the prozone phenomenon inherent to any antigen-antibody reaction.

CHANGING CLINICAL NEED FOR IMMUNOASSAY SYSTEM

Recently, clinical need of laboratory tests have been changed greatly, because of the increas ing governmental pressure to reduce the total medical cost throughout the world. Therefore, analytical tests are not only preformed in hospitals and/or independent laboratories of a large scale, but also may be required in a variety of circumstances; the home, health center, clinic, ambulance, ward or operating room. Thus, in addition to conventional large sophiscat ed fully automated instruments, the availability of new, simple to use, immunoassay technology is becoming an important factor to develop clinical laboratory devices as the "alternate site diagnostics". The challenge in designing new diagnostic tests is to produce a system that provides sensitivity, specificity, simplicity and speed of delivery appropriate to the clinical need. Thus, even a novel immuno-strip system has been developed, and it avoids all reagent additions/washings, and has automatic reaction timing, and yields results within several minutes of sample collection. However, a compact type of sensitive immuno-sensors must be developed for a satisfactorily small module of the immunoassay system in near future.

Many different subjects related to immunodiagnostics are also presented in the other sections of this proceeding, and in this section are included fluorescent immunoassay, latex agglutination immunoassay and recently developed fully automated enzyme immunoassay systems.

REFERENCES

1. H.H. Fudenberg, D.P. Stites, J.L. Caldwell and J.V. Wells, BASIC & CLINICAL IMMUNOLOGY, p. 11, Lange, LosAltos (1978).
2. H.E. Peacock and R.H. Tomar, MANUAL OF LABORATORY IMMUNOLOGY, p.7, Lea & Febriger (1980).
3. M. Heidelberger and F.E. Kendall, J.exp.Med. 65,647 (1937).
4. J. Oudin, Meth.med. Res. 5, 335 (1952).
5. G. Köhler and C. Milstein, Nature 256,495 (1975).
6. R.S. Yalow and S.A. Berson, Nature, 184,1648 (1959).
7. J. Haimovich and M. Sela, Science 164,1279 (1969).
8. R.K. Leute, E.F. Ullman, A. Goldstein and L.A. Herzenberg, Nature 236,93 (1972).
9. E. Soini and I. Hemmila, Clin.Chem. 25, 353 (1979).
10. J.S.A. Simpson, A.K. Campbell, M.E.T. Ryall and J.S. Wöoodhead, Nature 279,646 (1979).
11. A.Rembaum and W.J. Dreyer, Science 208, 364 (1980).
12. F. Adler and C.T. Liu, J. Immunol.,106, 1684 (1971).
13. S.J. Singer and A.F. Schick, J. Biophys. Biochem.Cytol., 9, 519 (1961).
14. M. Cais, S. Dani, Y. Eden, O. Gandolfi, M. Horn, E.E. Isaacs, Y. Josephy, Y.Saar, E. Slovin and L. Snarsky, Nature 270, 534 (1977).
15. S.L. Scharpe, W.M. Cooreman, W.J. Blomme and G.M. Laekeman, Clin. Chem. 22, 733 (1976).
16. G.Felmann, P. Druet, J. Bignon and S. Avrameas, IMMUNOENZYMATIC TECHNIQUES, American Elsevier, New York (1976).
17. E. Ishikawa, T. Kawai and K. Miyai, ENZYME IMMUNOASSAY, Igaku-Shoin, Tokyo (1981).
18. T.T. Ngo and H.M. Lenhoff, Appl.Biochem.Biotech., 6, 53 (1981).
19. P. Tijssen, PRACTICE AND THEORY OF ENZYME IMMUNOASSAYS, Elsevier, Amsterdam (1985).
20. T.T. Ngo and H.M. Lenhoff, Anal. Lett. 13, 1157 (1980).

Time-resolved fluorescence for immunoassays and DNA-probes

Erkki Soini, Ilkka Hemmilä and Patrik Dahlén

Wallac Oy, P.O. Box 10, SF-20101 TURKU, FINLAND

Fluorescent lanthanide chelates and their detection using time-resolved fluorometry for in vitro as well as for microscopic biospecific assays are reviewed, with reference to other fluorescent dyes and labelling materials. The minimum detectable dose of labelled components and the theoretical ultimate sensitivities of immunoassays and DNA-assays are discussed and compared with experimental results. It is concluded that the time-resolved fluorometry provides the highest potential sensitivity in immunoassays, and a sensitivity comparable to phosphorus-32 in DNA hybridization assays. It is also concluded that lanthanide chelates are a potential alternative for organic fluorescent dyes in microscopy and that they are most useful in multiparameter assays. The combination of organic fluorescent dyes and lanthanide chelates provides the highest separation efficiency between two assay parameters.

INTRODUCTION

Chelates of europium and terbium are potential alternatives to radioisotopic and non-isotopic labels in biospecific assays. Many lanthanides are fluorescent and have earlier been exploited in various fields (e.g. electroluminescence and lasers). The main advantages of using lanthanide chelates as fluorescence probes with biological material are the relatively high quantum yield, exceptionally large Stokes shift, narrow emission peaks, and optimal emission and excitation wavelength.

Owing to the natural fluorescence from various compounds in biological samples (such as serum proteins) and from the substrates (such as the cuvette, solution and solid matrix) conventional fluorescent probes suffer from serious limitations of sensitivity. With lanthanide chelates, however, it is possible to reduce the background level considerably by selective detection of long-decay fluorescence. The fluorescence decay time of lanthanide chelates is often in the order of 10...1000 µs, whereas the decay time of natural fluorescence in a typical biological sample is in the order of 1...20 ns. For this reason, the time-resolved fluorometer based on a pulsed- light source used with lanthanide chelates is potentially several orders of magnitude more sensitive than conventional fluorometry (ref. 1, 2).

Dissociation enhanced time-resolved fluoroimmunoassay

Studies on time-resolved fluoroimmunoassay (TR-FIA) were started in our laboratories in 1974. During the end of the 1970's the concept of using lanthanides as fluorescent probes was made practical and viable in cooperation with a number of collaborating laboratories, among whom Prof. Ekins and his collaborators played an important role (ref. 3, 4).

Time-resolved fluoroimmunoassay with dissociation-based enhancement of Eu fluorescence has been found reliable and practical for a number of clinical routine immunochemistry analytes and is known by the name DELFIA[R] (Dissociation Enhanced Lanthanide Fluoroimmunoassay) (Trade mark of Wallac Oy). Detailed descriptions of various methodological aspects of DELFIA can be found in a number of publications (ref. 5, 6, 7, 8, 9, 10, 11, 12, 13, 14).

Time-resolved fluorometry of directly fluorescent probes

A directly fluorescent lanthanide label requires that both the fluorescent and the chelating properties are incorporated into one ligand-lanthanide complex. When such a complex is bound to an immunoreactive component, completely new assay designs based on time-resolved fluorometry become real. An ideal requirement for the lanthanide chelate would be that it has a very high stability constant, it is water soluble, it has a suitable excitation spectrum with a high absorbance, efficient energy transfer to the chelated lanthanide ions, and it has to contain a functional group for covalent coupling to an immunoreactive component. It has, however, been difficult to combine these requirements in the same molecular structure, as those lanthanide chelates which are stable at high dilution are usually poorly fluorescent, and those which are highly fluorescent dissociate at high dilution.

In most of the reported immunoassays employing directly fluorescent lanthanide probes and time-resolved detection, terbium complexes have been used. Terbium ions have been bound to the immunocomponent via a bifunctional chelating agent as in the measurement of human serum albumin (ref. 15) and immunoglobulin G (ref. 16). Also specific ion binding sites on proteins such as transferrin have been utilized in an assay for gentamicin (ref. 17). In all these assays the detection sensitivity of the label is limited by the efficiency of the transfer of the excitation energy. Thus the labeling concept is suitable only for the assay of analytes for which high sensitivity is not required.

In the development of stable and fluorescent chelates the objective has been to incorporate suitable light-absorbing groups to strongly chelating structures. Efficient energy transfer from the absorptive aromatic structure to the chelated metal is possible only when there is a close contact between them. This is generally accomplished by using aromatic fenol derivatives (e.g. salicylates, fenols etc.) or nitrogen heterocycles (e.g. pyridines, bipyridine, o-phenanthrolines).

One example of such groups of stable and fluorescent Eu-chelates are phenyl-ethynyl-2,6-[N,N-bis(carboxymethyl)-aminomethyl]pyridines synthesized by Kankare et al. (ref. 18). These chelates were applied in nonseparation "space-resolved" assays: competitive solid-phase TR-FIA for hIgG and noncompetitive TR-FIA for MIgG. Similar Eu-chelates were utilized in two-site "sandwich" TR-IFMA for human choriogonadotropin (hCG) by measuring the fluorescence directly from coated surfaces (microtitration strips) (ref. 19). The assay sensitivity was 0.7 int.units/L and linear range extends to over 10,000 int.units/L of hCG.

This new directly fluorescent europium chelate was also used to localize rabbit IgG to human smooth muscle myosin in a histological section with Eu-labelled anti-rabbit IgG. The results obtained show that the antibody labelled with the europium chelate was seen in a conventional fluorescence microscope with a steady-state light source (ref. 20). This result encourages the development of a time-resolved fluorescence microscope because a significant improvement in the signal to noise ratio can be anticipated. These first results with europium chelate as a label in an immunocytochemical reaction show that it is possible to develop new fluorochromes for localization studies using a time-resolved fluorescence microscope, and a remarkable improvement in the sensitivity can be anticipated.

The good results of a similar experiment encouraged the development of a pulsed light time-resolved fluorescence microscope (ref. 21). In addition to normal immunohistochemical studies, in situ hybridization and various other tracer techniques are potential applications for these new fluorochromes. It would also be possible to satisfy the increasing need for double and multiple reactions for different molecules in the same sections by using fluorescent lanthanide chelates of europium, terbium and samarium simultaneously. Another important feature of lanthanide labels is their high atomic weight which will make it possible to identify the lanthanide label also in electron microscopy.

Derivatives of the stable and fluorescent Eu^{3+}-chelates, when coupled with haptenic antigens, can be used also for simple homogeneous quenching TR-FIAs applied e.g. for the measurement of serum thyroxine (ref. 22). A fluorescent and stable Tb-chelate was applied for a nonseparation homogeneous TR-FIA for a drug, theophylline (ref. 23). As opposed to the homogeneous thyroxine assay, where the fluorescence of Eu-labelled thyroxin is quenched on binding to anti-thyroxin, the fluorescence of Tb-labelled theophylline in this assay was enhanced on binding to anti-theophylline antibodies.

In the chelates described above diamino-tetraacetic acids were used to form the required chelating strength. Bicyclic cryptates are another chelating group which forms kinetically inert and stable chelates. Cryptate structures containing pyridines, bipyridines or o-phenanthrolines as excitation light collectors and mediators have been described by Matthis and Lehn (ref. 24, 25).

A different approach to form in situ fluorescent chelates is applied by Cyber-Fluor (Toronto, Canada). In their EuroFluorS™ chelate o-phenanthroline is used as the excitation light absorbing group, but the chelating moiety consists only of two carboxylic acids in addition to the two aromatic amines of the phenanthroline (ref. 26). In this system the chelate stability is confirmed by using a high excess of Eu^{3+} to saturate all the bound free ligands and form the fluorescent chelate. The fluorescence is read after the immuno-reactions directly from the dried surfaces (microtitration strips) with a front-surface fluorometer (ref. 27).

Multiparameter assays

In spite of their high quantum efficiency, organic fluorescent probes suffer from high background and poor separation efficiency in multiparameter assays. On the other hand, lanthanide chelates provide unique separation efficiency because of their special characteristics related to the very narrow emission peaks and different decay times varying from 1 µs to 1000 µs.

Hemmilä et al. (ref. 28) have reported on a double-label time-resolved immunofluorometric assay of lutropin and follitropin in serum using fluorescent lanthanides of europium and terbium. Another combination for double-label assays is europium and samarium (ref. 29). Sm forms fluorescent chelates with aromatic β-diketones and can be measured in a fluorescence enhancement solution as optimized for Eu^{3+} (ref. 4, 30). Sm has an emission wavelength at 643 nm, which is an advantage, but a relatively short decay time of 50 µs and a lower quantum yield.
The combination of organic fluorescent probes and lanthanide chelates offers the best separation efficiency. Fluorescein and rhodamine samples (decay times below 10 ns) in increasing concentrations have been measured in our laboratory with a time-resolved filter fluorometer with a delay time of 400 µs and window time 500 µs. With these instrument settings the signal from the short decay time fluorescent compounds with concentrations up to 10^{-3} mol/L and up to 10^{-5} mol/L, respectively, is zero and appears first at higher concentrations. With the same settings the instrument sensitivity for Eu-β-diketone in the DELFIA[R] "enhancement" solution is below 10^{-13} mol/L concentration. The time-resolved function can detect europium in the presence of a 10^8-fold excess of a short decay time fluorescent substance.

Low concentrations of fluorescein and rhodamine can also be detected in the presence of a high concentration of europium. This is based on the fact that europium emission does not reach its maximum during the short excitation pulse and only a fraction less than 0.1 % of the europium emission is detectable during the first microsecond, which is used for the detection of short decay time fluorescence from fluorescein or rhodamine.

Clusters of lanthanide chelates

Another method of improving the sensitivity is to combine a large number of label molecules as a cluster. Examples of this technique are the use of biotin-avidin, phycobiliprotein, polymers including latex particles and inorganic crystalline particles.
A general problem in combining fluorescent compounds in clusters is related to the average distance between the chromophores. If the distance is smaller than the absorption cross section of the chromophore, the absorption does not grow linearly with the number of chromophores.

A similar effect can be seen in fluorescence emission. With organic fluorescent compounds, which typically have a very narrow Stokes shift, the self-absorption becomes significant when chromophores are in clusters. As a consequence, the fluorescence efficiency decreases when the degree of conjugation increases (ref. 31).

Polystyrene or latex microspheres, which may contain thousands of fluorescent molecules, have been introduced as cell labels (ref. 32). The autofluorescence of a single cell, measured with a microscope fluorometer or a flow cytometer, is in the order of several thousands of fluorescein equivalents (ref. 33), and as a result the demonstration of minute amounts of macromolecules in cells and tissues by means of immunofluorescence is not always possible. Fluorescent clusters improve the detection sensitivity significantly because the photon emission is concentrated in particles providing strong signals in the presence of background fluorescence, autofluorescence and scattering from the biological object, substrate, or optics.

The use of phycobiliproteins (ref. 34) and polymer microspheres makes it possible to optimize the average distance between chromophores in order to avoid self quenching. Another way of making fluorescent clusters of a small size and avoiding self quenching is to choose fluorescent compounds with extremely long Stokes shift. In this respect lanthanide chelates offer a unique possibility as their Stokes shift is in the order of 200 - 300 nm. Consequently, they do not suffer from self-absorption, and the fluorescence efficiency increases linearly with the degree of conjugation with antibodies up to 25 chromophores per antibody. In theory it should be possible to build clusters of lanthanide chelates with a large number of lanthanide chromophores and to utilize the advantage of linearly increasing fluorescence.

Another approach using time-resolved fluorescence microscopy has been introduced by Tanke et al. (ref. 35, 36). Instead of chelates, they have investigated the possibility of using inorganic lanthanide crystalline phosphor with a particle size of 1 µm or less. These particles, combining a large number of chromophores, resist bleaching and emit long-decay-time fluorescence and are ideal for time-resolved fluorometry. Inorganic phosphors, however, may have a low extinction coefficient compared with organic structures and it is not yet clear whether they are competitive with lanthanide chelate clusters in time-resolved fluorometry.

Lanthanide chelates and nucleic acid labelling

The recent advances in the recombinant DNA technology have led to the possibility of using nucleic acid hybridization as a widespread method not only in molecular biology but also in fields such as diagnostic medicine. It is, however, apparent that before the DNA probe based technology can be generally applied in the clinical routine the radiolabels such as ^{32}P and ^{3}H have to be replaced by a non-isotopic detection system.

Some alternative labels have been developed based on for example biotinylated nucleotide analogs detected by streptavidin (ref. 37), haptens bound to nucleotides with immunological detection (ref. 38) and proteins cross-linked to the nucleic acid (ref. 39). The final detection principle in all these alternative procedures is the same: an enzyme catalyzed reaction and photometry. So far none of these procedures has been able to compete with radiolabeled probes in terms of assay simplicity and sensitivity.

The high specific activity of lanthanide chelates when measured by time-resolved fluorometry provides a sensitivity which gives the label technology great potential as a non-isotopic alternative in the field of nucleic acid hybridization. The available europium chelate labels, which are essentially non-fluorescent before dissociation and enhancement (ref. 4) are, however, not suitable to be used in hybridization procedures such as Southern blotting, Northern blotting and in situ hybridization. In these applications the primary label should preferably be fluorescent and the dissociation step must be avoided. In dot blot hybridizations, in which the denatured nucleic acid sample is immobilized on nitrocellulose or nylon membranes, the label dissociation and fluorescence enhancement technique can be used although it complicates the assay procedure.

In principle, as in the case of immunoassay, the dot blot filter hybridizations can be classified in direct and indirect procedures. Usually the direct assays are based on probes labeled with radioisotopes. The non-isotopic alternatives are still based on an indirect procedure, in which for example, a slightly modified specific probe is recognized after hybridization by a labeled compound such as streptavidin or a specific antibody. An indirect filter hybridization assay has been carried out using Eu-labeled antibodies and a DNA probe tagged with a hapten (ref. 40). After the hybridization and antibody incubations the washed filters were transferred into an enhancement solution to dissociate the europium ion and to form a new highly fluorescent chelate in solution. In these experiments with 1.2. kb single stranded probe the detection limit of Ad2 DNA was 5×10^5 molecules (20 pg DNA), which corresponds to 0.3 pg of actual target sequences. The sensitivity was improved 10-fold compared to the corresponding enzyme-labeled procedure. Positive results have also been obtained in indirect hybridization using a biotinylated nucleic acid probe and streptavidin labeled with europium (ref. 41).

Recently, a method based on the use of DNA probes labelled with chelator groups was published (ref. 42). In this method the hybridized probe was detected by attaching europium to the chelator group after hybridization and then measuring the attached europium in a time-resolved fluorometer. Although high sensitivity could be obtained, this method had some drawbacks. An extra step after hybridization was needed to chelate europium to the probe DNA. In addition, the chelation step was found to work incompletely thus resulting in a low signal and a low signal-to-noise ratio.

Because of the complexity of the indirect hybridization assays direct assays should be preferred, and that is why the nucleic acid probe molecules have to be directly labeled. Work on direct labeling is in progress in our laboratory, but besides the labeling chemistry the stability of the lanthanide chelates becomes critical because of the often quite demanding incubation conditions used in hybridizations.

Because of the chemical inertness of DNA we found it necessary to employ a two-phase procedure to modify DNA with stable europium chelates. First, single-stranded nucleic acid can be transaminated (ref. 43) to introduce reactive aminogroups (ref. 44). Subsequently, by employing an isothiocyanate analogue of the europium chelate, we were able to label transaminated DNA. After purification the transaminated λDNA was reacted with an isothiocyanate analogue of europium chelate. An excess of the chelate was used to drive the reaction to completion. After posthybridization washing, 200 μl of DELFIA^R enhancement solution was added to the microtiter wells. The resulting fluorescent Eu-chelate was measured in a time-resolved fluorometer.

The sensitivity of Eu-labelled probes is comparable to ^{32}P-labelled probes detected by liquid scintillation counting. This indicates that Eu-labelled probes together with time-resolved fluorometric measurement appear to provide one of the most sensitive nonradioactive hybridization methods. The sensitivity with the ^{32}P-labelled probe after autoradiography, however, was ten times better than with the Eu-labelled probe.

REFERENCES

1. E.Soini and I.Hemmilä, Clin. Chem. 25, 353-361 (1979).
2. E.Soini and H.Kojola, Clin. Chem. 29, 65-68 (1983).
3. T.Jackson, S.Dakubu and R.Ekins, Med. Lab. World, Sept. 23-28 (1983).
4. I.Hemmilä, S.Dakubu, V-M.Mukkala, H.Siitari and T.Lövgren, Anal. Biochem. 137, 335-343 (1984).

5. H.Siitari, I.Hemmilä, E.Soini, T.Lövgren and V.Koistinen, Nature 301, 258-260 (1983).
6. P.Halonen, C.Bonfanti, T.Lövgren, I.Hemmilä and E.Soini, in K-O. Habermehl (Editor), Rapid Methods and Automation in Microbiology and Immunology, Springer-Verlag, Berlin, 420-437 (1984).
7. U-H.Stenman, H.Alfthan, L.Myllynen and M.Seppälä, Lancet, 647-649 (1983).
8. M.U. Suonpää, J.T.Lavi, I.A.Hemmilä and T.N.Lövgren, Clin. Chim. Acta 145, 341-348 (1985).
9. J.U.Eskola, T.J.Nevalainen and T.N.Lövgren, Clin.Chem. 29, 1777-1780 (1983).
10. T.N-E.Lövgren, J. Steroid Biochem. 27, No. 1-3, 47-51 (1987).
11. E.Toivonen, I.Hemmilä, J.Marniemi, P.N.Jørgensen, J.Zeuthen and T.Lövgren, Clin. Chem. 32(4), 637-640 (1986).
12. J.U.Eskola, V.Näntö, L.Meurling and T.N.Lövgren, Clin. Chem. 31, 1731-1734 (1985).
13. E.Bertoft, J.U.Eskola, V.Näntö and T.Lövgren, Febs. Lett. 173, 213-216 (1984).
14. P.Helsingius, I.Hemmilä and T.Lövgren, Clin. Chem. 32, 1767-1769 (1986).
15. M.P.Bailey, B.F.Rocks and C.Riley, Analyst 109, 1449-1450 (1984).
16. J.E.Kuo, K.H.Milby, W.D.Hinsberg, P.R.Poole, V.L.McGuffin and R.N.Zare, Clin. Chem. 31, 50-53 (1985).
17. N.J.Wilmott, J.N.Miller and J.F.Tyson, Analyst 109, 343-345 (1984).
18. J.Kankare, H.Takalo and P.Pasanen, Fluorescent lanthanide chelates, Eur. Patent Appl. EP 203047 (1986).
19. I.Hemmilä and A.Båtsman, Clin.Chem. 34, 1163-1164 (1988).
20. E.Soini, L.Pelliniemi, I.Hemmilä, V-M.Mukkala, J.Kankare and K.Fröjdman, accepted for publication in J. Histochem. Cytochem, (1988).
21. H.J.Tanke, R.Runia, R. van der Geest, J.Bonnet and J.Slats, Abstracts for the XIII International Meeting of the Society for Analytical Cytology, Sept. 4-9, 1988, Breckenridge, Colorado, Supplement 2, p. 92 (1988).
22. I.Hemmilä, O.Malminen, H.Mikola and T.Lövgren, Clin.Chem. in press, (1988).
23. R.L.Hale and D.W.Solas, Eur. Patent Appl. EP 195 413, (1986).
24. G.Matthis and J.M.Lehn, Fr. Demande FR 2 570 703 (1986).
25. J.Marchand, Fluocis; a new analytical concept. Int.Symp. CIS, Paris, 29-30 janvier (1987).
26. R.A.Evangelista, A.Pollak, B.Allore, E.F.Templeton, R.C.Morton, and E.P.Diamandis, Clin. Biochem. 21, 173-178 (1988).
27. E.P.Diamandis, Clin. Biochem. 21, 139-151 (1988).
28. I.Hemmilä, S.Holttinen, K.Pettersson and T.Lövgren, Clin. Chem. 33/12, 2281-2283 (1987).
29. M.Saarma, L.Järvekülg, I.Hemmilä, H.Siitari and R.Sinijärv, J. Virol. Meth., in press (1988).
30. T.Shigematsu, M.Matsui and R.Wake, Anal. Chem. Acta 46, 101-106 (1969).
31. M.Goldman, Fluorescent antibody methods, p.131, Academic Press, USA, (1968).
32. R.S.Molday, W.J. Dreyer, A.Rembaum and S.P.S.Yen, J. Cell Biol. 64, 75-88 (1975).
33. J.F.Jongkind, A.Verkerk, W.J.Visser and J.M. van Dongen, Exp. Cell. Res. 138, 409-417 (1982).
34. D.C.Nguyen, R.A.Keller, J.H.Jett and J.C.Martin, Anal. Chem. 59, 2158-2161 (1987).
35. H.Tanke, J.Slats and J.Ploem, Pat. appl. PCT/NL86/00022.
36. H.J.Tanke, A.van Schadewijk, S.van Gelderen and B.Beverloo, Abstracts for the XIII International Meeting of the Society for Analytical Cytology, Sept. 4-9, 1988, Breckenridge, Colorado, Supplement 2, p. 32 (1988).
37. A.C.Forster, J.L.McInnes, D.C.Skingle and R.H.Symons, Nucl. Acids Res. 13, 745-761 (1985).
38. P.Tchen, R.P.Fuchs, E.Sage and M.Leng, Proc. Natl. Acad.Sci. USA 81, 3466-3470 (1984).
39. M.Renz and C.Kuez, Nucl. Acids Res. 12, 3435-3444 (1984).
40. A-C.Syvänen, P.Tchen, M.Ranki and H.Söderlund, Nucl. Acids Res. 14, 1017-1027 (1986).
41. P.Hurskainen, T.Hyypiä and T.Lövgren, Detection of nucleic acids by hybridization using time-resolved fluorescence, Proc. NOMBA Nordforsk Symposium Gene Technology in Basic and Applied Research, Savonlinna, Finland, May 27-29, 1984 (Abstracts), p.12 (1984).
42. A.Oser, W.K.Roth and G.Valet, Nucl. Acids Res. 16, 1181-1196 (1988).
43. R.Shapiro and J.M.Weisgras, Biochem. Biophys. Res. Comm. 40, 839-843 (1970).
44. D.E.Draper, Nucl. Acids Res. 12 989-1002 (1984).

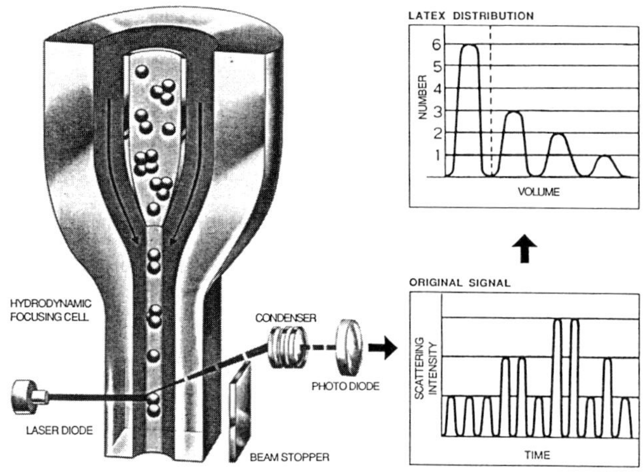

Fig. 1. Detection system of PAMIA

Agglutinated and unagglutinated latex particles flow one by one in the hydrodynamic focusing cell. Each of them is irradiated with a laser beam. Scattered laser light with latex particles is detected by the photodiode, and the pulses are discriminated according to the scattering intensity and then analyzed to provide latex distribution histogram. Using the histogram, the count of agglutinated latex particles (P: polymer) and the count of unagglutinated particles (M: monomer) are obtained and then the P/T is calculated according to the following formula:

P/T = P/(P + M)
P(Polymer): Count of agglutinated latex particles
M(Monomer): Count of unagglutinated latex particles
T(Total): Sum of P and M

The detection parameter P/T(%) correlates to the concentration of antigens or antibodies in test samples. The major advantage of using this parameter is that the use of the P/T can minimize the data variation caused by mechanical error resulting from several pipetting steps. This advantage results in higher reproducibility of test data than that of other latex immunoassay systems. Other advantages of using the P/T are presented as high sensitivity and wide dynamic range (Fig. 2). Figure 2 shows relative sensitivity of each detection parameter in alpha-fetoprotein assay. The value on the abscissa axis corresponds to the concentration of alpha-fetoprotein: 2 is equivalent to 10 ng/mL of alpha-fetoprotein, and 20 to 150 ng/mL. The relative sensitivity of parameter M increases linearly corresponding to the concentration of alpha-fetoprotein for 0 to 150 ng/mL (0 to 20 on the abscissa axis), reaches the peak value at the concentration of 250 ng/mL (30 on the abscissa axis), and then gradually decreases at higher concentrations. The relative sensitivity of parameter P undergoes at higher level for the concentration of 0 to 30 ng/mL (o to 5 on the abscissa axis), but it reaches its peak at 100 ng/mL (15 on the abscissa axis), then rapidly falls. The parameter P/T exhibits four times the sensitivity of parameter M at the concentration of 10 ng/mL and it has a sufficient sensitivity for the widest dynamic range.

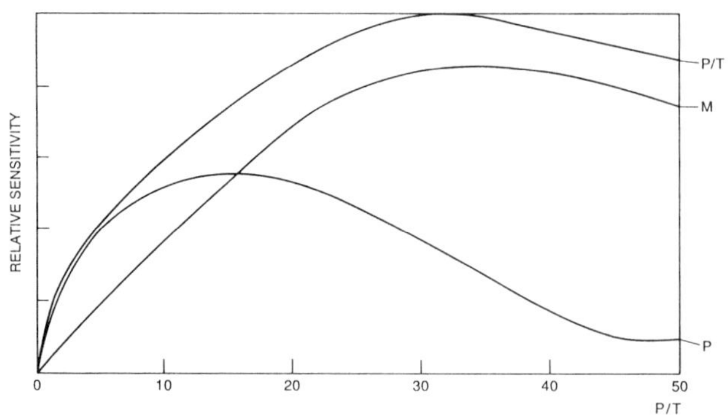

Fig. 2. Relative sensitivity of detection parameter P/T

In the immunoassays based on antigen-antibody reaction, it is necessary to eliminate the adverse effect of prozone phenomenon with antigen excess, for accurate determination of antigen concentration. The PAMIA system uses the two point measurement method to solve this problem. Figure 3 shows a reaction curve of alpha-fetoprotein for the range of 0 to 1,000,000 ng/mL (1g/mL). The T1 curve indicates the concentration-related change of P/T value with reaction times of 15 seconds, and T2 of 15 minutes. The T2 reaction curve reaches its peak at the concentration of 2,000 ng/mL, and the T1 value at this point is used as the threshold to detect antigen excess. Samples exhibiting higher T1 values than this threshold are considered to have higher concentrations than 2,000 ng/mL, even if their T2 values are lower than the T2 peak value at 2,000 ng/mL. Through the monitoring of T1 value for each samples, the PAMIA system prevents misreading a sample with antigen excess as a sample with a low concentration of antigens.

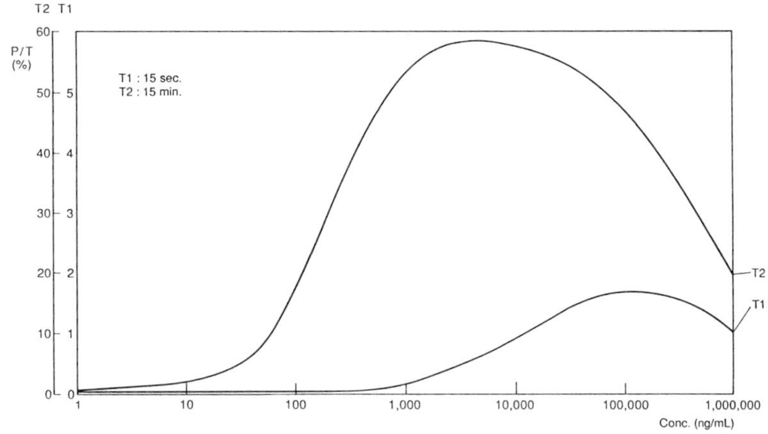

Fig. 3. Reaction curve of alpha-fetoprotein

The performance of PAMIA and RANREAM assay system is shown in Table 1. This system enables highly sensitive determination of these typical tumor markers, and is suitable for wide application to other tumor markers such as CA19-9 and CA125, thyroid hormone, viruses such as HBV and HIV, and other serum microproteins. Assay systems for these items are now under development.

The Immunochemical Analyzer PAMIA Series consists of two different models: the PAMIA-10, suitable for use in small laboratories, and the PAMIA-100, for large scale laboratory testing (Fig. 4). Table 2 shows the specifications of each model in the PAMIA Series.

TABLE 1. Performance of PAMIA and RANREAM

1.LINEARITY RANGE (ng/mL)	AFP CEA FRN B2M	2 - 1,000 1 - 250 2 - 1,000 5 - 200 (255 - 10,200)*	
2. REPRODUCIBILITY	AFP CEA FRN B2M	100 ng/mL 25 ng/mL 100 ng/mL 100 ng/mL (5,100 ng/mL)*	CV < 5%
3. OVERRANGE INDICATION	AT POINTS HIGHER THAN MAX. CONC. OF LINEARITY RANGE.		
4.CARRY-OVER	< 0.005%		

*Final concentration : B2M concentration is determined using the 1 : 51 diluted sample.

TABLE 2. Specifications of PAMIA

	PAMIA-10	PAMIA-100
1.SAMPLE VOLUME	10μL	
2.REACTION TIME	15 min	
3.THROUGHPUT	60 tests/hr	150 tests/hr
4.DATA STORAGE	160 samples	600 samples
5.LIGHT SOURCE	LASER DIODE (780nm)	
6.DETECTOR	HYDRODYNAMIC FOCUSING CELL & PHOTODIODE	
7.OTHERS	——	RANDOM ACCESS ON-LINE ID READER

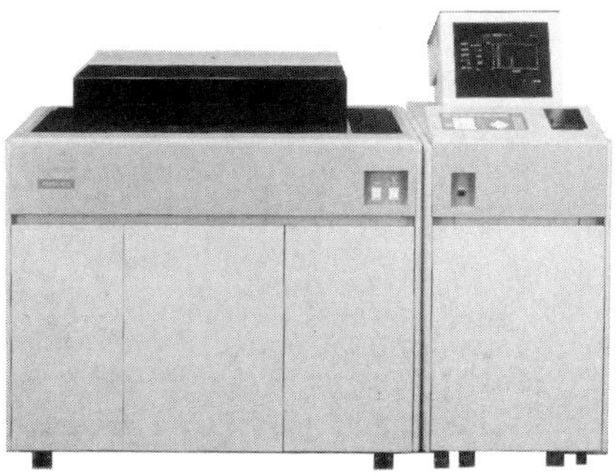

Fig. 4. PAMIA-100

In conclusion, this new immunoassay system consisting of PAMIA and RANREAM has many advantages such as the following.

• Providing accurate and reliable test results by using unique detection principles and highly specific reagent systems.
• Sensitive and precise measurement of serum microproteins such as carcinoembryonic antigen and alpha-fetoprotein.
• High sensitivity compared with RIA and EIA.
• Speedy data output, only 15 minutes.
• Multiple functions including data storage of standard curve and sample analysis, quality control program, self diagnosis before analysis, monitoring for carryover and antigen excess.
•Fully automated, operation-free analysis with high throughput of 150 test/h or 60 tests/h, starting after setting the reagents and test samples.

REFERENCES

1. J. M. SINGER & C. M. PLOTZ, Am. J. Med., 21, 888-892, 1956
2. R. HOIGNÉ, Helv. Med. Acta, 25, 422-429, 1958
3. C. L. CAMBIASO, A. E. LEEK, F. DESTEENWINKEL, J. BILLEN & P. L. MASSON, J. Immunol. Med., 18, 33-44, 1977

Magnetic micro-beads EIA by utilization of fully automated random access enzyme immunoassay analyzer, AIA-1200™

Masuo Inoue, Hidechika Hayashi, Hideo Suzuki, and Hiroshi Nakamura

Biotechnology Research Institute, TOSOH Corporation, 2743-1, Hayakawa, Ayase, Kanagawa 252, JAPAN

Abstract - AIA-1200™ has been developed for the automerization of heterogeneous enzyme immunoassay and has capabilities of multi-analyte and random access system (capable of analyte selection for each sample) and of 120 assays/hour throughput. This analyzer is designed for carry over less sampling from other patient's samples and for eliminations of background correction, enzyme reaction quenching step, and carry over from other assays' substrate by using so-called top-top rate measurement of fluorescence change. Enzyme immunoassay reagents are constructed of ferrite coated micro-beads for antibody solid phase support and of alkaline phosphatase labeled antibody or antigen for enzymatic amplification as lyophilized form in black plastic cups to enable one step heterogeneous enzyme immunoassay. This reagent pack concept facilitates to accelerate immune reaction and give accurate results by magnetic agitation of micro-beads to attain homogeneity of the reaction mixture. TSH assay showed good linearity through 125 μIU/ml and was found to have 0.07 μIU/ml of minimum detectable concentration. Within-assay precisions were 2.8-4.2% in three levels of samples. With two-site immunoradiometric assay, correlation was found to be y = 1.174x + 3.136, r = 0.970 (n = 144). T_3 and T_4 assays showed 3.7-7.0% and 2.5-7.7%, respectively, as within-assay precisions in three levels of samples. With other enzyme immunoassays of T_3 and T_4, correlations were found to be y = 1.121x + 0.079, r = 0.969 (n = 78) and y = 1.025x + 0.538, r = 0.964 (n = 75), respectively.

INTRODUCTION

The field of immunoassay has literally exploded in the last two decades, and there is no sign that this trend is slowing especially by the development of radio immunoassay (RIA, ref. 1). This technique

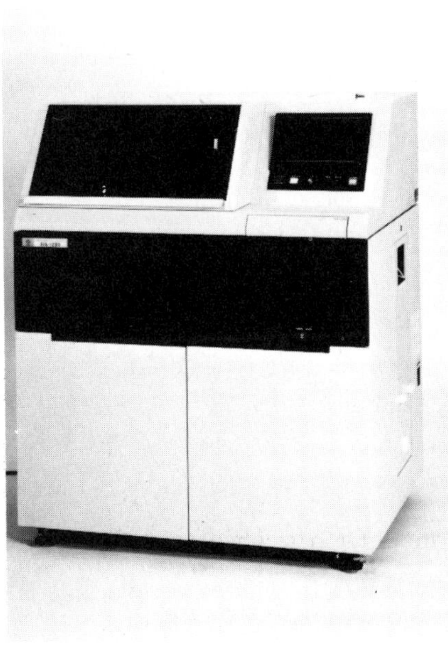

Fig. 1. AIA-1200™ enzyme immunoassay analyzer.

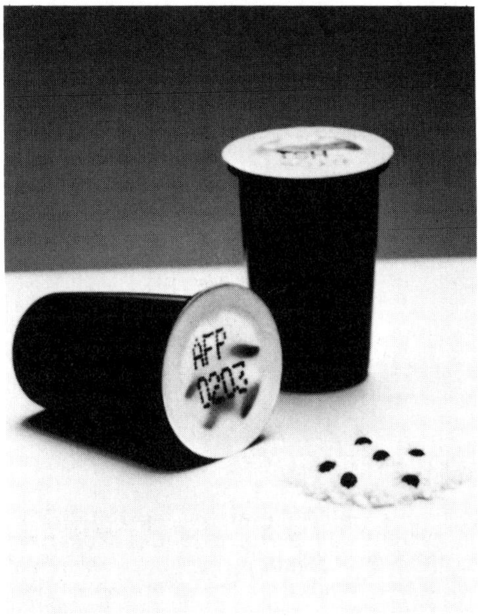

Fig. 2. Reagent packs, lyophilized antibody coated magnetizable micro-beads and conjugate.

has provided an extreme growth in detection and quantitation of trace components in biological fluid such as tumor associated antigens and hormones. Since RIA employs, however, radioisotopes which cause problems for transport, use, and disposal, its popularization has been limited. Meanwhile improvements in non-isotopic immunoassay has also been achieved. In recent years, many automated analyzers have been developed and opened the automerization in the non-isotopic immunoassay field, for example, immunonephelometry (ref. 2) by using laser or fluorescence in quantitation of relatively high concentrated plasma proteins, and fluorescence depolarization immunoassay (ref. 3) based on the principle of homogeneous immunoassay or homogeneous enzyme immunoassay by using enzyme-multiplied immunoassay technique (ref. 4) in quantitation of small molecule haptens. More recently, development of automated analyzer has also been activated in the field of heterogeneous enzyme immunoassay (EIA, ref. 5) which was proven to show similar sensitivity and reproducibility to RIA (ref. 6 and 7).

We, TOSOH Corporation, have recently introduced Fully Automated Random Access Enzyme Immunoassay System, AIA-1200™ (ref. 8) and its reagents, based on the principle of heterogeneous enzyme immunoassay in which analyzrer appearance and reagents are shown in Figures 1 and 2, respectively. The assay principle and characteristics of the system will be discussed. The assay results will also be discussed for TSH (Thyroid stimulating hormone, Thyrotropin), T_3 (Triiodothyronine), and T_4 (Thyroxin).

ASSAY PRINCIPLE

To establish high sensitive enzyme immunoassay system, heterogeneous EIA was chosen by using high affinity monoclonal or, in some cases, polyclonal antibodies for both sandwich and competitive immunoassays and by using ferrite coated micro-beads technology for solid phase support. In most cases, one step sandwich EIA is employed by using monoclonal antibodies recognizing at least two different epitopes. Preparation of antibody immobilized magnetizable micro-beads are attained by using polymer beads (1.5 mm in diameter) coated by ferrite and then polymers having a suitable functional group for antibody immobilization by chemical bond. By using this magnetizable micro-beads, magnetic agitation is achieved by the induction of external magnetic field movement throughout reaction to accelerate immune reaction and to attain homogeneity of the reaction mixture. Alkaline phosphatase (ALPase, E. C. 3.1.3.1) is used for enzymatic amplification for all chemistries by conjugation with antibody for sandwich assay or with antigen for competitive assay.

Lyophilization is achieved for both conjugate (ALPase labeled antibody or antigen) and antibody immobilized magnetizable micro-beads (usually 8-12 beads per assay) in a black plastic cup which is then sealed by aluminum foil to serve ready-to-use reagent pack. This black plastic cup serves as both immune reaction and enzyme reaction vessels in which this reagent pack concept makes the instrument and assay procedure very simple. This reagent pack concept is illustrated in Fig. 3.

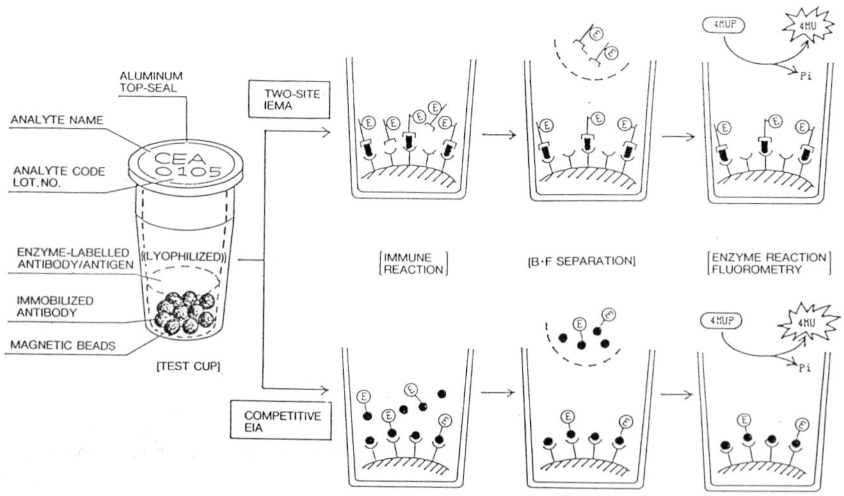

Fig. 3. Reagent pack concept.

SYSTEM CHARACTERISTICS

The analyzer is fully automated and has capability of random access enzyme immunoassay, in other words, the system can perform required chemistries for the specific sample out of any available chemistries the way sample required to be measured and can be added sample and/or chemistry reagent packs at any time. The system characteristics are summarized in Table 1.

TABLE 1. System characteristics

Type	Multi-analyte and random access
Analytes	Components in biological fluid (Tumor makers, hormones, etc.)
Method	Heterogeneous EIA with one-step sandwich or competitive assay
Assay throughput	120 Assays/hour, 1st: ca. 60 min., then 5 results/2.5 min.
Sample loading	100 Samples/disp. tips at a time
Reagent pack sorting	420 Reagent packs at a time
Sample programming	2000 Programs and/or 2998 tests
Reagents	
Reagent pack	Immobilized antibody on ferrite coated magnetizable micro-beads Alkaline Phosphatase (E.C. 3.1.3.1) labeled antibody or antigen
Sample	Serum, plasma, or urine (10–125 ul)
Reconstituent	Water with detergent (25–140 ul)
Washing solution	Buffered detergent
Immune reaction	37°C, 40 min. for all chemistries under magnetic agitation
Enzyme reaction	37°C, 2 min. for all chemistries Buffered 4-methylumbelliferyl phosphate (4-MUP) as substrate
Detection	Rate fluorescence change analysis Non-contact top-top measurement Excitation/emission: 365/450-500 nm
Calibration curve	Two to 6 points calibration 1St, 2nd, or 3rd order calculation
Work sheet	Output to display and/or printer

TABLE 2. Standard operation of patient samples

User attended steps

1. Enter test requests.
2. Load required chemistry trays.
3. Load patient samples and sample tips.
4. Initiate "START".

AIA-1200™ takes care of the rest

1. Reagent packs are randomly selected according to the load list and positioned in transport blocks. This is software-directed through system's touch screen.
2. An elevator transports blocks to the sampling station. Reagent pack foil seals are broken to prepare for reagent reconstitution.
3. Pipette tip attaches to the sampling arm. Then reconstituent and sample are aspirated and dispensed into a reagent pack to initiate immune reaction. This process eliminates cross-carry over from other patient's sample.
4. Transport block moves along the assay line where the temperature is maintained at 37°C. Antibody immobilized micro-beads are continuously agitated magnetically throughout reaction.
5. Two continuous washes and aspirations, followed by substrate addition. Five detectors read simultaneously 5 results.
6. Analyte concentrations are calculated based on the calibration curve stored in the system and results are collated on a printout providing all required patient results at once.

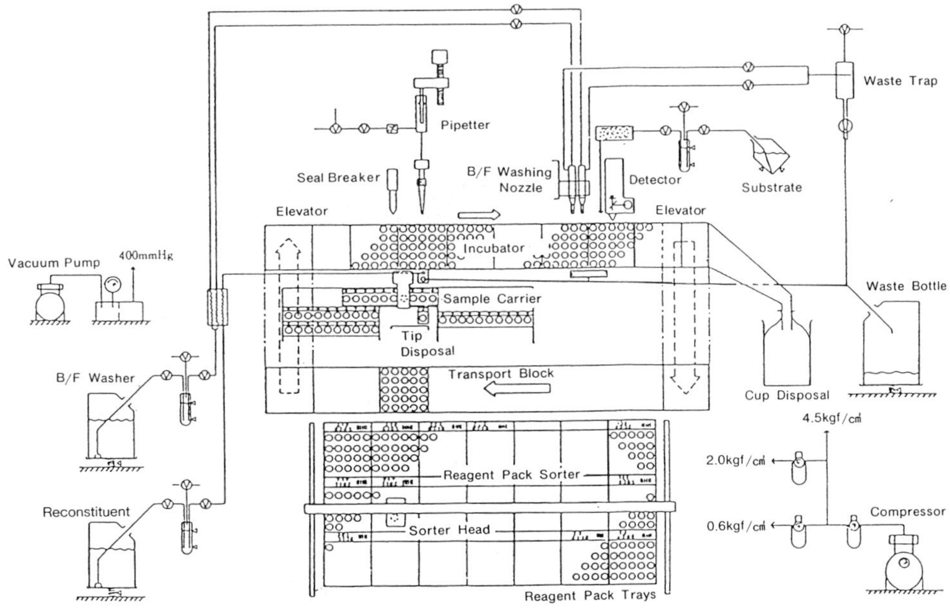

Fig. 4. AIA-1200 systems diagram.

The functions of each part are described below and system's diagram is shown in Fig. 4. Reagent pack sorter is consisted of reagent pack tray (holds 20 reagent packs and shows analyte's name, lot number, expiration date, and bar code) holder and sorter head which has bar code sensor, cup sensor, and cup transfer mechanism to transport blocks by using so-called magic hand under vacuum. This sorter checks analyte names and number of reagent packs to show the operator what kind of chemistry reagents and how many reagent packs are available. Reagent packs in a transport block are moved up to the seal breaker station where the aluminum top seals of each reagent pack are broken to prepare for reagent reconstitution. The transport block then moves to the sampling station. The sampling station consists of two major modules: sample carrier holder and pipetting mechanism. Sample carrier holds 10 sample cups and corresponding disposable pipette tips which are only used for each individual sample and this concept prevents contamination from other samples. After sample level sensor checked, pipetting arm attaches disposable pipette, aspirates required amount of reconstituent and then sample, and dispense to a reagent cup to initiate immune reaction. This simultaneous addition of sample and reconstituent initiates immune reaction at 37°C for 40 min. for all chemistries to facilitate random access for the system. Meanwhile, transport blocks move along the assay line incubator which controls immune reaction mixture at 37°C by using heater sheet panel and there are magnets underneath aligned moving back and forth for the external magnetic field movement to agitate immune reaction mixture by moving antibody coated magnetizable micro-beads. After exactly 40 min. immune reaction, two continuous washes and aspiration under magnetic agitation enables efficient bound and free conjugate separation (B/F separation). Right after B/F separation, about 220 ul of preheated substrate is dispensed in each cup and five detectors read simultaneously 5 results by rate measurement of fluorescence change at 37°C over a 100-second period for assured accuracy of results. This rate fluorescence measurement is obtained by irradiation of light (365 nm) from over the top of the cup and detection of emission light (450-550 nm) by the detector located over the top of the cup, so-called top-top rate fluorescence measurement, and therefore, eliminates corrections of the background, contamination by other assay's substrate, and reaction quenching step. The resulted rate fluorescence changes are converted to the analyte concentrations based on the previously stored calibration curves and printed out to the data sheet.

Standard operation of patient sample

Standard operation of everyday assay is quite simple and the only things operator should do is four simple steps and the system takes care of the rest for obtaining assay results as summarized in Table 2.

System performance

The system's performances, both analyzer and reagents, were evaluated for sampling precision, temperature and time dependences, and agitation rate dependence.

Sampling precision was firstly examined by using water and serum as shown in Table 3. Total volume of reconstituent and sample is in this case 150 ul. In the case of using water as sample, precisions are less than 1% and are quite satisfactory. In the case of serum, on the other hand, precisions are over 1% (1.32-1.74% in 10 replicates), but these results are satisfactory upon consideration of error in radiation dose measurements.

TABLE 3. Sampling precision (total volume = 150 μl).
Water solution was measured by Hitachi U-3200 (478mm) and serum solution was measured by Aloka ARC-300 (1 min.).

	5 μl	10 μl	50 μl	100 μl
ORANGE G. /WATER (Abs.)	0.5119	1.0174	0.4967	0.9736
	0.5147	1.0271	0.5017	0.9729
	0.5120	1.0224	0.5010	0.9765
	0.5204	1.0325	0.5013	0.9731
	0.5256	1.0288	0.5016	0.9726
	0.5214	1.0182	0.5006	0.9735
	0.5155	1.0249	0.5007	0.9733
	0.5223	1.02224	0.5009	0.9747
	0.5217	1.0300	0.5011	0.9735
	0.5187	1.0233	0.5008	0.9746
mean	0.5187	1.0247	0.5006	0.9738
SD	0.0047	0.0049	0.0014	0.0012
%cv	0.90	0.48	0.29	0.12
^{125}I/SERUM (cpm)	18112	36036	17532	36090
	18544	35921	17920	35580
	18690	34507	18189	35330
	18596	35705	18142	35258
	18653	35640	17579	35062
	18340	35344	18334	35552
	18914	35242	18335	35898
	19080	35165	18190	36257
	19037	35147	18248	36666
	18721	34945	17676	36130
mean	18666.9	35365.2	18014.5	35782.3
SD	299.6	467.4	313.2	508.5
%cv	1.61	1.32	1.74	1.42

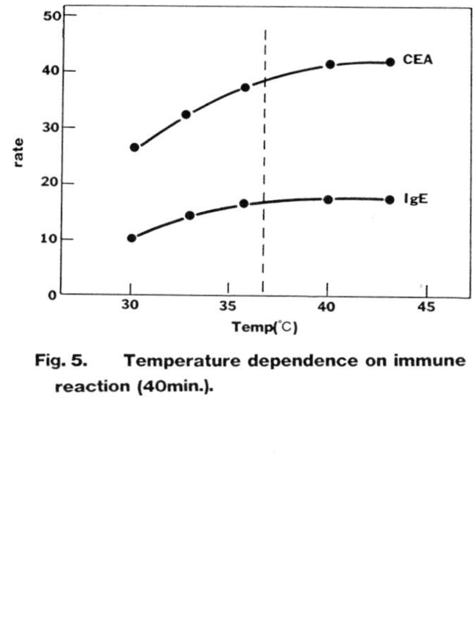

Fig. 5. Temperature dependence on immune reaction (40min.).

Temperature dependences on immune reaction (40 min.) are shown in Fig. 5. The result of temperature dependence from 30 to 43°C shows response increments, in other words, immune reaction rate increments, especially from 30 to 37°C, and temperature control becomes very important.

Time dependences on immune reaction (37°C) are shown in Fig. 6. After 4 hours, antigen-antibody reaction becomes equilibrium. But after only 40 min. reaction, 40-60% of the reaction took place. Therefore, time control also becomes very important. These time and temperature controles, however, can be easily obtaincd by the analyzer.

Agitation rate dependences on immune reaction (37°C, 40 min.) are shown in Fig. 7. Up to about 60 cycles/min. agitation rate, response, in other words, immune reaction rate increases according to the agitation rate. But over 60 cycles/min., response becomes nearly constant. Therefore, 85

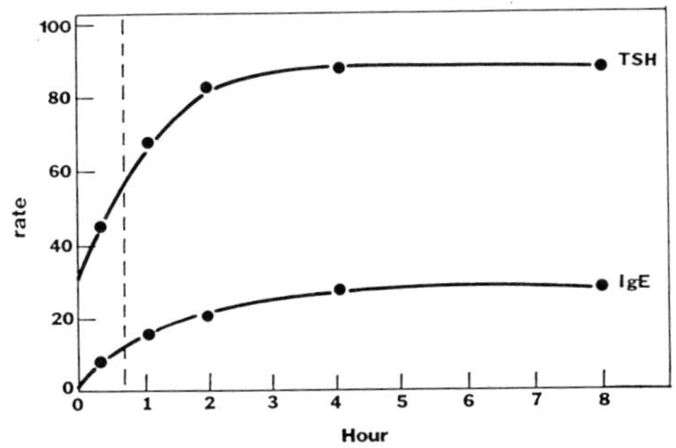

Fig. 6. Time dependence on immune reaction (37°C).

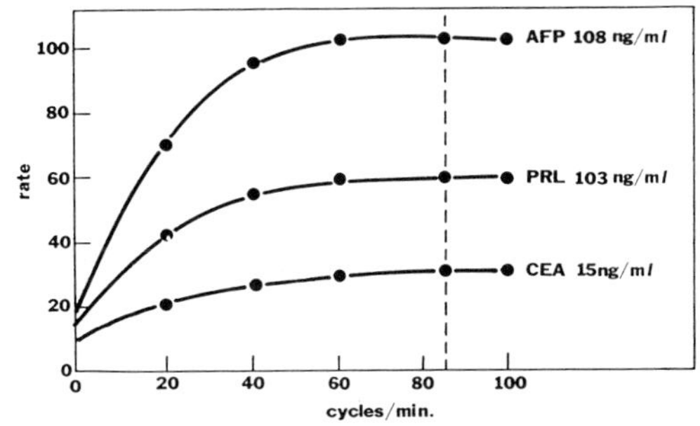

Fig. 7. Agitation rate dependence on immune reaction (37°C, 40min).

cycles/min. of agitation rate was chosen. Figure 7. also shows the agitation effect of immune reaction mixture by magnetizable micro-beads up to about 5 times.

ASSAY PERFORMANCE

To evaluate total system, AIA-1200™ analyzer and reagents, assay performances of TSH, T_3 and T_4 were examined. In the case of one step sandwich assay, only one washing step is required and assay process becomes simpler whereas two step sandwich assay requires one extra washing and conjugate addition. High dose hook effect (pro-zone phenomena) becomes, however, very critical in the case of antigen excess as far as one step sandwich assay is concerned. This effect were examined for AFP (Alpha-fetoprotein), IgE (Immunoglobulin E), Ferritin, and TSH. The results were satisfactory and showed detector range over (DO, more than ca. 700 of fluorescence rate response) as shown in Table 4. In most of one step sandwich assays, two points calibration (zero and positive calibrators) is used for conversion of rate response to concentration in the case which shows calibration curve linearity throughout the dynamic range.

In the case of competitive assays, only sample and reconstituent addition is required to initiate immune reaction since both antibody and conjugate (ALPase-T_3 or -T_4) are lyophilized in a cup. Six points calibration (zero and five positive calibrators) is used to obtain calibration curve (B/B_0, ratio of bound to free ligand, on the vertical axis instead of rate response, in semi-logarithmic plot) and conversion equation of rate response to concentration by using logit-log third equation.

TSH assay
Two monoclonal antibodies having K values of 10^{10}–10^{12} l/mol are used for capture and tracer antibodies. In this assay, 12 antibody bound magnetizable micro-beads are used, sample is 100 ul, and reconstituent is 50 ul. Since calibration curve linearity exceeds more than 125 μIU/ml, dynamic range was set to 100 μIU/ml and calibrators zero and 50 μIU/ml are used for two points calibration to get calibration curve and conversion equation as shown in Fig. 8.

Table 4 High dose hook effect

Concentration was calculated from assigned (*) value.
DO represents detector range over.

Analyte	concentration	Response (rate)
AFP	245000	DO
(ng/ml)	24500	DO
	2450	DO
	245*	207.2
	24.5	22.4
IgE	150000	DO
(IU/ml)	15000	DO
	1500	327.4
	150*	38.5
FERR	140000	DO
(ng/ml)	14000	DO
	1400	250.2
	140*	33.3
TSH	6477	DO
(μIU/ml)	648	DO
	64.8*	94.5
	6.5	11.5

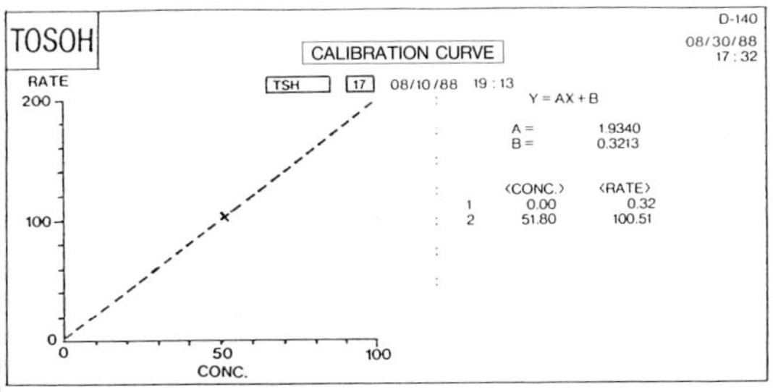

Fig. 8. Calibration curve for TSH.

TABLE 5. Within-assay precision of TSH (μIU/m*l*)

No.	(LOW)	(MID)	(HIGH)
1	5.44	25.49	46.18
2	4.91	24.96	48.18
3	5.29	24.12	46.88
4	5.35	26.46	45.66
5	4.94	25.23	47.34
6	4.84	24.83	48.40
7	5.18	24.18	40.38
8	5.13	27.38	45.30
9	5.25	25.48	48.53
10	5.40	24.85	47.17
11	5.20	25.20	47.75
12	5.38	24.19	48.12
13	4.93	25.95	48.31
14	4.86	24.34	46.18
15	5.20	24.63	47.15
16	5.13	25.58	45.04
17	4.91	24.89	46.41
18	4.79	25.18	47.90
19	4.98	24.99	48.46
20	5.14	24.70	46.35
21	5.37	22.63	48.41
22	5.32	24.24	49.47
23	5.08	22.65	46.98
24	5.08	24.09	46.62
MEAN	5.13	24.84	47.38
SD	0.20	1.03	1.31
%CV	3.8	4.2	2.8

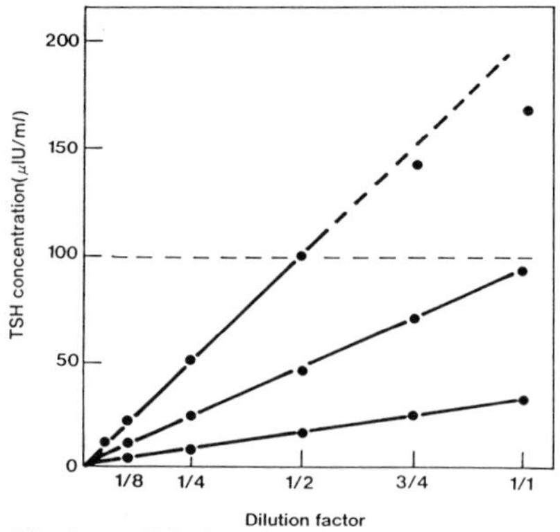

Fig. 9. Dilution linearity tests of TSH over dynamic range.

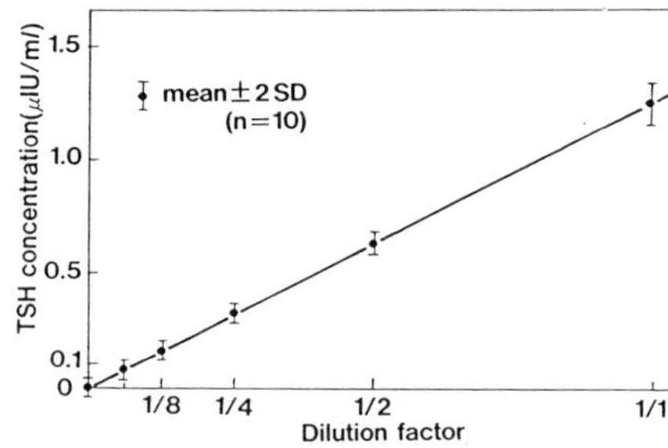

Fig. 10. Dilution linearity test of TSH at lower concentration.

Within-assay precisions were examined and are showned in Table 5. The results showed good precisions for low (5.13 μIU/ml), medium (24.84 μIU/ml), and high (47.38 μIU/ml) concentrated samples at cv (co-efficient of variation) = 3.8, 4.2, and 2.8%, respectively, by 24 assay replicates for each concentration.

Sample dilution linearities were then checked for three different concentrated patient samples by using specimen diluent which is a part of reagent and showed no detectable TSH contained. Good linearity relationships were obtained in all samples within the dynamic range of 100 μIU/ml as shown in Fig. 9. Dilution linearity test was again examined at lower concentration, less than 1.5 μIU/ml, to show good linearity relationships as shown in Fig. 10.

Minimum detectable concentration was evaluated by using 2 SD (standard deviation) method and serial dilution method to show 0.04 and 0.07 μIU/ml, respectively, as shown in Fig. 11. From these results, minimum detectable concentration of TSH assay can be concluded as at least 0.1 μIU/ml.

Correlation with two-site immunoradiometric assay (Two-site IRMA) is shown in Fig. 12. to give a good correlation, y = 1.174x + 3.136, correlation co-efficient, r = 0.970, number of samples. n = 144.

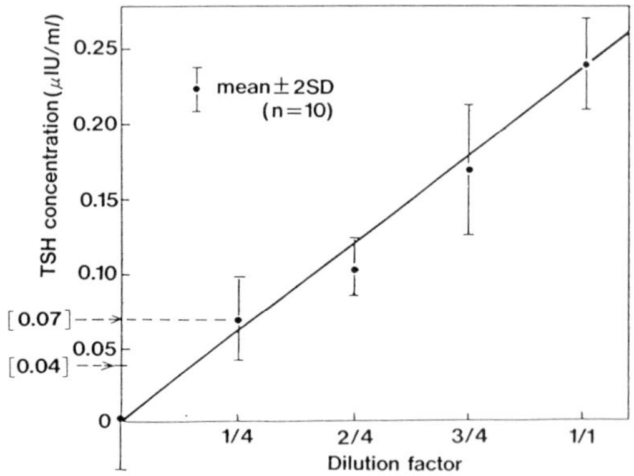

Fig. 11. Minimum detectable concentration of TSH reagent pack.

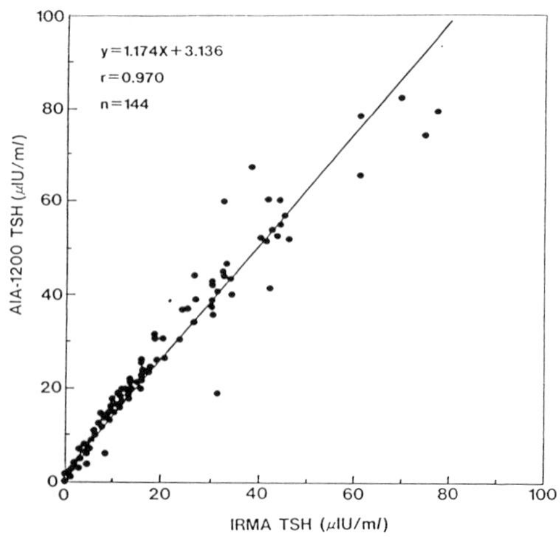

Fig. 12. Carrelation of TSH reagent pack immunoradiometric assay (IRMA).

<u>T_3 and T_4 assays</u>
In these competitive assays, polyclonal antibodies are used for capture antibodies. In these hapten assays, 12 antibody bound magnetizable micro-beads are used, samples are 75 ul for $T_3$and 10 ul for T_4 and reconstituents are 75 ul for T_3 and 140 ul for T_4. Dynamic ranges are set to 6.4 ng/ml and 24 ug/dl for T_3 and T_4, respectively. Calibration curves of typical T_3 and T_4 are shown in Figures 13 and 14, respectively.

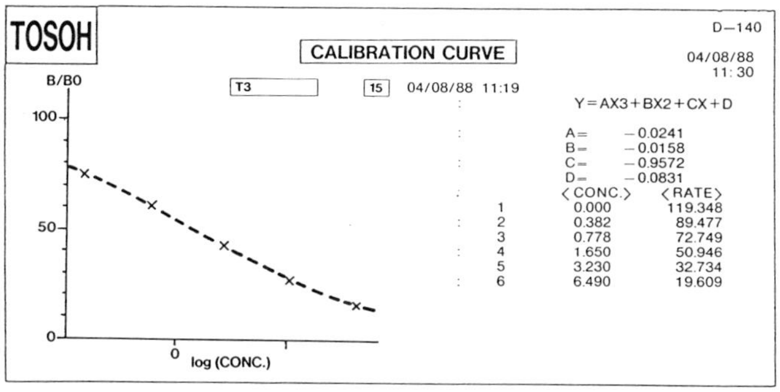

Fig. 13. Calibration curve for T_3.

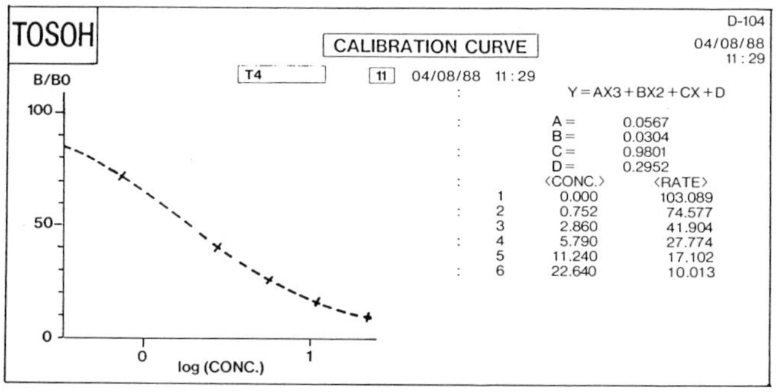

Fig. 14. Calibration curve for T_4.

Within-assay precisions were examined and are shown in Tables 6 and 7 for T_3 and T_4, respectively. The T_3 results show good precisions for low (0.820 ng/ml), medium (1.279 ng/ml), and high (3.378 ng/ml) concentrated samples at cv = 7.0, 5.4, and 3.7%, respectively, by 20 assay replicates for each concentration. The T_4 results show also good precisions for low (3.69 ug/dl), medium (7.13 ug/dl), and high (14.63 ug/dl) concentrated samples at cv = 7.7, 5.7, and 2.5%, respectively, by 20 assay replicates for each concentration.

TABLE 6. Within-assay precision of T_3 (ng/ml)

No.	(LOW)	(MID)	(HIGH)
1	0.79	1.26	3.47
2	0.73	1.20	3.27
3	0.85	1.30	3.58
4	0.81	1.30	3.43
5	0.86	1.24	3.55
6	0.75	1.23	3.25
7	0.72	1.27	3.33
8	0.83	1.25	3.37
9	0.86	1.27	3.44
10	0.87	1.34	3.61
11	0.77	1.27	3.23
12	0.82	1.20	3.23
13	0.87	1.24	3.28
14	0.88	1.33	3.42
15	0.90	1.34	3.25
16	0.79	1.50	3.24
17	0.88	1.20	3.38
18	0.72	1.29	3.26
19	0.87	1.32	3.52
20	0.87	1.23	3.44
MEAN	0.820	1.279	3.378
SD	0.0588	0.069	0.126
%CV	7.0	5.4	3.7

TABLE 7. Within-assay precision of T_4 (μg/dl)

No.	(LOW)	(MID)	(HIGH)
1	4.15	6.77	14.16
2	3.87	7.32	14.46
3	3.96	6.63	15.15
4	3.87	7.79	14.83
5	3.92	7.89	14.92
6	3.58	6.68	14.50
7	3.81	6.52	14.74
8	3.49	7.25	15.36
9	3.47	7.02	14.87
10	3.45	7.36	15.00
11	3.52	7.22	14.20
12	3.27	7.04	14.31
13	3.37	6.75	14.14
14	3.72	7.10	14.88
15	3.58	7.70	14.80
16	3.44	7.32	13.97
17	4.18	7.37	14.55
18	3.57	6.93	14.45
19	3.34	6.48	14.66
20	4.14	7.35	14.74
MEAN	3.69	7.13	14.63
SD	0.28	0.41	0.36
%CV	7.7	5.7	2.5

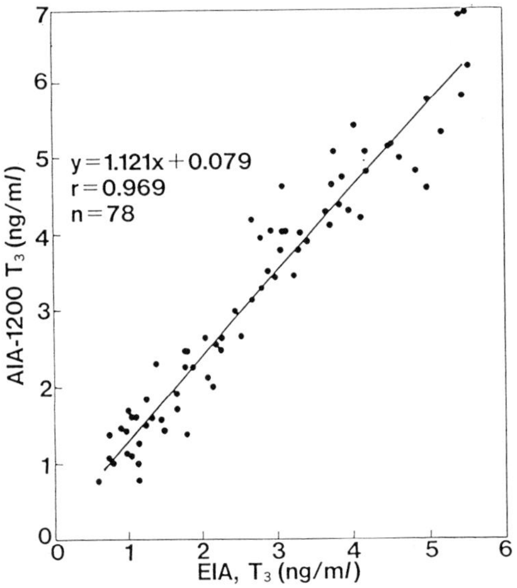

Fig. 15. **Correlation of T_3 reagent pack with other enzyme immunoassay kit.**

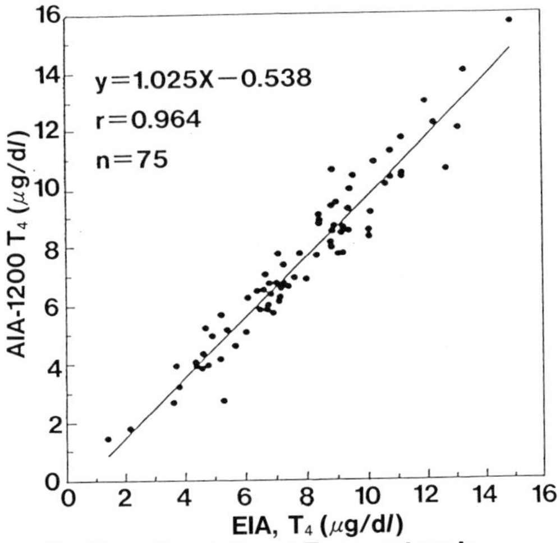

Fig. 16. **Correlation of T_4 reagent pack with other enzyme immunoassay kit.**

Correlation with other enzyme immunoassays are shown in Figures 15 and 16 for T_3 and T_4, respectively, to give good correlations, $y = 1.121x + 0.079$, $r = 0.969$, $n = 78$ for T_3 and $y = 1.025x - 0.538$, $r = 0.964$,
$n = 75$ for T_4.

CONCLUSION

The heart of this AIA-1200™ Fully Automated Random Access Enzyme Immunoassay System is the reagent pack concept and innovation of new technology in clinical chemistry. Construction of reagent pack configurations allows high sensitive enzyme immunoassays by using heterogeneous technique with magnetizable micro-bead solid phase technology. This system has been developed to maximize the usage of this unique configuration of reagent packs: assay automerization, random access, carry over less sampling, rate fluorescence analysis, lot stable calibration curves, and user friendly and powerful computer software.

This system redefines the future of immunochemistry which offers rapid and high sensitive measurement of trace components in the biological fluids such as tumor associated antigens, hormones, and viruses within one hour and is expected to contribute to automation, reliability, speediness, and less labor for detection and quantitation in clinical chemistry laboratories.

REFERENCES AND NOTES

1. T. Chard, An Introduction to Radioimmunoassay and Related Techniques, p. 41, Elsevier Biomedical Press, Amsterdam (1982), in a series of "Laboratory Techniques in Biochemistry and Molecular Biology".
2. J. C. Sternberg, Clin. Chem. 23, 1456 (1977).
3. M. E. Jolly, S. D. Stroup, and H. J. Wang, ibid. 27, 1575 (1981).
4. K. E. Rubenstein, R. S. Schneider, and E. F. Ullman, Biochem. Biophys. Res. Commun. 47, 846 (1972).
5. B. K. Van Weeman and A. H. W. M. Schuurs, FEBS Letters 43, 215 (1974)
6. P. Tijssen, Practice and Theory of Enzyme Immunoassays, p. 329, Elsevier Science Publishers B. V., Amsterdam (1985), in a series of "Laboratory Techniques in Biochemistry and Molecular Biology".
7. J. H. Carter, J. Clin. Immunoassay 7, 64 (1984).
8. H. Hayashi. H. Suzuki, S. Iwasaki, S. Mitsuhisa, and H. Nakamura. Toyosoda Kenkyu Houkoku 31, 45 (1987).The name 'AIA-1200' is a registered trade mark in Japan. The following technical terms appeared in this article is only tentative : Fully Automated Randon Access Immunoassay Analyzer (or System), reagent pack, reconstituent, and washing solution.

The Abbot IMx^{TM}—an automated immunochemistry system based on microparticle capture technology

J. Smith, J. Mitchell, M. Fiore, S. Safford, T. Doan, G. Barnes, K. Zeng, M. Ulanday, K. Burns, R. Nelson, C. Grandone, D. Smiter, V. Yue, T. Gunderson, K. Chirko, and D. Berry

Abbott Laboratories, Diagnostic Division, Abbott Park, IL, 60064

Abstract - We describe a new clinical laboratory system, the IMx™, to automate immunoassay testing. The IMx employs two analytical technologies to process immunoassays: a novel technology known as Microparticle capture Enzyme Immunoassay (MEIA) for high molecular weight analytes and fluorescence polarization immunoassay (FPIA) for low molecular weight analytes. MEIA technology is a fast, highly sensitive and specific assay methodology. The key innovative elements of the technology include a submicron solid phase for accelerated kinetics, an efficient separation procedure, and an ultrasensitive detection method. The IMx instrument is able to process a carousel of up to 24 samples in 30-40 minutes using approximately 150 ul of serum per test. Calibration curves are stable for at least two weeks. No sample pretreatment is required and sample dilutions are performed automatically. The instrument is microprocessor based and uses a robotic arm and rotating carousel to process the assays. A front surface fluorometer is used to quantitate the enzymatic generation of flourescent product at a rate proportional to the concentration of the analyte. Performance of the alpha-fetoprotein (AFP) assay on IMx shows within-run coefficients of variation of less than 4% at sample concentrations greater than or equal to 2.9 ng/ml. Assay sensitivity, defined as two standard deviations above the zero standard, is less than 0.4 ng/ml. Correlation of the IMx AFP assay with the Abbott AFP-EIA Monoclonal Assay was excellent (r = 0.987, y = 0.332 + 0.970x, n = 2278).

INTRODUCTION

The last few years have seen the beginning of an evolution in immunoassay testing from manual testing procedures characterized by labor intensive and time consuming techniques as well as poor reproducibility to highly automated systems which provide calibration stability, short reaction times, reduced hands-on time, and improved assay precision. We have developed a user-friendly benchtop instrument, the IMx™ that completely automates immunoassay testing. The IMx can process a batch of 24 samples in 30 to 40 minutes with no operator intervention. Two separate analytical technologies are employed for processing immunoassays: a new technology known as microparticle capture enzyme immunoassay (MEIA) for high molecular weight analytes and fluorescent polarization immunoassay (FPIA) for low molecular weight analytes. FPIA is the same technique used in the Abbott TDx™ analyzer for measuring the concentrations of many therapeutic drugs and some hormones (ref. 1,2). The incorporation of both technologies into a single instrument greatly enhances the immunoassay testing capabilities of the IMx.

PRINCIPLE

The MEIA technology is based on three key features: a miniturized solid phase, and efficient separation procedure, and an ultrasensitive detection method. The MEIA solid phase consists of submicron polystyrene latex particles which are coated with a capture molecule specific for the analyte being measured. Due to the small size of the microparticles, the MEIA solid phase has a very large surface area which results in a high antibody binding capacity. The total surface area of the particle available for reaction is 6.11 cm^2, compared to only 1.27 cm^2 for the 1/4" bead (ref. 3). Additionally, the diffusion distance between analyte and solid phase is approximately 100 times smaller for the microparticle assay than for the corresponding 1/4" bead assay. Together, these factors result in increased assay kinetics and decreased assay incubation times, permitting assays to be completed in 30 to 40 minutes. An additional benefit of microparticle technology is that suspensions of microparticles can be handled as liquids, thus making assay protocols easily automatable.

Separation of the microparticles from the reaction mixture is accomplished via "microparticle capture" by a glass fiber matrix (ref. 4). This technology relies on the high affinity of protein-coated microparticles for inert glass fibers. When a suspension of microparticles is passed through a thin glass fiber matrix, the microparticles are retained by the matrix while excess reagent and interfering substances flow through and are easily removed. The effective pore size of the glass matrix is several times larger than the microparticle diameter, resulting in rapid flow and efficient separation, as well as decreased susceptibility to clogging by viscous samples.

Detection of the immune complex on the glass fiber matrix is accomplished with an alkaline phosphatase-labelled conjugate that catalyzes the hydrolysis of the substrate, 4-methylumbelliferyl phosphate (4-MUP) to its highly flourescent product, 4-methylumbelliferone (4-MU). The rate of formation of MU on the glass fiber matrix is proportional to the concentration of analyte in the sample.

The MEIA technology can be used in either a "sandwich" or a competitive ligand format, and with one-step or two-step reaction sequences. In a typical two-step sandwich format, antibody-coated microparticles are incubated with sample to form the Ab-Ag complex. An aliquot of this reaction mixture is transferred to the glass fiber matrix for separation of the microparticle-bound analyte. An alkaline phosphatase-labelled antibody conjugate is added to form the second half of the sandwich complex. In the competitive format, the enzyme-antibody conjugate is replaced with an enzyme-analyte conjugate, but the reaction sequence is the same. Excess conjugate is removed by rinsing the matrix with on-line buffer. Substrate is then added and the fluorescence measured.

IMx ANALYZER

The IMx analyzer automatically performs all the steps required for analysis of a patient sample: counting the samples, identifying the assay to be run, warming the reagents and reaction cells to the appropriate temperature, pipetting reagents and sample, diluting samples (if required), timing incubations and other assay steps, washing away unbound conjugate, detecting and quantitating the fluorescent signal, and processing the data to yield a useful result.

An assay sequence is initiated by loading the appropriate number of reaction cells into a carousel. Approximately 150 ul of sample and controls (run in singlecate) or calibrators (run in duplicate) is added to the sample well of each of the reaction cells. No sample pretreatment is required. The carousel is then placed in the analyzer and the appropriate reagent pack loaded into the reagent block. The door is closed and the RUN button pressed. The instrument then begins a preparation process in which all stepper motors are "homed", the type of carousel and its "lock" status are identified, the reagent pack barcode is scanned to determine the assay to be run, and the carousel- and reagent-heating systems begin warming reagents and reaction cells to the appropriate temperatures. When this sequence is completed, the assay protocal is started. Fluorescent signals measured at the end of the assay protocol are converted to rates which are then converted to concentrations by comparison to a stored standard curve. A printed report is generated with key assay values flagged if out of range. The assay sequence is aborted if certain control variables are not within specification.

The IMx system (Fig. 1) consists of a benchtop analyzer; MEIA reagent packs and reactions cells; FPIA reagent packs, sample cartridges and cuvettes; and calibrators and controls. The analyzer itself is comprised of a 24-position MEIA carousel or a 20-position FPIA carousel, MEIA front-surface fluorometer, FPIA optics system, reagent heater block, air heater system, diluent heater system, pipetting arm which includes reagent barcode reader, fluid delivery system, on-line MEIA and FPIA buffers, waste container, keyboard and display, thermal printer, user-interchangeable system and assay software modules, MEIA lamp power supply, and the necessary electronics to operate the instrument (ref. 5).

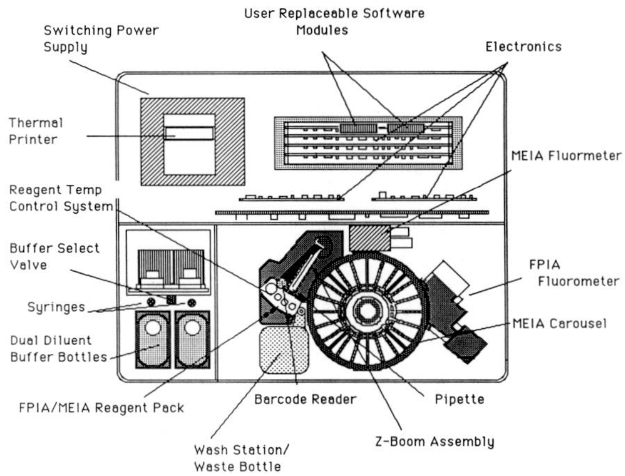

Fig. 1. Major components of the IMx analyzer.

A very key part of the IMx system is the MEIA reaction cell. Within this single unit occur the immunochemical and substrate reactions necessary to quantitate the analyte. It is composed of a sample well, pre-dilution well, incubation well, and glass fiber matrix with blotter. The reaction cell is not assay specific and can be used with all MEIAs.

The pipette/fluid delivery system transfers fluids from reagent bottles to reaction cells and from well to well within a cell. It consists of a robotic arm that moves both horizontally and vertically, and positions the pipette arm over the reagent bottles, reactions cells, and wash stations. The pipette itself is a teflon-coated stainless steel tube. Fluid levels are sensed by measuring electrical conductivity between the pipette tip and an external electrode.

Carryover between samples and reagents is minimized by washing the pipette/electrode assembly in a specially designed two-compartment wash station. The outer area is used to discard excess sample and reagent remaining in the probe, while the inner area is used to wash both the inside and outside of the probe. The use of a separate waste disposal prevents contamination of the rinsing area, thereby minimizing carryover. We tested sample carryover in the IMx using hCG as the model assay. Using a wash volume of 2.0 ml between each sample aspirate, we were able to detect only 1-4 mlU/ml hCG in a zero sample run immediately after a high sample of 1.3 X 10^6 mIU/ml.

To achieve reproducible EIA performance, temperature must be controlled precisely during all incubation steps of the assay. The IMx relies on three separate systems for temperature control: 1) a closed-loop heating block to control the temperature in the reagent vials at 35.0 $\pm$ 0.5 C; 2) a flow-through heating block which controls the diluent temperature to 35.0 $\pm$ 0.5 C; and 3) a forced-air heating system to control reaction cell temperature to 34.0 $\pm$ 0.7 C.

MEIA reaction cells and FPIA cuvettes are heated in their carousels by forced air from below the carousel (Fig. 2). Ambient air is drawn in by a fan and forced over a heating element, past a thermistor and up towards the carousel where it bathes the reaction cells and cuvettes. An analog circuit compares the thermistor temperature to a setpoint determined in the software. In this way, the CPU can control heater system output to minimize warm-up time at the beginning of a run and maintain constant air temperature during a run, regardless of changing ambient conditions. During a run, temperature is controlled by reading an additional remote thermistor placed in the air flow in the immediate vicinity of the reaction cells. The temperature at the remote thermistor is compared to a setpoint determined during temperature calibration. The IMx employs a single-point calibration procedure that relates a manual measurement of the temperature of an aliquot of diluent buffer in a well of the reaction cell (at equilibrium) to the temperature measured at the remote thermistor. The CPU controls the air heater circuit in response to readings at the remote thermistor to implement closed loop control at the remote thermistor location. Because the equilibrium temperature at this location corresponds to the liquid temperature of the reaction cell (previously established during the calibration procedure), closed-loop control of the reaction mixture is also achieved. A temperature calibration is stable for a minimum of one week.

The detection system used in the IMx is a front surface fluorometer that selectively excites and measures emission from 4-MU in the presence of 4-MUP. Concentrations of 4-MU as low as 100 nM can be detected in the presence of 1.2 mM 4-MUP, with a dynamic range up to 3000nM 4-MU.

The fluorometer (Fig. 3) consists of a low pressure mercury arc lamp, an excitation bandpass filter and dichroic beamsplitter, focusing/collection lens, photodiode, photodiode filter, emission longpass filter, emission bandpass filter, photomultiplier tube, and signal-processing electronics. UV light emitted by the mercury lamp is filtered by the excitation bandpass filter to produce energy predominantly at 365 mm to excite 4-MU. This filter also limits light transmission below 345 nm to <0.01%, thereby minimizing excitation of 4-MUP. Light transmitted through the excitation bandpass filter strikes the dichroic beamsplitter which is reflective at 365 nm and transmissive at 448 nm. A portion of UV light passes through the dichroic beamsplitter, through the UG-1 filter glass and strikes a photodiode. The signal received at the photodiode is representative of the energy sent to the reaction matrix and is used to normalize fluorescent rate read data. This signal is also proportional to the lamp current and is used to control lamp intensity to within 5% over the lifetime of the lamp. The 365 nm light reflected from the dichroic is focused through a lens onto the reaction matrix. The lens also serves as the collector for 448 nm light emitted from the surface of the matrix during a read. The emitted light passes through the dichroic and additional longpass and bandpass filters before reaching the PMT. In this way, stray 365 nm excitation energy and 387 nm energy due to 4-MUP emission are minimized. The entire fluorometer system resides inside the thermally controlled environment of the analyzer so that thermal drift is minimized.

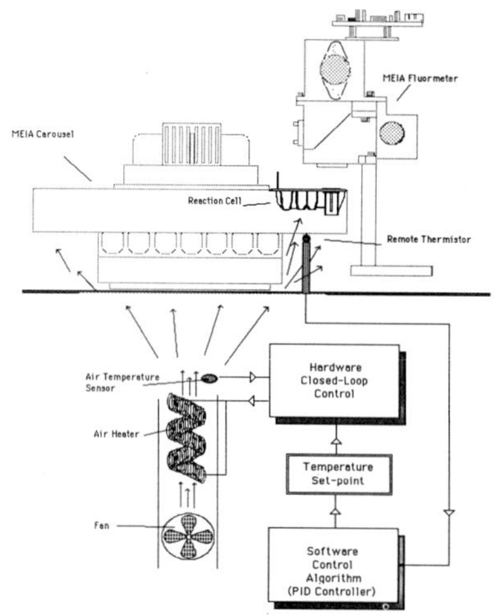

Fig. 2. Schematic representation of reaction-cell temperature control scheme

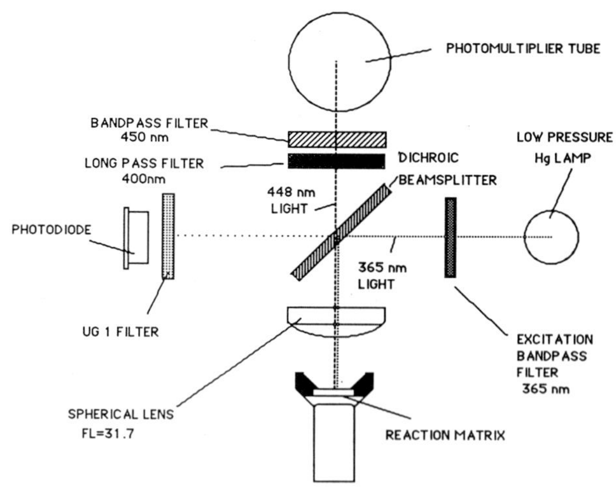

Fig. 3. Optical schematic of front-surface fluorometer.

The fluorometer is calibrated using a set of six stable fluorescent standards (three concentrations in duplicate) which consist of specially constructed reaction cells loaded with discs containing specific amounts of an inorganic Europium phosphor in a durable ceramic matrix. The fluorescent intensities of the calibrators were chosen to cover the entire dynamic range of fluorescent signal possible in an assay. PMT gain is varied to set the signal of the middle fluorescent standard to its nominal calibrated value. A linearity check is then performed to verify that the PMT is still operating in the linear region over the entire range of assay fluorescence values at the new gain setting. Optics calibrations are stable for a minimum of one week.

IMx ASSAY PERFORMANCE

The IMx assay for alpha-fetoprotein (AFP) is an example of a typical sandwich-type protocol (ref. 6). In the first step of the assay, sample is incubated with a suspension of anti-AFP antibody-coated microparticles. After the binding of sample analyte to the capture antibody is complete, an aliquot of the mixture is transferred to a glass-fiber matrix. The microparticles absorb to the glass fibers while excess sample is removed by washing with on-line diluent. A second antibody, labelled with alkaline phosphatase, is added and incubated on the matrix. After incubation, the matrix is again washed to remove excess conjugate. Separation of excess sample and reagents is rapid (<3s) and efficient (requiring <200 ul of wash solution). Substrate (4-MUP) is then added to the matrix for detection and quantitation. The concentration of analyte is directly proportional to the rate of fluorescence emitted from the surface of the matrix. The fluorescence rate is measured and compared with a calibration curve stored in the instrument to obtain the concentration of AFP. Calibration curves for AFP, as for all IMx assays, are stable for a minimum of two weeks.

The sensitivity of the IMx AFP assay was calculated to be less than 0.4 ng/ml. This sensitivity is defined as the concentration at two standard deviations above the 0 ng/ml calibrator, and represents the lowest measurable concentration of AFP that can be distinguished from zero. The assay shows no interference from lipemic specimens with up to 1126 mg/dl of triglycerides, icteric specimens with up to 50 mg/dl of bilirubin, or hemolyzed specimens with up to 800 mg/dl of hemoglobin. Concentrations of total protein in specimens can vary from 5.4 to 16 g/dl without significance effect.

AFP assay precision data, obtained from three separate clinical sites, is summarized in Table 1. Within run coefficients of variation are based on replicates of three, while within and between lab CVs are projected for singlecate testing. Six human serum panels ranging in concentration from 2.9 to 250 ng/ml of AFP were tested. Within run CVs were approximately 4% or better, while within lab CVs were all less than 7% and between lab CVs less than 10%.

TABLE 1. IMx AFP reproducibility

PANEL	MEAN AFP (ng/ml)	WITHIN RUN % CV	WITHIN LAB % CV	BETWEEN LAB % CV
A	2.90	4.2	6.7	9.2
B	10.26	3.3	4.8	4.9
C	40.45	2.9	4.5	6.4
D	68.80	3.3	4.8	5.1
E	150.28	3.4	5.2	5.2
F	249.67	3.6	6.4	8.1

Data from 3 sites.
Within run CV's are based on replicates of 3.
Within and between lab CV's are projected for singlecate testing.

The Imx AFP assay offers an optional dilution protocol with a 1:3 dilution for sample concentrations greater than the 0-350 ng/ml dynamic range. Correlation of the dilution protocol with the neat protocol (manual dilution) using 133 specimens with concentrations of AFP up to 1050 ng/ml, was excellent (r = 0.996, y = -1.4 + 1.01x, see Fig. 4). An extended correlation was also performed in which 191 specimens with concentrations up to 60,000 ng/ml were manually diluted and analyzed with both protocols. Excellent agreement was again seen, with a correlation coefficient of 0.994, slope of 1.00 and intercept of 31.7 ng/ml.

The performance of the IMx AFP assay was compared to the Abbott AFP EIA monoclonal assay using specimens of varying types. The overall correlation observed was excellent (r = 0.987, y = 0.332 + 0.970x, n = 2278, see Fig. 5). A breakdown of the correlation data into individual specimen types and concentration ranges is presented in Table 2. Equally good agreement was seen in each group of patient samples tested.

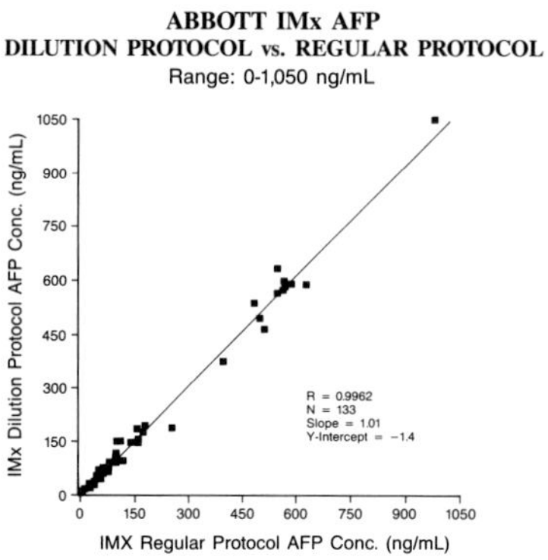

Fig. 4. Correlation of IMx AFP dilution protocol vs. neat protocol.

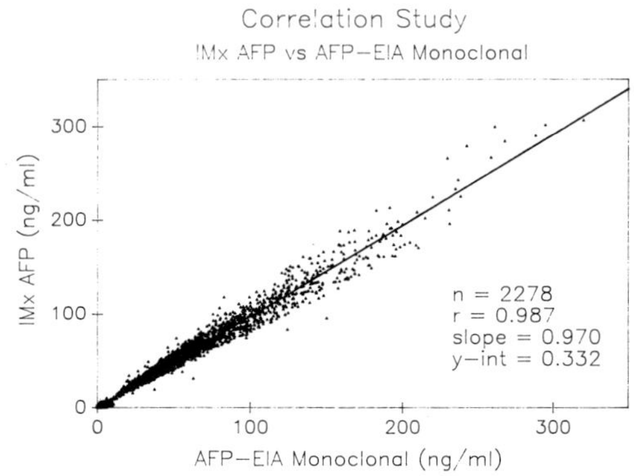

Fig. 5. IMx AFP patient correlation: IMx AFP assay vs. Abbott AFP EIA monoclonal assay

TABLE 2. IMx AFP correlation summary: IMx AFP assay vs. Abbott AFP EIA monoclonal assay

Specimen Type	N	Corr. Coef.	Slope	Y-Intercept
Overall				
0-500 ng/ml	779	0.9927	1.03	-1.7
0-5,000 ng/ml	810	0.9948	0.96	0.0
0-500,000 ng/ml	859	0.9957	0.94	-588
Malignants				
0-500 ng/ml	215	0.9943	1.04	-1.0
0-5,000 ng/ml	245	0.9940	0.96	4.0
Testicular Cancer				
0-5,000 ng/ml	112	0.9912	1.01	2.2
Liver Cancer				
0-5,000	24	0.9969	0.93	-9.1
Maternal Serum				
0-350 ng/ml	1697	0.9742	0.98	1.7
Amniotic Fluid				
0-65 ng/ml	1361	0.9759	0.99	0.0

REFERENCES

1. S.R. Popelka, D.M. Miller, J.T. Holen and D.M. Kelso, Clin. Chem. 27, 1198-1201 (1981).
2. M.E. Jolley, S.D. Stroupe, K.S. Schwenzer, et al., Clin. Chem. 27, 1575-1579 (1981).
3. L.B. Bangs, Boston: Seragen Diagnostics Inc. (1985).
4. W.E. Brown, Clin. Chem. 33, 1567-1568 (1987).
5. M. Fiore, J. Mitchell, T. Doan, et al., Clin. Chem. 34, 1726-1732 (1988).
6. G. Barnes, T. Danna, C. Miceli, D. Massie, V. Loos and N. Shaw, Clin. Chem. 33, 919 (1987).

Robotics in clinical laboratory medicine

Robin A Felder,Ph.D.*, James Boyd,M.D., John Savory,Ph.D., Keith Margrey,M.E., Dorothy Vaughn,B.S., and Antonio Martinez,B.S.

*Assistant Professor of Pathology, Associate Director of Clinical Chemistry and Toxicology, Department of Pathology, The University of Virginia, Charlottesville, Virginia, 22908.

ACKNOWLEDGMENTS

Supported in part by Perkin Elmer Corporation, Norwalk, CT.

Advances in the flexibility and availability of robotic systems are beginning to have a major impact on the organization of laboratory medicine. The availability of such devices promises to revolutionize the concept of the clinical laboratory and to usher in a new era in laboratory testing. Clinical laboratory robots can take many forms, but the two configurations that have shown the most promise are robotic arms and programmable pipetting devices. Although robots require a large initial investment, they are cost-effective because they do not take breaks, can work unattended and can perform tasks late into the evening without showing signs of fatigue. Implementation of laboratory robotics requires a large initial investment, careful planning, attention to detail, and specialized training of staff and skilled support personnel in order to be successful. There are three basic configurations of robots: the cartesian robot with 3 degrees of freedom, the cylindrical robot with four degrees of freedom, and the jointed robot which has the highest degree of flexibility with 5 degrees of freedom. Robotic locomotion is a recent improvement in robotic design which is made possible by linear tracks. Several hospitals have used robots successfully in the clinical laboratory for the implementation of complex procedures. Other laboratories are investigating the concept of using robots for simple repetitive tasks, such as sample preparation and introducing samples into analyzers. The benefits of the latter approach include abbreviated development time and procedures which are less prone to failure. The use of clinical laboratory robotics appears promising in reducing the cost of laboratory testing by the automation of tests that have up until now been highly labor-intensive. In addition, robotic automation offers the prospect of improved patient care through shorter test turnaround times gained by placing the robotic lab close to the patient bedside.

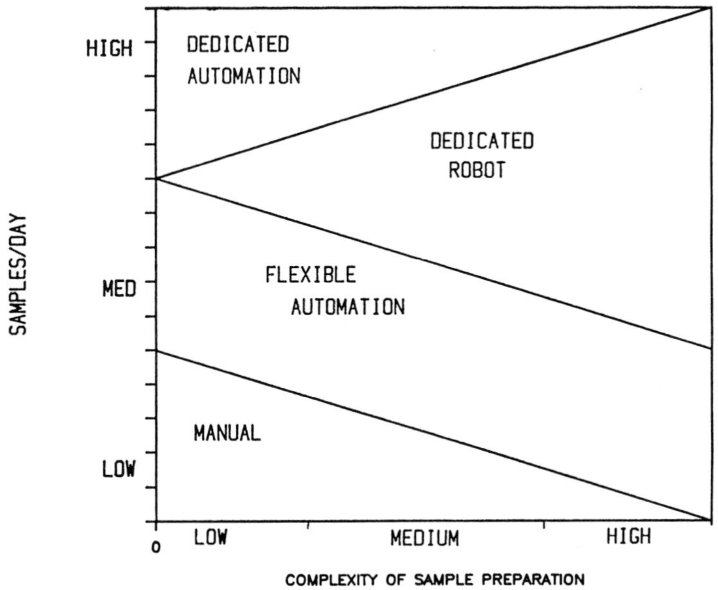

Fig. 1

INTRODUCTION

Many clinical pathologists have viewed the arrival of the laboratory robotic assistant as being many decades into the future. As you will see from the examples presented later in this presentation, laboratory robots are currently in use in several clinical laboratories. We are looking at the first examples of robotic implementation as the beginning of a new generation in laboratory medicine that may be as influential as the introduction of the autoanalyzer in the 1960s. While the laboratory robot is being welcomed as the ideal labor replacement technology by laboratory administrators, robots are viewed with fear as labor replacements by laboratory technologists. An understanding of this emerging technology will demonstrate that they will be valuable assistants in the laboratory. The purpose of this paper will be to define laboratory robotics, describe some commercially available robots, and review the state of the art in clinical laboratory robotics.

There are four main areas of the clinical laboratory that lend themselves to robotic automation: obtaining the specimen, sample delivery to the laboratory, sample processing and cataloguing, and sample delivery to the automated method, or sample analysis. Today it is feasible to automate virtually all aspects of sample handling except perhaps venipuncture. It will be many years before a robot will be produced with sufficient sensor technology to perform venipuncture, and then there may be additional problems with patient compliance. All other aspects of the laboratory are robot compatible, yet some areas are better suited for robots than others.

Sample complexity can be related to the numbers of samples to be analyzed with respect to the best method of laboratory automation (Fig. 1).

Manual methods are best suited to samples of low complexity and low sample numbers. On the other hand, automated analyzers are the best choice when very large numbers of samples of rather simple complexity must be analyzed. Robotics can perform analysis that are simple or complex, although their utility increases with sample complexity. Furthermore, since present day robotics operates at a slower pace than a laboratory technologist, small to medium sample number are best suited for robotic automation. Robotic systems must be built to handle peak load demands, such as those encountered in most clinical laboratories. Unfortunately, this often results in an idle robot during low demand periods. However, robotic labor is less expensive than manual labor.

There are 5 major reasons to consider robotic automation; greater productivity, improved precision, reduced errors, reliable documentation, safety, and increased job satisfaction. Robots can operate 24 hours a day unattended, and therefore, can produce more work than a comparable manual laboratory. In most robotic laboratories today there has been an improvement in the precision of laboratory results and a reduced error rate associated with analyses performed by robot. This is a result of elimination of two of the main sources of operator error, fatigue and inattention. There is often a similar reduction in transcription errors because most robotic laboratories have electronic transfer of information. In today's clinical laboratory there is the constant threat of human retrovirus contamination. Robots can reduce the number of technologist contacts with patient specimens therefore improving laboratory safety. Many of the mundane jobs of the laboratory can be automated by robot freeing up technologists for the more complex analytical methods. This should result in increased job satisfaction as technologists use more of their professional skills.

Many factors must be considered before purchasing a robot. The complexity of robot movement should be matched to the demands of the analytical method. The range of movements of a robot can be measured in terms of degrees of freedom and the actual performance envelope (APE). For a fixed base robot, at least 6 degrees of freedom are needed to orient an object in a 3 dimensional space. Three degrees of freedom are necessary to locate the center of gravity in the X, Y and Z planes, and 3 degrees of freedom are necessary to orient the object around its center of gravity. Robot motion can be described in terms of joints. Cartesian robots have three joints that extend in and out of the coordinate plane (prismatic joints). Cartesian robots have 3 prismatic joints, cylindrical robots have 2 prismatic joints and 1 rotational joint, and a fully articulating robot has no prismatic joints but 3 angular joints and 1 rotational joints. Increased APEs have been attained by placing robots on linear tracks which travel the length of the laboratory bench either attached to the laboratory bench or mounted suspended on the ceiling (Fig. 2). Other factors which describe robot motion are resolution, repeatability, accuracy, acceleration, speed and load capacity.

A robot at work interacts with a variety of peripheral devices

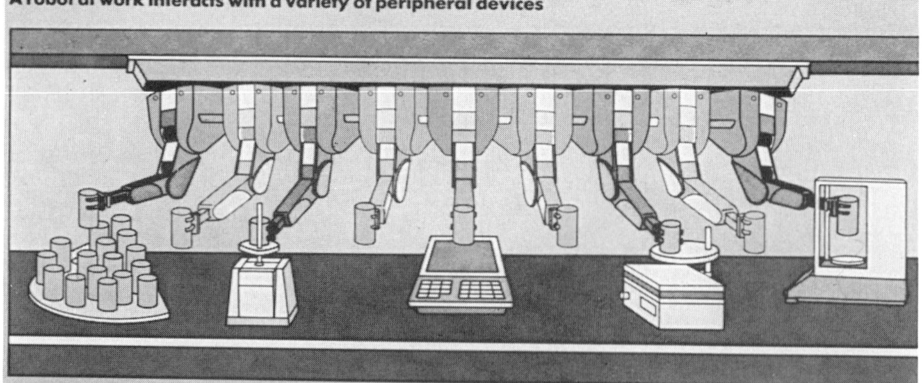

A robot suspended from an overhead track travels the length of a laboratory bench, driven by computer as it moves from one peripheral device to another. For laboratories designed along rectilinear lines, the robot takes up no benchtop space, a plus in small or crowded areas.

Fig. 2

Three basic types of robots are commercially available (Fig. 3). Pipetting stations are cartesian robots that have been adapted for liquid handling. Since pipetting stations cannot move objects around the laboratory bench they cannot officially be designated as robots. Cylindrical robots are available which can operate from the center of a laboratory bench and exchange gripper hands when analytical needs change. Finally the most sophisticated laboratory robots available today are the jointed robots displaying the widest range of motions.

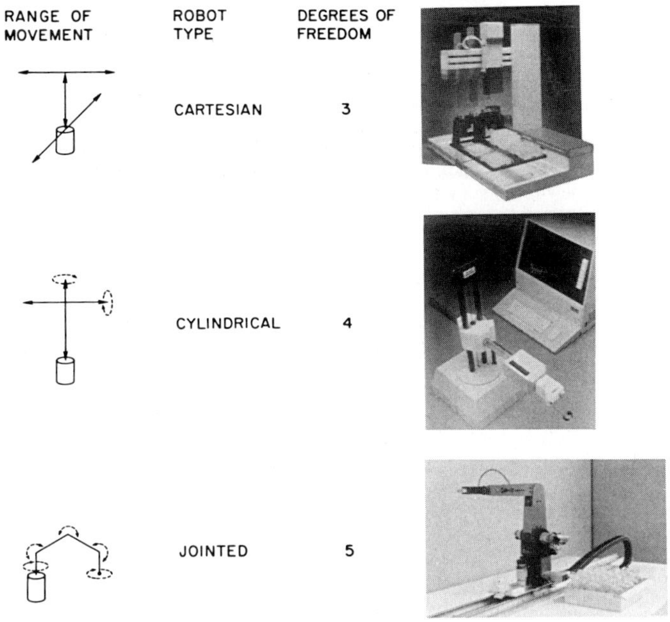

Fig. 3

Robots operate in conjunction with a variety of peripheral equipment. Components of a robot system can be subdivided into: the robot, controlling hardware, software, interfaces, and peripheral equipment. The robot itself possesses actuators (hands), position encoders, sensors and teaching devices (pendants). Generally, peripheral devices for robots are arranged in a circular pattern with the robot being at the center. A complete system is composed of robot hands designed for the analytical method, peripheral devices such as pan balances and mixers and pipettes, and finally interfaces to send the resulting data to a central computer facility.

Software design has had a major impact on the availability of robot technology to the average laboratory. Behind simple commands like "GO TO MIXER", are complex algorithms controlling each robot joint movement. A typical robot program is displayed below (Fig. 4). Robotic software is designed as a combination of a high level robot language and robot driver routines which interact with the robot controlling language (Fig. 5).

Programming a robot for specimen preparation

Program language	**What the robot will do**
PROCEDURE SAMPLE	
SPEED 5	Set speed
JUMP_ADM	Jump over instrument in path (avoid collision)
AT_PANEL	Position in front of autodiluter control panel
PRESS_ENTER	Press enter (initializing pipetter)
AT_PANEL	Move hand away from panel
JUMP_ADM	Return to rack jumping over instrument in path
RAKIN 1	Get first tube from input rack
JUMP_ADM	Return to pipetter jumping over instrument in path
AT_PIP	Position below pipetter
UP 20	Move up 20 mm
PIP_ON	Dispense
PIP_OFF	Switch off power to pipetter
DOWN 20	Move down 20 mm
JUMP_ADM	Return to rack jumping over instrument in path
RAKIN 1 BACK	Return tube to rack
END PROCEDURE	

Fig. 4

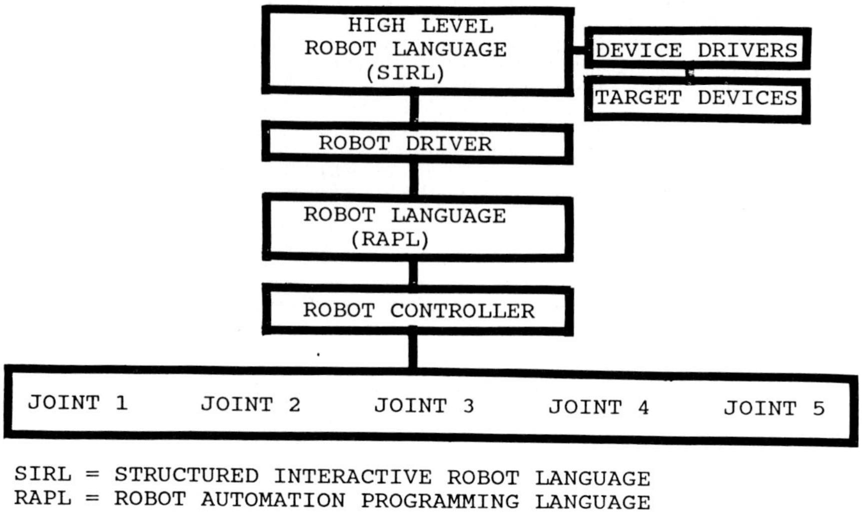

Fig. 5

Several laboratories have used robots in the clinical laboratory with a high degree of success. Relatively little robotics applications exist in the clinical environment compared to the industrial setting. It has been estimated that there are between 1000 and 1500 robots in use in the 75,000 industrial analytical laboratories in the U.S.A. (ref. 1) while in the clinical laboratories there are only 4 or 5 examples or working robotics systems. It is not readily apparent to laboratory managers how current robots can perform all the quality control steps currently performed by medical technologists to assure an error free laboratory. The modern clinical laboratory is not an assembly line production with a continuous stream of identical samples that can be processed in a similar manner. Each clinical sample is an irreplaceable record of the health of a patient at the time of sample collection. Consequences of incorrect clinical analysis are sufficiently grave to make robotic automation a distant possibility in the minds of most laboratory managers. Pioneers into the robotic automation of the clinical laboratory have realized the necessity for fail safe operation of all components of the robotic system and have incorporated redundant measures to assure correct results.

Dr. Pippinger (ref. 2) at the Cleveland Clinic Foundation has successfully incorporated several Zymate robotic systems into a laboratory performing antidepressant drug extractions and HPLC analysis. Medical technologists are necessary to prepare reagents and to place necessary supplies at designated locations within reach of the robot and to evaluate the quality of the final results. However, the robot completes the drug extractions and sample injection using a specially designed injection hand into the chromatograph. For several years these robots have been performing their repetitive tasks with only minor malfunctions.

Dr. Godolphin (ref. 3) at the Vancouver General Hospital has automated a highly complex steroid receptor analysis using a Zymate robotic system. Samples for estrogen receptor analysis are placed in a rack by the technologist following which the robotic lab adds reagents, incubates the specimens and centrifuges the resulting reaction mixture. Completed samples are placed in scintillation vials by the robot for radioactive measurements in a beta scintillation counter. Dr. Godolphin is also evaluating the automation of sample processing at the receiving end of the clinical laboratory. Using a combination of robotics and single tube centrifuges allows him to serially processing samples as they enter the laboratory. Sample processing is currently the rate limiting step in most clinical laboratories. The "Labot" serial centrifuge will be eventually incorporated into a robotic sample handling system which should not only speed up laboratory productivity but also reduce risk of AIDS and hepatitis exposure.

Castellani (ref. 4) reported recently the use of a robot to perform preparative immunologic precipitations of samples with final placement in a rotor for subsequent analysis. This robotic system which consisted of a Zymate robot and a Cobas-Bio rotor (Roche Diagnostics, Nutley, N.J.), was the first literature reported system combining a clinical analyzer and a laboratory robot. However, the placement of the rotor into the analyzer and the transfer of data to the laboratory computer was performed manually.

Friedman (ref. 5), has used a Zymate robot to dilute and transfer samples for blood grouping in the blood bank. For this task a Zymate robot was used which featured exchangeable pipette hands. The robot was also used to orient samples for bar code reading. This system had the robot configured as a pipetting device. After the robot performed the liquid handling, an operator would proceed with the manual aspects of the test. Many manufacturers of programmable pipetting devices are marketing them as robots that can perform serology or transmissible disease testing. While not true robots, since they cannot move objects around the bench surface, they can be programmed for a wide variety of liquid handling tasks. One manufacturer of blood banking automation (Flow Laboratories) markets a robot which is interfaced to a variety of microplate handling devices (pipettes, readers, washers, centrifuges). The entire device is enclosed in a protected hood, obviously designed to reduce operator exposure to contaminants. The IROBAL is the most integrated approach to robotics marketed to date and is well suited for the endocrinology laboratory.

To date the clinical laboratory with the greatest degree of robotics sophistication is that of Sasaki at the Kochi Medical School in Japan (ref. 6). Many of the labor intensive laboratory procedures have been automated in his laboratory using a variety of robots and fixed automation devices. Sasaki's work will presented as part of this Congress.

For high throughput operations a combination of programmable mechanical devices may be used. Two robots working in tandem can pass work completed in one area to a second step in another area. At the University of Virginia we are investigating the use of a programmable pipetting station in combination with a robotic arm to increase laboratory efficiency (ref. 7). The analysis of glycated hemoglobin is an example of solid phase extraction; a manually intensive analytical method commonly in use in many laboratories. Extraction of glycated hemoglobins was accomplished by automatic transfer of samples to extraction columns, washing, and then elution into spectrophotometer tubes using a custom designed trolley system. After the eluates were collected, a robotic arm placed them into a spectrophotometer equipped with a sample changer and automatic data reduction system. Results were comparable by the manual and robotic procedures. While one analytical method is being processed by the pipetting station the robot will be preparing reagents for the next analytical run. Total front to back automation is possible with the advantage of serialized batch throughput.

Another commercial system is available which combines a programmable pipetting station, a microplate reader, laboratory balance, incubator and robot into an integrated device (Synchron Instruments, Etten-luer, Netherlands). A cylindrical robot on a linear track allows 5 degrees of freedom. Electronic communication is provided through multiplexed RS-232 interface boards residing in two microcomputers. This integrated approach to robotics is the first example of its kind to date.

All of the robotic applications in clinical laboratories to date have automated relatively complex analytical methods. At the University of Virginia we are investigating the use of robotics to perform whole blood analysis in small laboratories located next to the patient bedside (ref. 8). The details of this project will be presented elsewhere in this Congress.

Although the feasibility of using laboratory robots in clinical laboratories is apparent, data documenting the failure rate of laboratory robots or their supporting computational hardware and software have been scarce. As more clinical laboratories incorporate robotics we will have a more complete understanding of their impact on patient care.

The changes facing medical technologists today, brought about by the introduction of robotics, are not unlike those which occurred after the introduction of automated analyzers. Robot technology, like the autoanalyzer, is being met with a combination of skepticism and trepidation over the potential loss of jobs (ref. 9). The introduction of autoanalyzers increased instead of decreased the demand for jobs in the clinical laboratory (ref. 10). Robotics can also be expected to either maintain the current demand or increase the demand for jobs in the clinical laboratory. Introduction of laboratory robotics will further redefine the role of the medical technologist to emphasize new skills. Many of the entry level jobs will be concerned with method development and trouble shooting or maintenance of robotic systems. Less time will be spent processing and delivering samples to analyzers. A more technically competent medical technologist with training in the analytical sciences will be required for the modern laboratory. This trend towards a more professional career should increase job satisfaction through increased demand for skill on the job.

Training programs in robotics and computer systems will be an obvious need. In a recent survey of robotics educational programs conducted by Eslami (ref. 11) it was found that there are approximately 68 educational institutions (48 of which are in the U.S) offering advanced educational courses in robotics and robotics related engineering. The greatest increase in the number of educational institutions on this list occurred in 1983 when there was a perceived need to provide the burgeoning field with robotics qualified graduates. There have been fewer than 25 graduates with Ph.D.'s from institutions with robotics programs each year over the last four years. Of all respondents to the survey none of the investigators had a research interest in clinical laboratory robotics. There is a need for training programs which will produce technologists at the masters or Ph.D. level who can design and implement robotic systems for clinical laboratories. Very few clinical laboratories have educational programs with personnel who are qualified to teach courses on robotics or computer-related applications. Medical technologists of the future must receive at least a modicum of training in this emerging field to be competitive for existing jobs.

The difficulty in assessing the impact of robotics comes from the difficulty in measuring the reduced costs associated with this type of technology. It is anticipated that the savings brought about by robotics will be a more indirect influence on overall hospital operating costs rather than a direct reduction in the manpower necessary to operate a clinical laboratory. For example, robotic technology will allow the operation of remote laboratories close to the critically ill patient resulting in faster turnaround in critical care analysis such as blood gas and electrolyte results. The improved patient care brought about by rapid sample analysis with subsequent more accurate diagnosis should shorted the time spent in the hospital for some patients. There has been an overall decrease in the turnaround time and a reduced transcription error in reporting tests, however the cost benefit of these improvements are difficult to assess.

SUMMARY AND CONCLUSION

Planning a robotic laboratory requires careful evaluation of many interacting factors, such as: benefit to the patient, cost of the robot, development time, and throughput desired. The initial cost of the robotic hardware is usually relatively small compared to the cost of peripheral devices, engineers and training of laboratory staff.

Medical technologists are usually wary of cost saving measures especially those which involve the reduction in the number of employees. Education of the laboratory staff about the implementation and operation of robotic arms will help to reduce the anxiety felt by technologists over potential loss of employment. The future role of laboratory technologists will become one of method development and technical support for robotic devices. However, training centers for clinical laboratory robotic technology will not come close to meeting demand.

Robotic technology can be best utilized through cooperation between administrators, directors and medical technologists. The net result will be more efficient health care delivery at a reduced cost to the patient.

REFERENCES

1. B. Fowler, American Laboratory, 62-70 (1988).

2. C. Pippinger, Med Lab Observer 5, 4-11 (1985).

3. W. Godolphin, J.A. McEwen and R.M. Bohl. Proceedings of the 12th Canadian Medical and Bioengineering Conference, 1st International Federation of the Pan Pacific Symposium, 178-179, (1986).

4. W.J. Castellani, F.V. Lente and D. Chou, Clin Chem 32, 1672-1676 (1986).

5. L.I. Friedman and M.L. Severns, Vox Sang 51, Suppl. 1, 57-62 (1986).

6. M. Sasaki and Kataoka, Japan J. of Medical Technology 16, 228-231 (1988).

7. R.A. Felder, W.D. Holman, M.M. Wu, J.R. Spina, H.M. Barnwell and A. Martinez, Advances in Laboratory Automation Robotics, in press, Zymark, Massachusetts (1989).

8. J.C. Boyd, R.A. Felder, K.S. Margrey, A. Martinez aand J. Savory, Clin Chem 33, 1560-1561 (1987).

9. W. Godolphin, Advances in Laboratory Automation Robotics 3, p. 553, Zymark, Massachusetts (1986).

10. M. Walter, Medical Lab Sci 44, 378-382, (1987).

11. W. E. Snyder, Newsletter of the IEEE Council on Robotics and Automation 1, 7-18, (1987).

Critical care testing using unmanned robotic facilities

James C. Boyd, Robin A. Felder, John Savory, Keith S. Margrey, Antonio Martinez, Dorothy Vaughn

Department of Pathology, Box 214, University of Virginia Medical Center, Charlottesville, VA 22908

Abstract - In confronting increasing pressure to reduce health care spending, many laboratories have centralized their services to conserve resources, but this has adversely affected their ability to supply testing with a rapid turnaround (<5 minutes). Our laboratory is addressing this problem by developing robotically operated unmanned laboratories that are located in close proximity to critical patient care areas. Each laboratory is equipped with a multi-jointed robot (Perkin Elmer Corp.), a whole blood electrolyte analyzer (DuPont) and blood gas analyzer (Corning Diagnostics), and a touch-screen computer terminal (IBM PS/2 50) for interaction with the user. Following introduction of a blood sample into the laboratory by a user terminal session, control of the blood analysis is maintained by the robot computer (IBM-PC) through programmed robot motions and commands to the blood analyzer via a programmable bi-directional interface developed in our laboratories. The robot computer and user interaction terminal computer are linked via a 3Com local area network (LAN) to a central file server for data storage and access to patient demographic information. All robotic laboratory results will be passed to a central monitoring area for review by laboratory technologists before being released for clinical use. Unmanned, robotically-controlled laboratories are a technically feasible and promising alternative for the provision of rapid-turnaround critical care testing in areas remote from the main laboratory.

INTRODUCTION

Economic reform of health care delivery in the U.S. fostered by soaring medical costs has forced clinical laboratories to reexamine their efficiency and the best use of available manpower. In confronting economic constraints many laboratories have chosen to centralize their services to conserve on labor and equipment resources, but this has adversely affected their ability to supply testing with a rapid turnaround (<5 minutes). Such rapid turnaround is frequently desired for a small repertoire of tests by physicians caring for critically-ill hospitalized patients, but, it is difficult to provide without a means of rapid specimen transportation to the laboratory. The use of human messengers for specimen transportation has been found to be slow and too expensive. A few institutions have had success in using pneumatic tube or conveyor belt systems to provide rapid specimen delivery to a central laboratory facility but not without high cost and occasional breakdowns.

The alternative model to a centralized laboratory for providing rapid turnaround testing is the use of a series of small satellite laboratories that are located in close proximity to the patient care areas they serve. A major advantage of the satellite laboratories is their accessibility. A disadvantage is the inefficient use of personnel that are required to staff these laboratories full-time, 24 hours per day. Decentralization may also raise doubts about the quality of laboratory results. Monitoring the quality of analyses provided by satellite laboratories is often difficult, especially when the satellites are operated by hospital departments other than the central clinical laboratories. In addition, facilities such as small blood gas laboratories located within operating rooms are frequently exempt from inspection by official hospital accreditation agencies.

FULLY-AUTOMATED ROBOTIC LABORATORIES

In designing laboratory services for a 600 bed replacement hospital that is under construction at the University of Virginia, we followed the alternative model by developing a series of satellite laboratories in proximity to critical care patient units whose functions will be monitored in a central facility called satellite central. These laboratories are being designed to provide a limited menu of whole blood tests including electrolytes, blood gases, and hemoglobin, and will be operated by remote control using laboratory robots (refs. 1,2,3). Our approach, if successful, will allow the advantage of rapid turnaround testing to be realized without a large increment in the personnel required for laboratory operation. In addition, patient and quality control data generated by the satellite laboratories will be constantly monitored by the Central Clinical Laboratories. The Central Clinical Laboratories will be responsible for maintenance and repair of the analytical instruments and robots in the satellite laboratories.

Our approach of performing only whole blood analyses in the network of satellite laboratories contrasts with the current usage of robotic systems for performing complex assays. Whole blood analyses have traditionally required little technologist manipulation, but have had high labor costs because of the large amounts of time spent by technologists waiting for specimens to analyze. In operation, we envision the delivery of a sample by any member of the clinical staff to the nearest robotic laboratory. Each laboratory will be equipped with a user interaction station similar in design and function to an automated bank teller machine. After the user chooses the analyses required from a touchscreen menu and places a patient sample into a depository, the robot will automatically introduce the sample into the appropriate analytical instrument. All quality control functions and calibration cycles will be triggered automatically by the controlling software of the robot computer. Patient results will be passed electronically to a central monitoring station staffed by trained medical technologists. Here, all results generated in the satellites will be checked and verified by the technologist for transmission to the host central laboratory computer system. The software of this host computer will do comparisons of the data with established normal ranges and previous results on the same patient. Technologists in the satellite central monitoring station will be able to electronically order repeat analysis or to request the introduction of a quality control specimen and even instrument repair by the robot.

ROBOTIC LABORATORY DESIGN

Although there are several commercially available robotic arms that can be utilized for handling laboratory specimens, our proposed application exceeded the supplied capabilities of all systems we evaluated. Considerable design and creativity were required for development of robot motion-control software, the computer interfaces needed for robotic control of laboratory instruments, and the user interaction station functions. Our development was carried out using a Perkin-Elmer Masterlab robot arm and IBM-PC computer for robot and instrument control. The final configuration of our laboratories is represented diagrammatically in Fig. 1.

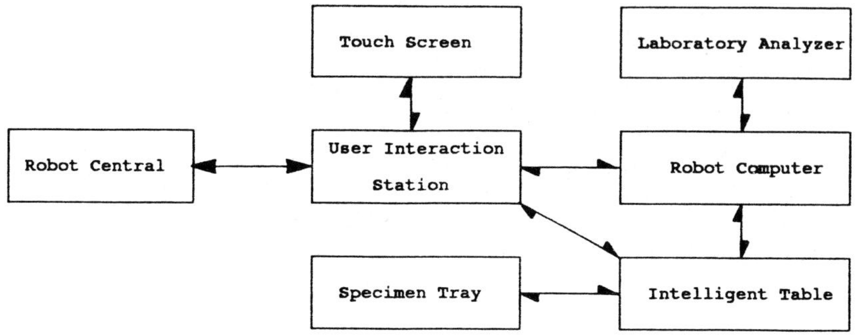

Fig. 1. Robot Laboratory Configuration

Four different computers are utilized in carrying out the satellite laboratory functions. The first computer, an IBM-PC is utilized for robot motion control and instrument control. The second, an IBM PS/2 50, is used for user interaction station functions, touchscreen control, and packaging of patient results for transmission to satellite central. The third, an Intel 8085 microprocessor is used for control of several devices on what we call an "intelligent table," including the sample tray, a syringe volume detector, a dropped syringe detector, and a syringe capping/uncapping station. The fourth, an IBM PS/2 80 is utilized as a network file-server. All computers are interfaced with one another via serial RS-232C communications or a 3Com Plus ethernet network.

To enable computer control of the laboratory analyzers, a programmable bi-directional interface was developed in our laboratories. The interface, an Intel 8085 microprocessor with associated programmable read-only memory and serial interface controller chips, was mounted on a circuit board that plugged directly into the chassis of each laboratory analyzer. The interface allowed direct access to the data bus of the instrument and, thus, to all instrument front panel and monitoring functions. The interface permitted software initiation of all calibration cycles, chamber evacuation, washes, and sampling mode as well as retrieval of patients' results, calibration results, and initialization of instrument settings for the patient's temperature and hemoglobin concentration and for the barometric pressure, time and date. The interface was designed to follow a uniform communications protocol so that the same series of commands could be issued, for instance, to calibrate or run a sample on any instrument. To facilitate the uniform command protocol, personality cards were designed for each instrument being interfaced that translated uniform protocol commands to instrument-specific commands.

Programs to control the robot were written in Perkin Elmer Robot Language (PERL) on the IBM-PC computer. PERL is very similar to the BASIC computer language, but it incorporates commands to allow easy control of robot movements. Programs in PERL on the IBM-PC allowed integration of the instrument functions with the robot movements. To enhance the gripper of the robot, we added photo-diode detectors that allowed the robot control program on the IBM-PC to determine whether the robot had actually gripped a tube. Gripper sensors supplied with the robot allowed sufficiently accurate measurements of container size to detect whether the robot had grasped an improperly sized specimen container.

There were several design considerations involved in developing the user interaction station. First was the creation of touch screens that allowed easy entry of patient and test selections by the naive user. Second was the development of an interrupt-driven serial interface with the robot controller computer to allow independent operation of the two computers without one having to "wait" for the other to finish a specific operation before it could receive a message. Third was the establishment of database that received and stored demographic information on the patients served by the robot laboratory, and, that allowed limit and delta checks to be performed on patient results. Programs to control the user interaction station were written in the "C" computer language. Screen display was accomplished using the SayWhat screen display software (The Research Group, San Francisco, CA). A Edmark touchscreen with EZTouch software (Edmark, Bellevue, WA) fitted to the monitor of the IBM PS/2 50 computer was utilized for user input of touch selections.

The touch screens, as presently designed, require the user to enter a security authorization code. Help screens are available to assist with using the system. Patients in the patient care areas local to the robot laboratory are presented in menus to the user. Selection of the patient is made by moving a light bar up or down the menu of patients. If the patient is not in the demographic database of the user-interaction station, the user may enter demographic information by using a keyboard display on the touchscreen. Once the patient information has been gathered by the system, a test selection screen is presented to the user. Test selections are made by touching "toggle-switches" on the touchscreen display. Representative screens showing this process are shown in Figs. 2 and 3.

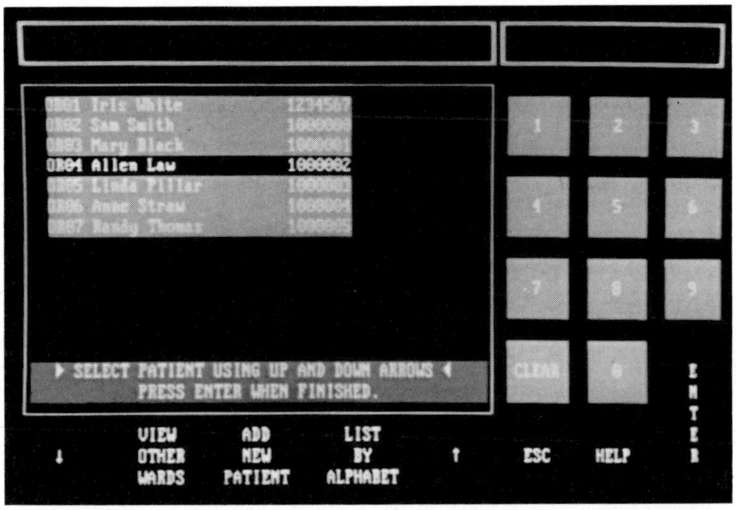

Fig. 2. Touchscreen display showing patient selection from menu.

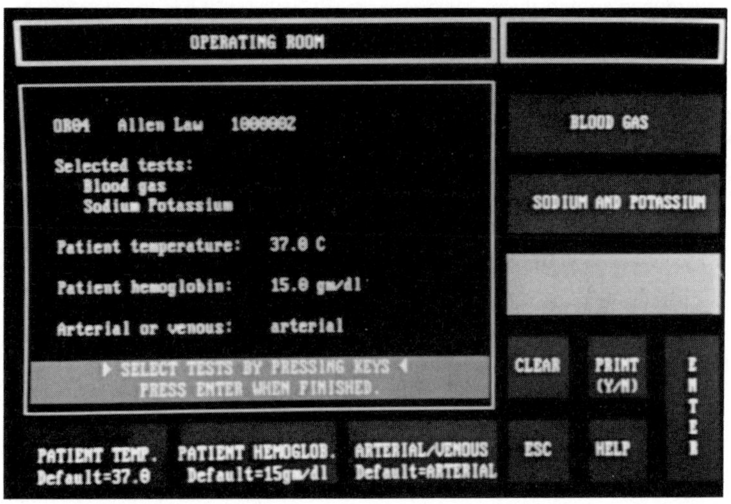

Fig. 3. Touchscreen display showing test selection.

Following user identification of the patient and what tests are desired, the sample is placed into the sample tray by the user and subsequent specimen handling is carried out entirely by the robot. The robot arm grasps the sample syringe, it removes the airtight cap from the end of the syringe, activates the appropriate laboratory analyzer for analysis, and introduces the sample into the instrument. For the Corning 178 blood gas analyzer the last step is the most critical and exacting, in terms of positioning the syringe tip properly into the small orifice of the blood gas analyzer. The average overall time required to complete one assay with the robot arm is 215 seconds, whereas, the average assay time with human introduction of the sample is 130 seconds. Various fail-safe operations have been programmed into the robot control programs to allow the robot to detect and recover from such errors as failed sample introduction into the laboratory analyzer, insufficient sample in the syringe, and improper specimen container.

RELIABILITY OF ROBOTIC ANALYSIS

We evaluated the reliability of robotic specimen handling by comparing results of robotically controlled analyses of 300 blood gas specimens with manually controlled analyses of those same specimens in a routine laboratory environment. All robot functions were carefully monitored and any flaws in its operation were noted. Twenty-three of the specimens had insufficient sample volume to be analyzed both ways. The excellent comparison data between the specimens introduced by hand and by the robot are shown in Figs. 4, 5, and 6. However, the robot had difficulty in successfully handling several "as received" specimens without human intervention. The foremost problem was the presence of specimen labels and/or surgical tape wrapped around the syringes that frequently stuck to the robots grippers and caused the sample to be mishandled. Thus, we have given careful consideration to setting standards for specimen preparation prior to introduction into the remote robotic laboratories.

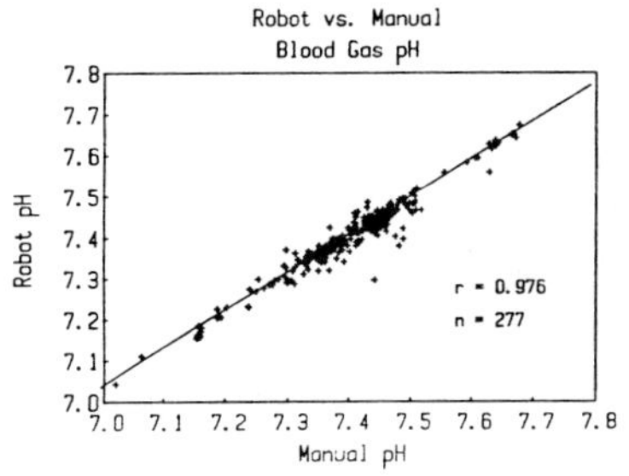

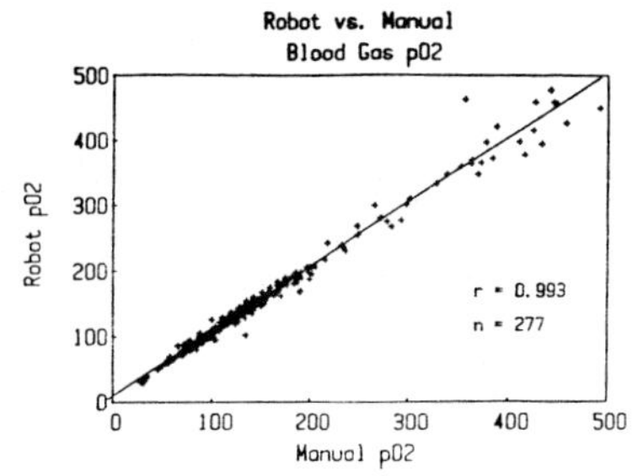

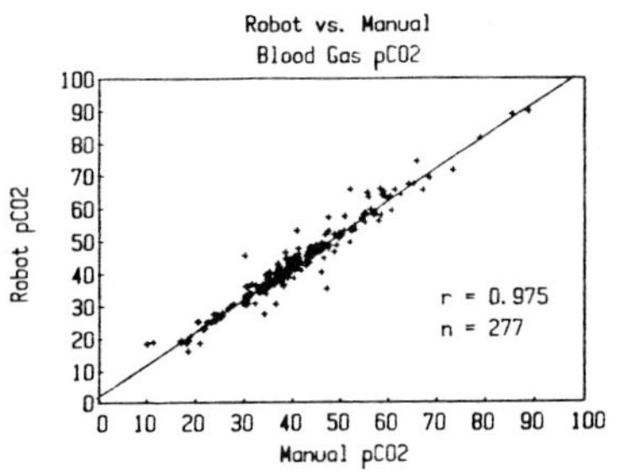

Figs. 4, 5, and 6. Blood gas pH, pO_2, and pCO_2 as determined by a robotic laboratory compared with a laboratory technician.

Initially, these laboratories will accept only specimens in 3 ml. syringes that have been properly capped, and have no labels or surgical tape wrapped around them. Specimen identification will be accomplished by the user-interaction station computer recording the specimen tray location of the patient sample syringe.

DATA HANDLING

Once patient results have been generated in the robot laboratory, they are passed by computer to the central robot laboratory monitoring station (satellite central) where a technologist is stationed and responsible for patient data monitoring, quality assurance, and troubleshooting. Facilities are available to allow the technologist to institute remote maintenance activities such as recalibration or the initiation of a wash cycle.

The information flow from the robot laboratory goes from the robot controller computer to the user interaction station computer which stores the information in a file on the ethernet file-server. The technologists in satellite central have access to this file through their computerized monitoring station which is one of the nodes on the 3Com ethernet network. Once the results have been reviewed and verified, they will be passed on to the Sunquest laboratory information system installed at the University of Virginia, and from there to the Technicon medical information system (MIS) that has terminals and printers in each nursing station. Each passage of data from one computer to another has involved the development of a separate interface. The interfaces between the robot central monitoring station and the user interaction stations, and the interface to the Sunquest laboratory information system are still being developed.

SUMMARY

Based upon our data and experience in operating this system, we conclude that robotic specimen handling is feasible in a remote, unmanned laboratory facility for whole-blood analyses. Several areas remain that are still being addressed including the detection and correction of clots and bubbles in samples, the design of a positive specimen identification system, the development of a refrigerated specimen rack for storage of specimens prior to and following analysis and a sophisticated computer-computer interface to allow the remote monitoring of each self-contained robotic laboratory by a trained technologist. More human observation of the system will be required to make fail-safe software allowances for operational problems that we have not as yet experienced.

We can also conclude that robotic specimen handling is facilitated by the use of bi-directional programmable instrument interfaces that allow direct computer access to all instrument front panel functions. Such facilities are rare in present laboratory instruments, but could easily be made available by instrument manufacturers. In addition, the reliability of robotic specimen handling can be improved by including fail-safe error detection routines in the robot controller software, and by equipping the robot with enhanced sensing capability such as optical detectors on the hand. As an alternative approach for operating a series of remote satellite laboratories, robotic specimen handling appears to hold much promise.

REFERENCES

1. R Felder, J Boyd, J Savory, Med Lab Prod 2, 18-19 (1987).
2. JC Boyd, in Proceedings of the Advances In Clinical Testing Conference, 1987, Biomedical Business International, Macmillan, Tustin CA, pp 6-1 - 6-16.
3. JC Boyd, RA Felder, KS Margrey, A Martinez, J Savory, Clin Chem 33, 1560-1 (1987).

How to make and manage clinical laboratory systems using robotic facilities

Masahide SASAKI, M.D.

Department of Clinical Laboratory, Kochi Medical School,
Okocho, Nankoku City, Kochi Prefecture, Japan.

Abstract - In order to solve staffing problems and to protect the technologists from dangerous samples such as AIDS, laboratory robots were invented and connected with the CONVEYOR BELT SYSTEM (ref. 1,2) by the technologists working at our laboratory.
We have been successful in making 2 types of robotic facilites for 8 serological tests, such as HIV, HTLV-1 antibody, etc. and for 16 blood transfution tests, such as ABO blood typing, etc..

INTRODUCTION

The robot consists of a basic robot, peripheral instruments and personal computer. As a basic robot, we chose the RT 3000 type made by SEIKO Watch Co. and we invented a variety of peripheral instruments, such as pipetters and grip-hands and radially installed these instruments to the top of the robotic arm. We also adapted a personal computer to control both the robotic arm and the peripheral instruments, serving as the link between data gathering from and to the hospital main computer (ref. 3-5).

In this paper, we would like to introduce the outlines of the robotic systems and show their effectiveness for the laboratory management.

THE BASIC ROBOT AND IT'S PERFORMANCE

The outline of the basic robot and the performance are shown in photo.1 and table 1.

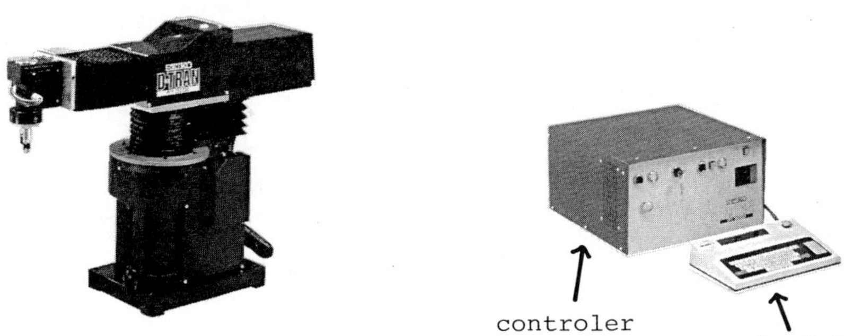

Photo. 1. Main robot, SEIKO RT 3000 type.

The SEIKO robotic arm is driven by direct current servo motors. The robot constantly monitors its position using optically encode monitors, which are installed in each joint. Each drive system maintains a positional accuracy of less than 0.025mm under normal operating conditions. Adding these mechanical accuracies, all articulating arms are covered with bellows type covering in order to protect from the dust which is produced by the robotic operations.

TABLE 1. The specifications of RT 3000 ROBOT.

4 directions	Movement	Movement speed	Analytical ability
Wrist rotation Wrist pitch Elbow joint Shoulder joint	± 999° 300mm 290° 120mm	150°/sec 750mm/sec 90°/sec 360mm/sec	0.005°/p 0.025mm/p 0.003°/p 0.012/p
Mixed mass speed	—	1400mm/sec	—

Reproducibility of positional accuracy	Carrying weight	Weight of main robot
± 0.025 mm	5 kg	108 kg

INVENTED PERIPHERAL INSTRUMENTATION

1) Devised the manipulators.

We put a round aluminum plate (r=20cm) on the top of the arm of the robot and attached 3 kinds of pipettes and hand grippes to the plate, so that robotic arms mechanically designed like a windmill would be better suited to their operation. The pipettes attached to the aluminum plate are Digital Multi-channel Pipette (Titertek Inc.) for dividing reagents. Multistepper 20/50 (Titertek Inc.) for stepwise dilutling of samples and Electronic Digital Pipette EDP-250X (Ranin Co.) for sampling. We also attached a micro plate holder to the aluminum plate and taxed our ingenuity to get this equipment to run by compressed air.

2) Automatic regent supplying equipment.

During the measurement procedures for serological tests, there are some fears that the antibody or antigen from the red cells or gelatine particles used as reagents will break down due to the mechanical mixing force. Thus, we especially invented an automatic supplying reagent container which can gently mix and continuously supply the reagent to the pipette in the refrigerator (Fig.1).

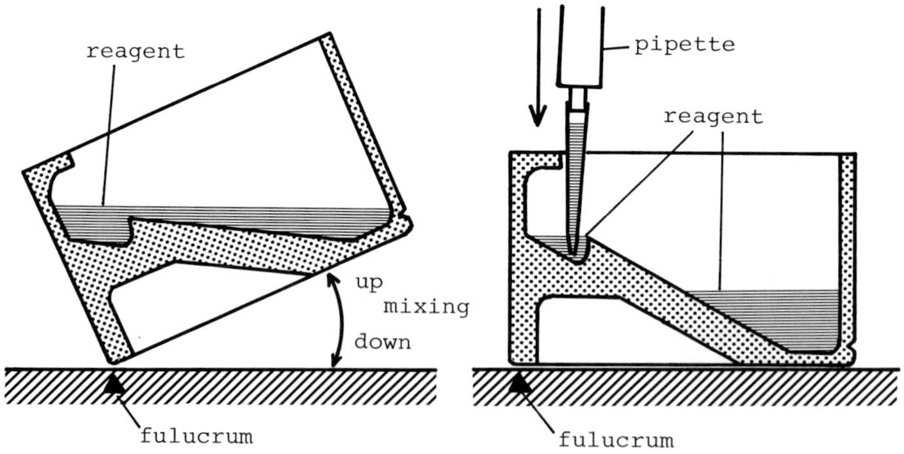

Fig. 1. An automatic supplying reagent container.

3) Automatic centrifugal machine

As for blood typing, the technologists used to use the centrifugal procedure in order to more clearly obtain blood aggregation by the reaction of antigen and antibody between the red cells. However, we made a special centrifugal machine which can maintain a constant speed of 1000 r.p.m. and can stop the rotor at the same position in order to pick up the samples easily. With this invention, we were successful in getting the arm of the robot to automatically put in or take our the blood typing tray from the centrufugal machine.

4) Other invented equipment.

We also contrived the following equipment.
(1) The cooking devices for holding and mixing the microplate or blood typing tray.
(2) Microplate supplying machine.
(3) The disposable tip supplying machine which can select the number of tips and attach them to the pipette automatically.
(4) The sample tube controler to determe the order of the test tube.
(5) The blood typing tray supplying machine.
(6) The revolving type incubator which can turn round just like a revolving stage for incubating the blood typing tray.

ROBOT APPLICATION FOR SEROLOGICAL TESTS.

One of the robots was made for serological tests, and can measure 8 tests at the same time, such as HTLV-1 antibody, HIV antibody, Thyroid, Microsome, TPHA Syphilis, Anti streptokinase, Rheumatoid arthritis,Mycoplasma, Anti DNA and Toxoplasma test. The robot functions to automatically select each test component acording to the order from clinical doctor sent through the computer (Fig. 2).

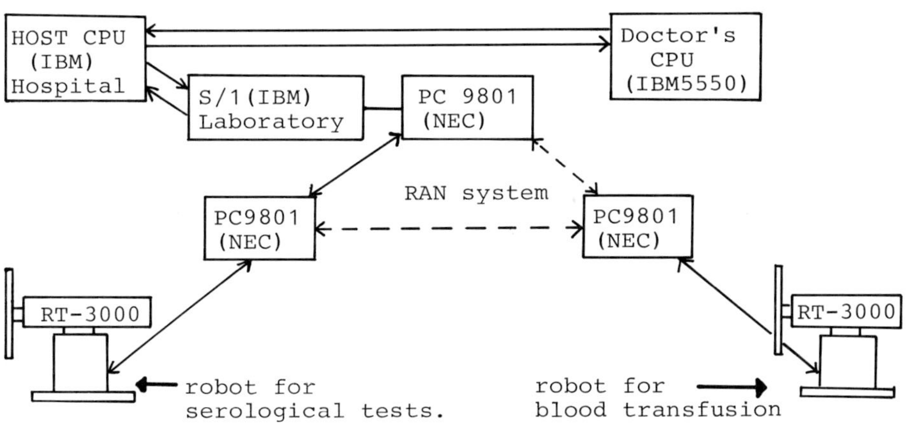

Fig. 2. The organization of the communication system between the computers and the robotic system. (---incomplete line)

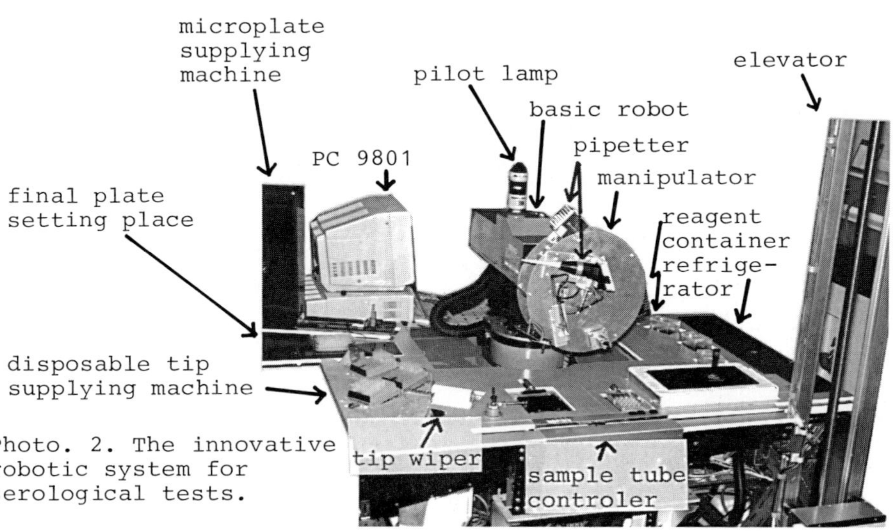

Photo. 2. The innovative robotic system for serological tests.

1) Arrangement of the invented equipment.

We radially installed 3 kinds of pipetters and a micro plate holder as manipulators to the top of the robotic arm and set up peripheral instruments such as the cooking device, the microplate supplying machine, the disposable tip supplying machine and the sample tube controler around the robot (Photo. 2). This robot also taxed our ingenuity in getting it to interact with the controlling computer to perform routine tasks.

2) The operative process for serological tests.

The operation prosess is shown in Fig. 3. Most robotic movements are just the same as those performed by technologists. For example, the robotic arm can wipe the top of the pipette (disposable tip) on the edge of the microplate hole, mimicking the technique of the technologist after the samples or reagents are delivered.

APPLICATION FOR BLOOD TRANSFUSION TESTS.

The robot made for blood transfusion tests can treat 16 components, such as ABO blood typing, cross matching tests, Rh factor and another 8 components for identification tests of the donor's blood (HTLV-1 antigen, HIV antibody, Hbs antibody, Hbs antigen, TPHA Shiphilis test, Total protein concentration, serum albumin concentration and GPT activity).

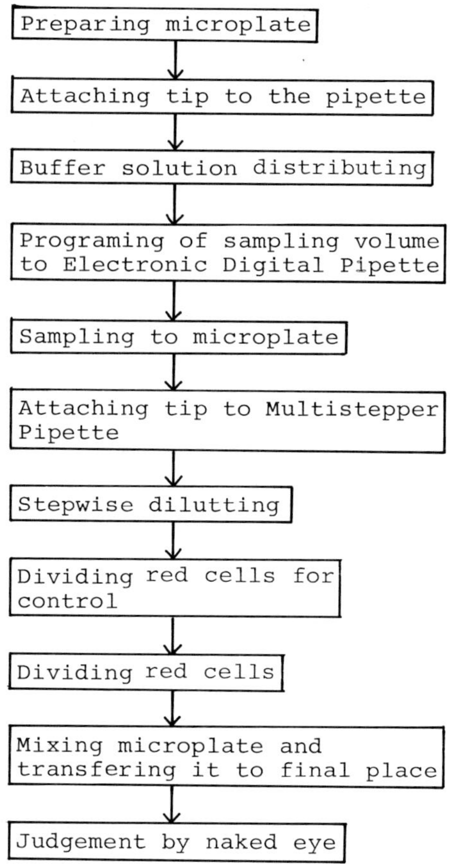

Fig. 3. The operative process for serological tests by the robotic system.

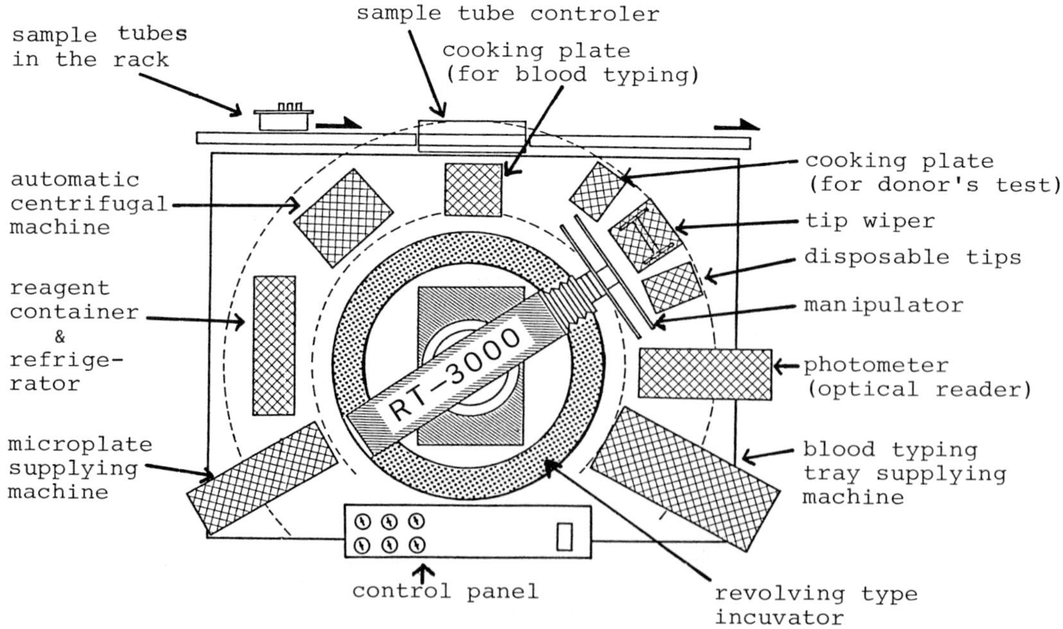

Fig. 4. Arrangement of the equipment for blood transfusion robot.

1) Arrangement of the equipment.

Adding to the peripheral instruments for the serological robot system, we invented other kinds of instruments and attached them to the robot for blood transfusion tests.
In the process of cross matching test for blood transfusion, it is neccessary to incubate the test reaction at 37°C, for 15min. and to centrifuge within 1min. at 1000rpm. For these reasons, we specially invented a revolving type of incubator, an automatic centrifugal machine and a hinged-shape blood typing tray and set them up around the robot. Fig. 4 shows the arrangement of the invented equipment for blood transfusion tests.

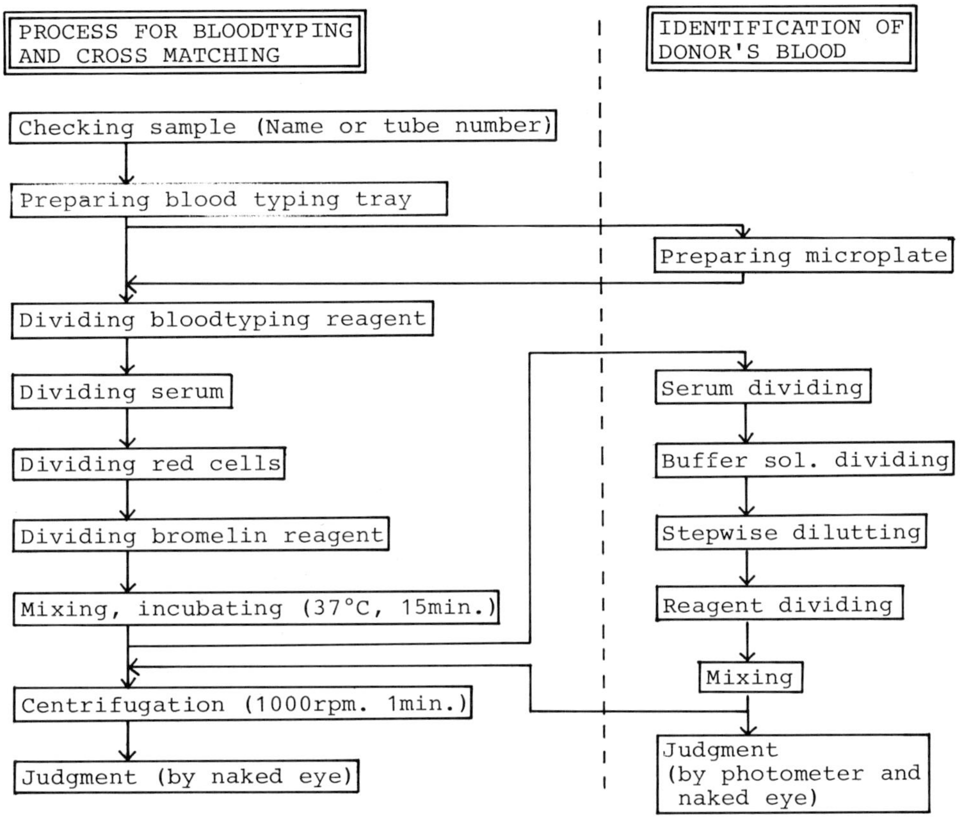

Fig. 5. The operative process for blood transfusion tests by the robotic system.

2) The operative process for blood transfusion by the robotic system.

The steps for the operation are shown in Fig. 5. In consequence, introducing the robotic system the blood transfusion tests has simplified the jobs of the technologists so that they only separate serum and blood cells, put the sample rack on the conveyor belt and read the results of the blood typing.

REFERENCES

1. M. Sasaki, Jpn. J. Clin. Pathol., Japan 32:119-126 (1984).
2. M. Sasaki, H. Sonobe, S. Koresawa, M. Nishida, JJCLA, Japan 10:82-90 (1985).
3. M. Sasaki, Jpn. J. Clin. Pathol., Japan 35:1072-1078 (1987).
4. K. Ogura, M. Sasaki, H. Kataoka, M. Nishida, JJCLA, Japan 12:613-618 (1987).
5. M. Sasaki, H. Kataoka, J. Med. Tech., Japan 16:228-231 (1988).

How useful the trace metal analyses are in diagnosis and therapy

Yukio Tanaka

Montreal Children's Hospital, Montreal, Quebec H3H 1P3, Canada

Abstract - Analyses of many trace metals have entered the repertoire of routine clinical analyses in many hospital laboratories. They are used to detect trace metal-related diseases (eg. copper in Wilson's disease and Menkes' kinky hair syndrome and zinc in acrodermatitis enteropathica), toxic metal poisoning (eg. lead, mercury, cadmium, aluminum), and trace metal deficiencies (eg. zinc, copper,selenium, manganese), and to monitor certain medical treatments (eg. lithium, gold, platinum or copper and lead in chelation therapy). In addition to these routine analyses, other trace metals such as molybdenum and chromium, as well as those mentioned above are being analyzed as a part of clinical research, the outcome of which may become useful in diagnosis and therapy in near future. Selection of proper samples (blood plasma, blood cells or urine) is essential in order to obtain clinically useful information. Utmost care must be taken to prevent sample contamination. However, it is also important to try to extract clinically valid information from "invalid" (contaminated) samples because those "invalid" samples may be the only samples obtainable. Because of the sensitivities required for trace metal concentrations in clinical samples and the speed demanded by clinical situations, atomic absorption spectrophotometers (both flame and flameless) are most widely used. Interferences from co-existing bulk elements such as calcium and sodium and background absorption from matrices must be controlled in order to obtain accurate results. Single-element determinations normally suffice; however, simultaneous multi-element analyses would be very useful in such cases as nutritional monitoring of patients on total parenteral nutrition. Many interesting observations have been made in animal experiments in the past. Efforts should be made to duplicate these observations in human subjects in order to make trace metal analyses even more useful in medicine.

INTRODUCTION

Only a decade ago, trace metal analyses were considered to be "special" among clinical tests and just a handful of hospital laboratories performed analyses of such metals as copper, zinc, and lead. Other trace metals, for example selenium, manganese, and aluminum, were only analyzed as a part of research projects and hospital laboratories were rarely involved in these analyses. In recent years, however, analyses of many trace metals have been firmly established as a part of "routine" clinical tests because of remarkable progress made in the field of trace metals in clinical medicine. At the same time, difficulties in trace metal analyses, namely sample contamination and interferences from specimen matrices, have become better understood by the analysts, and analytical results today are highly reliable. It is the purpose of this short review to examine the usefulness of trace metal analyses as clinical tests.

AREAS IN WHICH TRACE METAL ANALYSES ARE USED FOR DIAGNOSIS AND THERAPY

L. Detection of genetic diseases related to trace metals

Wilson's disease (hepatolenticular degeneration) (ref. 1) is a rare hereditary disease and is characterized by abnormal deposits of copper in many organs, particularly in liver and central nervous system. Patients with this disease normally become symptomatic (either hepatic or neuro-psychotic) as a young adult and have very low serum copper as well as ceruloplasmin levels, grossly elevated urinary copper excretion, and hepatic copper contents. For the diagnosis of this disease, blood samples are normally sent for analyses of serum copper levels first. It should be remembered, however, that serum copper levels are easily affected upwards by a number of factors including oral contraceptives. Therefore, low serum copper levels in Wilson's disease patients may be elevated to low normal levels in these cases; on the other hand, urinary copper concentrations are only affected by certain liver diseases including Wilson's diseae. Therefore, the first sample should be the urine instead of blood for detection of this disease. Patients with this disease are decoppered with penicillamine and urinary copper levels are measured to follow the treatment. This chelating agent also carries other trace metals, particularly zinc, into urine; therefore, it is advisable to monitor the extent of zinc loss in these cases.

Menkes' kinky hair syndrome (ref. 2), a fatal genetic disorder affecting baby boys, is characterized by growth and mental retardation, abnormal steely hair, hypothermia and seizures. The patient's serum copper and ceruloplasmin are extremely low. Recently, in autopsy samples of a Menkes' disease patient, manganese was found to be distributed in the body differently from normals (ref. 3); this is an interesting observation in view of seizures in Menkes' disease patients and "deficient" levels of blood manganese in some epileptic people.

Acrodermatitis enteropathica (ref. 4) is a rare autosomal recessively inherited disease and normally occurs in babies of Iranian, Armenian, or Italian origin. The patients become symptomatic soon after weaning from breast feeding. Features of this disease include characteristic dermatitis, alopecia, and very low serum zinc levels, due to malabsorption of this element.

Sickle cell anemia is not diagnosed by trace metal analyses, but this hematologic disease is characterized by high urinary zinc and low serum zinc (ref. 5).

2. Toxic metal poisoning cases

Intoxication with lead occurs very often among occupationally exposed workers and children who ingest lead-containing stuff (pica) (ref. 6). Blood lead levels and free erythrocyte protoporphyrin are most often, and most conveniently, analyzed to determine the body burden; in acute intoxication, however, the latter may still be normal. Whole blood lead levels are traditionally measured for diagnosis of poisoning. In lead-poisoned patients, anemia with low hematocrit is common and their blood cells where nearly all of blood lead is present are diluted with plasma containing virtually no lead. Therefore, packed blood cell lead levels should reflect the body burden better than whole blood levels. In chronic exposure cases, patients are often subjected to an EDTA challenge test for assessment of body burden, and their urinary lead excretion is measured. When lead-poisoned patients are treated with chelating agents, urinary excretion of lead is monitored. In addition to this, such essential metals as copper, zinc, and manganese are also carried away into urine. These metals should be monitored particularly in those patients whose pre-chelation status of these metals was only marginal.

Massive mercury poisonig epidemic has occurred in Japan (Minamata disease) (ref. 7) and in Iraq (ref. 8), both via mercury-contaminated foods. In addition, cases of accidental occupational exposure among workers and children who swallowed mercury-containing button batteries are known. Mercury determinations are done by the cold-vapor atomic absorption method.

Cadmium poisoning occurred in Japan from eating contaminated rice (Ouch-ouch disease) (ref. 9) and occasional accidental poisoning cases including ingestion of button batteries containing cadmium are also known.

Patients with renal insufficiency ingest a large amount of aluminum-containing ant-acids in order to control their phosphate levels, and as a result accumulate toxic quantities of aluminum (ref. 10). Accumulation of aluminum in hemodialysis patients from contaminated dialysis water has also occurred. Analyses of serum aluminum in these patients are now performed in much greater frequencies in hospital laboratories than before. A desferroxamine challenge test has been used to assess the body burden of aluminum.

3. Nutritional deficiencies

Occurrence of nutritional zinc deficiencies in man is well documented (ref. 11). More recently, zinc deficiency cases among patients receiving total parenteral nutrition (TPN) has been observed in 1960's and addition of zinc and other essential metals to TPN solutions are now carried out routinely (ref. 12). Although serum (or plasma) zinc is normally measured in these patients on TPN and those whose zinc status must be assessed, it is not clear to this date if serum zinc levels can accurately indicate the information sought. It is known that some clinically zinc deficient patients have serum zinc levels which are low but still within the normal range. This may be due to partial hemolysis of blood cells which contain much more zinc than serum. It may be quite possible that in zinc deficient state blood cells may be very fragile, causing partial hemolysi during blood collection procedures, either venus or skin puncture. It should also be kept in mind that in practice of routine clinical setting blood samples are taken into an evacuated tube!

Nutritional copper deficiency has been recorded among premature babies on milk-based formulae, babies and children with chronic diarrhea, and TPN patients. In addition, copper deficiency anemia and conditions in association with hypoproteinemia due to copper losses in various diseases are known (ref. 13).

An endemic disease called Keshan disease in China is a dietary selenium deficiency syndrome which originates from low selenium contents in the soil of the region and low selenium levels in the crop (ref. 14). A selenium deficiency syndrome similar to Keshan disease was also reported in North America (ref. 15). It is interesting to note that the syndrome is not observed in the part of New Zealand where the selenium levels in the soil and the blood of the residents are low. A fatal selenium deficiency case was recorded in a TPN recipient (ref. 16). It is also interesting that the incidence of certain types of cancer was linked to dietary selenium intakes (ref. 17).

It is generally believed that manganese deficiency in human beings can not occur because our diet generally contains sufficient quantities of manganese. Perhaps our total manganese intakes with food may appear to be enough to rule out possible manganese deficiency in man; however, how much of the total manganese can be absorbed and how much of the absorbed manganese can be utilized as a nutrient are the questions which are not answered to this date. It is also possible that some individuals can not absorb manganese normally or excrete excess amounts of manganese. Therefore, it is too naive to believe that manganese deficiency can not occur in man because our dietary intake is sufficient.

In fact, "deficiency" levels of blood manganese have been observed among epileptic children (ref. 18). The "deficiency" level was defined as below the mean minus two standard deviations of the normal levels. Similarly low blood manganese levels were also found among adult epileptics (ref. 19 and 20).

Hurley et al. (ref. 21) demonstrated that manganese-deficient rats produced offspring with ataxia and enhanced susceptibility to convulsions caused by electroshock. In man, however, manganese deficiency has been described in only one case, in which an adult on a metabolic study was considered to have become manganese-deficient because this metal was inadvertently omitted in his diet. Unfortunately, this "manganese deficiency" was not supported by determining the manganese levels in his body fluids or tissues.

In 1976, a blood sample of a 12-year old epileptic boy was analyzed for lead, as requested by his physician, to rule out lead poisoning as a cause of his conditions; however, his blood lead level was very low. Because of the animal experiment by Hurley, his blood was analyzed for manganese. It was found to be only 6.5 μg/L whole blood, much lower than the levels found in neurologically normal children (15.1 ± 4.1 μg/L, mean ± 1 S.D.). A number of children with chronic convulsive disorder were therefore tested for their blood manganese levels. These were found to be generally lower (9.4 ± 3.5 μg/L) than those in normal children but showed considerable overlap with the range found in the latter. A great number of abnormalities have been cited as the etiology of convulsive disorders. It is therefore probable that a majority of convulsive children examined may have one or more causative abnormalities other than manganese. It may be assumed that convulsive children, whose blood manganese levels are less than 7.0 μg/L (mean minus two standard deviations of normal children), are "deficient" in this metal and, perhaps, ssusceptible to convulsions. <u>Based on this assumption</u>, convulsive children with the "deficient" levels of manganese had a level of 5.2 ± 1.2 μg/L. Low magnesium status can cause seizures, but this patient's blood magnesium level was normal, so were the magnesium levels of manganese "deficient" convulsive children. At that time, it was not known if whole blood manganese levels reflect the body burden of manganese. Hurley et al. (ref. 22) stated later that the blood manganese appears to be a valid reflection of tissue manganese level and may be useful as an indication of manganese nutriture.

It was also found that newborn babies have much higher blood (ref. 23) and erythrocyte (ref. 24) manganese levels than older children and adults, and that the high blood manganese levels in newborns decline steadily until the age of 12-18 months when the levels reach those of older children and adults (ref. 25).

It is not known at this time whether the low manganese levels in the blood of some epileptics are due to nutritional deficiency. However, as shown by Hurley (ref. 21), manganese supplementation to deficient rats lessens high susceptibility to convulsions; therefore, the nutritional status of manganese in these patients may be of great importance.

4. Therapeutically used metals

Lithium has been used successfully in the treatment of manic-depressive psychosis patients for suppression of their manic phase. Because of its high toxicity, even at a slightly above the upper limit of its therapeutic range (0.5-1.5 mmol/L serum), it is necessary to monitor lithium levels of patients regularly. In interpreting the results of serum lithium levels, it is necessary to know when the last dose was given because of the short biological half-life of lithium. Patients with toxic side effects are seen quite often; in most cases the lithium levels are around 2 mmol/L but this author has seen up to 7 mmol/L in a very severe but non-fatal intoxication case.

The current trend is to measure both the plasma and packed blood cell lithium levels in the patients. Normally, the cell lithium level is $\frac{1}{4}$ to $\frac{1}{2}$ of the plasma level depending on the dosage and duration of therapy. In some patients, however, the blood cells accumulate excessive amounts of lithium.

Gold compounds have been used to treat rheumatoid arthritis patients for many years. Gold levels in serum are often monitored because of the toxic reactions, primarily dermatitis in milder cases and severe renal damage with impaired creatinine clearance. The relationship between the efficacy and toxicity of these substances and plasma gold levels is not well understood, and it appears difficult to predict appearance of the toxic side effects.

Cisplatin, a platinum complex, has been used successfully as an anti-cancer agent. It is also highly toxic, causing renal damage, and magnesium leaks out into urine. As a result, low serum magnesium levels are seen often in these patients. Frequent monitoring of serum and urinary magnesium levels is indicated. A very interesting attempt is being made to suppress the nephrotoxicity of cisplatin with selenium and some trace metals which induce metallothionein (ref. 26).

5. Research

A number of elements are being investigated with various objectives. Many of them will have direct applications in the clinical laboratory medicine for diagnosis of diseases. Only a few examples of these possibilities can be mentioned here.

Since the discovery of chromium as an essential metal involved in the carbohydrate metabolism, the research on chromium suffered a great deal mainly because of extreme difficulties in analyses. Only in the last several years, serum chromium became reliably measurable by the flameless atomic absorption method. Even today, analysts can not relax during sample procurement and analyses, or the results would be useless because of sure contamination! Nevertheless, the chromium research is progressing steadily (ref. 27) and concrete results will be seen in near future.

Molybdenum did not attract much attention of investigators in the past. This metal is known to be an antagonist of copper; therefore, the relationship between these two metals would be of great interest in diseases in which copper metabolism is abnormal. A genetic disease with molybdenum deficiency has been described (ref. 28). One of the difficulties regarding molybdenum is its analyses by atomic absorption because of carbide formation in the graphite tube.

Two recent findings on mangasese have been mentioned earlier in relation to Menkes' disease and convulsive disorder. In addition, manganese appears to be involved in carbohydrate metabolism. Several reports on animal experiments are available (ref. 29) and at least one investigation deals with a diabetic boy (ref. 30). Vigorous investigations on this aspect of manganese are expected.

ANALYSES OF TRACE METALS IN CLINICAL SAMPLES

1. Sample procurement: problems of contamination

Since samples must be procured using a device, contamination of various devices used means contamination of the samples which come in contact with the devices. Selection of suitable devices and their cleanness are very important.

There are a number of blood collection tubes available, but tubes used for trace metals are those without any anticoagulant, with heparin, or with EDTA. In this author's experience, heparinized tubes are, in general, cleaner than those with EDTA. EDTA in the tube will extract metals from the glass and stopper after collection of blood. EDTA also extracts metals from the erythrocytes into the plasma, therefore, the sample can be used only for determination of whole blood levels of trace metals. Evacuated tubes prepared specifically for trace metals, for example Bectron-Dickinson's Royal Blue top tubes, are better than anything else. However, these special tubes are NOT contamination-free, particularly with ultra-trace metals such as manganese in plasma, for which specially washed tubes are needed. Evacuated plastic tubes for blood collection have recently become available.

Stainless steel needles used for blood collection are also the source of contamination for elements such as chromium and manganese. It is necessary to wash off the contaminants with blood prior to collecting specimen for ultra-trace metals, or alternatively, a plastic cannula must be used.

Our "routine" procedure of blood collection, keeping it as economica as possible, is as follows: a "butterfly" to which a plastic syringe is attached is inserted into a vein and a sufficient quantity of blood is drawn slowly into the syringe for all the tests other than ultra-trace metals, then the syringe is removed from the butterfly and blood is allowed to drip into an acid-washed plastic tube for ultra-trace metals. A part of the blood collected in the syringe is placed in a Becton-Dickinson's Royal Blue tube with sodium heparin and is used for trace metals such as copper and zinc either in plasma and packed cells. The packed blood cells in the heparinized tube, after washing with a physiological saline solution prepared from ultra-pure sodium chloride, can be used also for such metals as manganese because of its high concentrations in the cells. If necessary, the clot of blood in the acid-washed tube can be transferred into a pyrex tissue grinder and hemolyzed completely after adding a tiny drop of Triton X-100. Syringes and Royal Blue tubes are regularly checked for contamination. It is absolutely essential to draw blood slowly into the syringe and to let blood drip into the tube in order to prevent contamination of plasma/serum from the blood cell metals by partial hemolysis; manganese and zinc are very much higher in concentration in the cells.

Urine samples should be collected, preferably directly, into acid-washed plastic bottles. A wide-mouth, recutangular plastic bottle (2 L capacity) is particularly suitable both for men and women. Cleanness of the genital area, particularly in women, is important to prevent contamination of the urine. Use of a squeeze bottle with deionized water is advisable. Plastic urine collection bags which can be attached to a baby and infant can be flushed out with deionized water (or with a dilute acid solution first, if necessary) prior to application. Twenty-four hour urine samples are often collected for zinc determination. It is absolutely important to avoid contamination with seminal fluid, whcih contains very high amounts of zinc. Urine samples may be contaminated with blood from menstruation; the extent of contamination can be estimated by measuring the venous blood of the patient for iron and the element in question.

Stool samples should be collected in plastic containers. No standard procedure for stool trace metal analyses exists; the following is our stool handling procedure. Timed stool collection is placed in a beaker and deionized water is added until the whole mixture can be stirred using a magnetic stirrer (up to 10 cm-long magnet is available). When the mixture is thoroughly mixed and becomes homogenous, several 5 mL aliquots are taken into acid-washed test tubes and then freeze-dried. From the dry weights of the aliquots and the total volume, the amount of total solid matter is calculated. The freeze-dried stool is then processed as any other solid samples.

Autopsy and biopsy samples are weighed (either wet or dry), placed in an acid-washed pyrex test tube, which is then sealed after addition of an appropriate amount of 2N ultra-pure nitric acid, and the tube is heated in a boiling water bath until the content is completely degraded. Hair, nail, and freeze-dried stool samples can be processed in a similar way. In this way, the blank reading is always quite low since no concentrated acid is used as is done in wet ashing method. The background absorption in the atomic absorption determination is corrected by the Zeeman effect.

After samples are collected and pre-treated, they are processed for analyses mainly using only plastic wares. All the tubes and pipet tips should be acid-washed when ultra-trace metals are analyzed. It is better to washed them immediately before use; storing acid-washed plastic wares is a dangerous practice. For ordinary trace metals, clean plastic wares without acid-washing are sufficient. When handling samples for ultra-trace metal analyses, all samples should be handled in a laminar flow chamber. Similarly, all reagents used for ultra-trace metals should also be prepared in the laminar flow chamber.

ANALYSES

In clinical laboratories, the speed with which the samples are processed, and the results are sent out to the clinicians, is very clitical. For this reason, any analytical method which requires unacceptable length of time to produce results, no matter how accurate they are, is not suitable. For trace metal analyses, atomic absorption spectrophotometry can satisfy the speed requirement of clinical tests. Unfortunately, atomic absorption instruments are relatively inexpensive and many people who have no or very little knowledge on this technique purchased an instrument, sent a technician to the manufacturer's training course, and produced and published numbers (but not results) in the past.

There are mainly two problems in the atomic absorption methods, particularly in the flameless techniques; namely interferences from the sample matrices and background absorption. The former should be overcome by the use of the method of standard additions. The latter can be overcome by a few different ways. The first method using a continum light source (denterium and tungsten halide lamp) works well under the optimum conditions; however, the lamps will age and they have to be replaced from time to time. Application of the Zeeman effect to the atomic absorption (ref. 31) is a major advance in the analyses of clinical samples. Thanks to this method, most of sample pretreatment procedures became obsolete and the time required to complete analyses became much shorter in many instances. The most recent Smith-Hieftje method uses the self-absorption of hollow cathode lamp; this method is not applicable to certain elements with little self-absorption and requires special hollow cathode lamps whic can withstand drastic changes of lamp current.

Finally, the simultaneous, multi-element atomic absorption (Hitach Z-9000) in conjunction of application of the peak width method for quantitation (ref. 31) is the latest major advance which will be discussed in Dr. Yasuda's paper.

REFERENCES

1. C.A. Owen, Jr., Wilson's Disease. The Etiology, Clinical Aspects, and Treatment of Inherited Copper Toxicosis, Noyes Publ., Park Ridge, NJ (1981).
2. D M Danks, P.E. Campbell, B.J. Stevens, V Mayne and E. Cartwright, Pediatrics, 50, 188-201 (1972).
3. Y. Tanaka, unpublished results.
4. E.J. Moynahan, Bull. Soc. Fr. Derm. Symph. 80, 54 (1973).
5. A.S. Prasad, E.B. Schoomaker, J. Ortega, G.J. Brewer, D. Oberleas and F.J Oelshlegel, Clin. Chem. 21, 582 (1975).
6. J.Quarterman, Trace Elements in Human and Animal Nutrition, 5th Ed (W. Mertz, ed), p. 281, Academic, Orlando, FL (1986).
7. T. Tsubaki and K. Irukayama, Minamata Disease, Kodansha, Tokyo (1977).
8. F. Bakir, S F. Damluji, L. Amin-Zaki, M. Mutadha, A. Khalidi, N.Y. Al-Rawi, S. Tikriti, H.I Dhahir, T.W. Clarkson, J.C. Smith, and R.A Doherty, Science 181, 230 (1973).
9. K. Tsuchiya, Keio J. Med., 18, 195 (1969).
10. A.C. Alfrey, Trace Elements in Human and Animal Nutrition, 5th Ed (W. Mertz, ed), p.399, Academic, Orlando, FL (1986).
11. A.S. Prasad, Zinc Deficiency in Human Subjects (A.S. Prasad, A.O. Çavdar, G.J. Brewer, and P.J. Aggett, eds.), Liss, New York, NY (1983).
12. Expert Panel Guidelines for Essential Trace Element Preparations for Parenteral Use, J. Am. Med. Ass. 11, 205 (1979).
13. B.L O'Dell, Clinical, Biochemical and Nutritional Aspects of Trace Elements (A.S. Prasad, ed), Liss, New York, NY (1982).
14. K. Ge, A. Xue, J. Bai and S. Wang, Virchows Arch. A: Pathol. Anat. Histol., 401, 1 (1983).
15. P J. Collip and S.Y Chen, N. Engl. J Med. 304, 1304 (1981).
16. C.R. Fleming, J T Lie, J T McCall, J.F O'Brien, E E Baillie and J L. Thistle, Gastroenterology, 83, 689 (1982).
17. G N Schrauzer and D A White, Bioinorg. Chem. 8, 303 (1978).
18. Y. Tanaka, C L. Dupont, and E. Harpur, Am. Chem. Soc., National Meet. Abst., Chicago, IL (1977).
19. P.S Papavasiliou, S.T Miller, V. Rosal, Y.Y. Wang and R B. Aronson, Neurology, 29, 1466 (1979).
20. G.F Carl, C.L. Keen, B B Gallagher, M.S Clegg, D B. Littleton, D.B. Flannery and L.S Hurley, Neurology, 36, 1584 (1986).
21. L.S. Hurley, D.E. Wooley, E. Rosenthal, P.S. Timiras, Am. J Physiol., 204, 302 (1963).
22. C L. Keen, M.S. Clegg, B. Lonnerdal and L.S. Hurley, N. Engl. J Med., 308, 1230 (1983).
23. U. Callegarini, J.M. Chiu, and Y. Tanaka, 10th Int. Congr. Clin. Chem., Abst.Mexico City (1978).
24. S. Hatano, Y. Nishi, and T Usui, Am. J. Clin. Nutr., 37, 457 (1983).
25. C.L. Dupont and Y. Tanaka, 10th Int. Congr. Clin. Chem., Abst., Mexico City (1978).
26. N. Imura, A. Naganuma, M. Satoh and J-T. Chen, Essential and Toxic Trace Elements in Human Health and Disease (A S. Prasad, ed), p. 443, Liss, New York, NY (1988).
27. R.A Anderson, Trace Elements in Human and Animal Nutrition, 5th Ed. (W. Mertz, ed.), pé 225, Academic, Orlando, FL (1987).
28. J.L. Johnson, W.R. Waud, K V. Rajagopalan, M. Duran, F.A. Beemer and S K. Wadman, Proc. Natl. Acad. Sci., 77, 3715 (1980).
29. C.L. Keen, B. Lonnerdal, and L.S. Hurley, Biochemistry of the Essential Ultratrace Elements (E. Frieden, ed.), p. 89, Plenum, New York, NY (1984).
30. A.H Rubenstein, N.W. Levin and G.A. Elliott, Lancet, 2, 1348 (1962).
31. H. Koizumi and K. Yasuda, Spectrochim. Acta, 31B, 523 (1977).

Coupled LC-AAS system for trace metal analysis of biological samples

Shozo Nomoto*, Kazuyoshi Yamauchi*, Moritoshi Satou*,
F. William Sunderman, Jr.**,

*:Division of Clinical Chemistry, Shinshu University School of medical Technology, Matsumot, 390 Japan.
**:Department of Laboratory Medicine, University Connecticut School of Medicine, Farmington, CT. 06032 U.S.A.

This report describes two newly developed methods to measure trace metals in blood plasma or serum. The method consists of two parts: sample fractionation with a Fast Protein Liquid Chromatograph (FPLC) and analysis with a flame type or a nonflame type of Atomic Absorption Spectrometer (AAS). They were coupled either directly (direct coupling system) or manually (semi-direct coupling system). The former, coupled FPLC and flame type AAS, was quit effective for zinc bound protein analysis, and the latter, coupled FPLC and nonflame type AAS was for nickel containing protein.

The analysis through them brought some new and unexpected infomation on the binding condition of alpha2-macroglobulin and the metals as follows :
1. The metals bound to alpha2-macroglobulin were exchangeable in vitro.
2. Maximum zinc binding capacity of alpha2-macroglobulin was 700 to 1000 ug of Zn/g of alpha2-M. The zinc binding capasity of alpha2-macroglobulin was approximately twenty times greater than that of albumin.
3. Approximately one third of the zinc binding capacity of alpha2-M was normally occupied with zinc in vivo.

Introduction

It was 1970 when we first detected nickel-containing metalloprotein in rabbit serum through protein fractionation by colun chromatography and atomicabsorption-spectrophotometric analysis. A subsequent study led us to isolation of human nickel-containing metalloprotein named "nickeloplasmin" in 1971. The metalloprotein was a macroglobulin with approximate molecular weight of 700,000 Da, and immuno-electrophoretically belong to alpha2-macroglobulin and was a glycoprotein positive for periodic acid-Schiff reaction.

Even existence of nickeloplasmin itself, however, became doubted afterward, became there appeared no report which confirmed our results with the methods of our own for 15 years. We then reinvestigated the protein, in summer of 1987, successfully confirming its presens. The methods used in 1987 consisted of (a) A high-performance liquid chromatography (HPLC) for protein fractionation and (b) Zeeman electothermal atomic absorption spectrophotometry for nickel determination. The results were much more clear with the new method than with the previous one. Today I would like to present several features of our newly designed system of 1987, comparing to our old system of 1973.

Method and materials.

Table 1 is a comparison of the old and new systems. Both system are devided into two parts: the first part is column chromatographic fractionation of protein and the second is detection of nickel by atomic absorption spectrophotometer. As shown above left in the table. The old system fractionated proteins with column chromatography using Sephadex G-200 and DEAE cellulose. In the new system we used FPLC with Superose-6 and Mono-Q as a column-medium. Not only the new system achieved better results, but also it was more than 20 times faster than the old system.

		Old system	New system
Mediums for Column Chromatography	Gelfiltratio	Sephadex G-200	Superose 6
	Ionexchange	DEAE-cellulose	Mono-Q
Detection of Nickel	pretreatment of sample	Digestion, Chelation, Extraction	none
	atomyzatio by	Flame or Graphite-furnace	Graphite-furnace

Table 1. Comparison of Old and New systems in columun-chromatographic part and nickel-detection part.

The second part of the system, nickel determination, are demonstrated below in the table. The old system required pretreatment for the fractionated samples befor analysis it by atomic absorption spectrophotometer. The procedure of pretreatment includes (a) sample digestion with acid-mixture and heating, (b) neutralization and pH adjustment of the digested sample with ammonium hydroxide solution, (c) chelation of nickel in the sample with ammonium pyrrolodine dithiocarbamate (APDC), and (d) extraction of the chelate with mathylisobuthlketon (MIBK) (1, 2). On the other hand, samples from the new chromato graphic system can be injected directly into the graphite furnace of atomic absorption spectoroscopy.

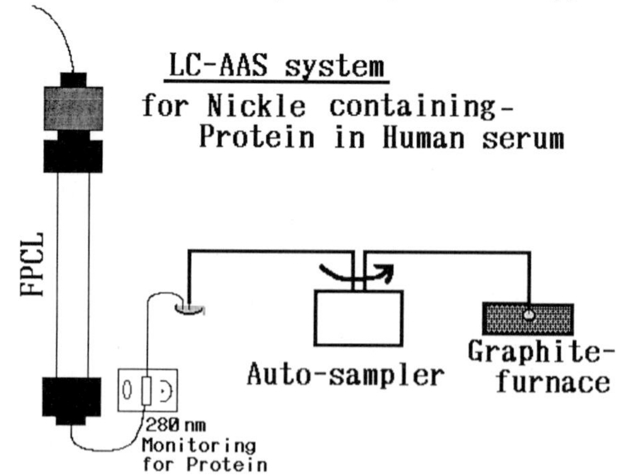

Figure 1

Figure 1 is a picture showing the whole apparatus for the new system. Tris-buffer 100 mmol/L containing sodium nitrate 50 mmol/L, pH 7.7 was used as a eluate for gel-filtration chromatography. Tris-buffer 50 mmol/L containing sodium nitrate 75 mmol/L and 1000 mmol/L, pH 7.7 were used as a gradient- elution system for ion-exchange chromatography.

The most remarkable merit of the new system was elimination of a process of sample pretreatment, which was produced by following two factors.

1. Use of high performance atomic absorption spectrophotometer furnished with a Zeeman-effect-background correction mechanism.
2. Use of sodium nitrate instead of sodunm chlorid or sodum sulfate to control the ion-strength of the eluate for ion-exchange column chromatography. As is generally known, sodium chloride or sodium sulfate is most widely used in grdient-buffer system for usual protein fractionation. Therefor I should like to explain this second point a littel detailedly.

Sodium nitrate has its own advantage and disadvantage, when applied to this nickel protein analysis. The disadvantage is high absorbance of the light at the wave-length of 280nm, which usually used protein monitoring at column chromatography. It thus is widely accepted that sodium nitrate is unsuitable for a constituent of eluate for the column chromatography. The advantage is absence of interference at the nickel detection with an electrothermal atomization apparatus. Nickel can not be measrued by electrothermal atomic absorption spectroscopy when the sample contains excess amount of sodium chloride or sodium sulfate. This is because sodium chloride or sodium sulfate generates huge background signals at the sample atomization. Sodium nitare caused almost no such interference at the sample atomization in the graphite furnace. The advantage of sodium nitrate completely overweigh its disadvantage, when the sample is applide to a new superb instrument. We did fortunately try to use sodium nitrate against a common sense in protein fractionation, obtaining a very good result.

Results

As illustrated in figure 2, elution patterns obtained by gel-filtration chromatography on "Superose 6" showed three Ni-containing fractions (peaks "A", "B", and "C"). Recovery of nickel in these chromatographic fractionations was two to three times the amount of the original serum samples, indicating that certain serum constituents extracted nickel from the buffer, chromatogrphic medium, and/or FPLC apparatus during the fractionation. Peak "A" (sample 3) contained alpha2-macroglobulin; peak "B" (sample 5) contained albumin, β- , and γ-globulins, based upon agarose gel electrophoresis (figure 3). Peak "C", whic eluted beyond the bed-volume (Vt) of the gel filtration column, contained the serum ultra-filtratable constituents (e.g., amino acids) that bind nickel.

Ion-exchange chromatography of peak "A" on "Mono-Q" medium separated three protein peaks ("A1", "A2", and "A3"), of which only one ("A3") contained nickel (figure 4). Peak "A3" migrated as a single protein band on SDS-acrylamide gel electrophoresis, and was identified as alpha2-macroglobulin by immunoelectrophoresis.

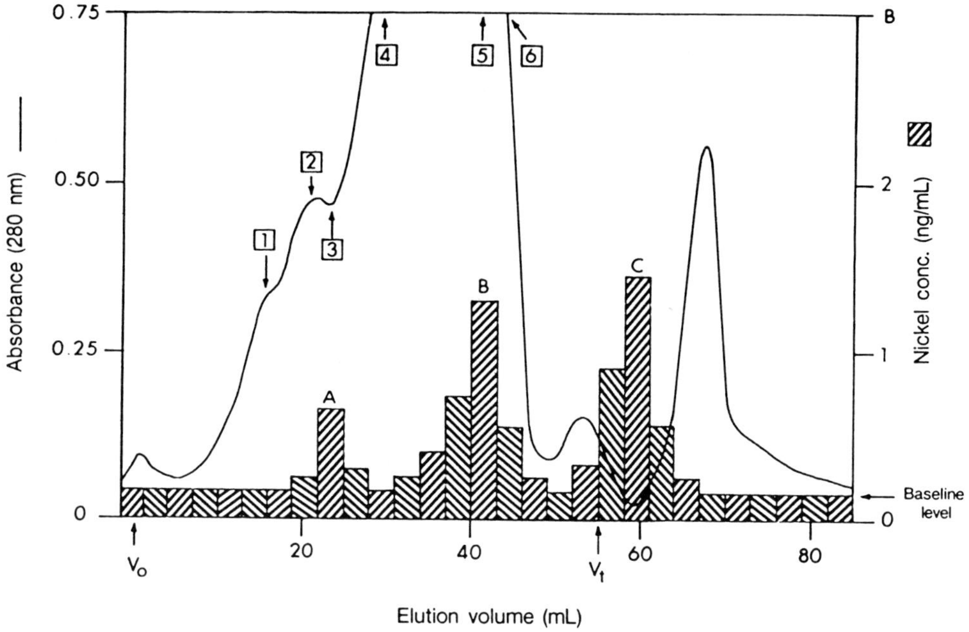

FIGURE. 2. Chromatographic profiles of Ni and A_{280} nm in effluent from a gel-filtration column of "Superose 6" (void volume V_o; bed volume V_t). The starting material was human serum (2 mL). Three Ni-containing peaks ("A", "B", and "C") were detected. The fractions labelled 1, 2, 3, 4, 5, and 6 correspond to samples analyzed by agarose gel electrophoresis (see figure 2).

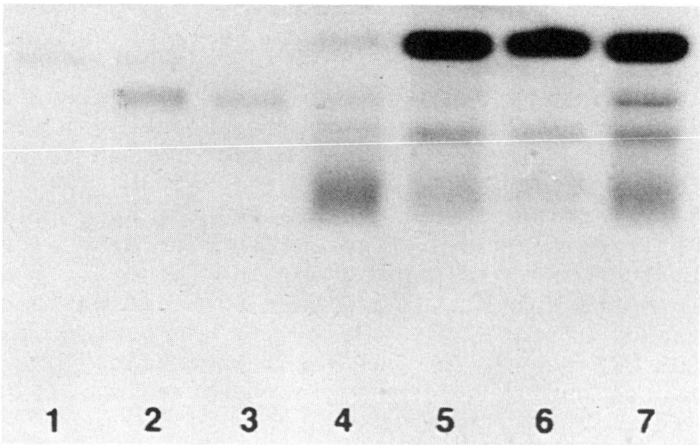

FIGURE 3. Electrophoretic fractionation of serum protein fractions on agarose gel, stained with Coomassie blue. The samples in lanes 1 to 6 are fractions 1 to 6 obtained by gel-filtration chromatography (see figure 1). Fraction 1 contained no detectable proteins; fractions 2 and 3 contained α-globulins; fraction 4 contained predominantly β- and γ-globulins; fractions 5 and 6 contained albumin, with some β- and γ-globulins. The sample in lane 7 is the starting material (human serum).

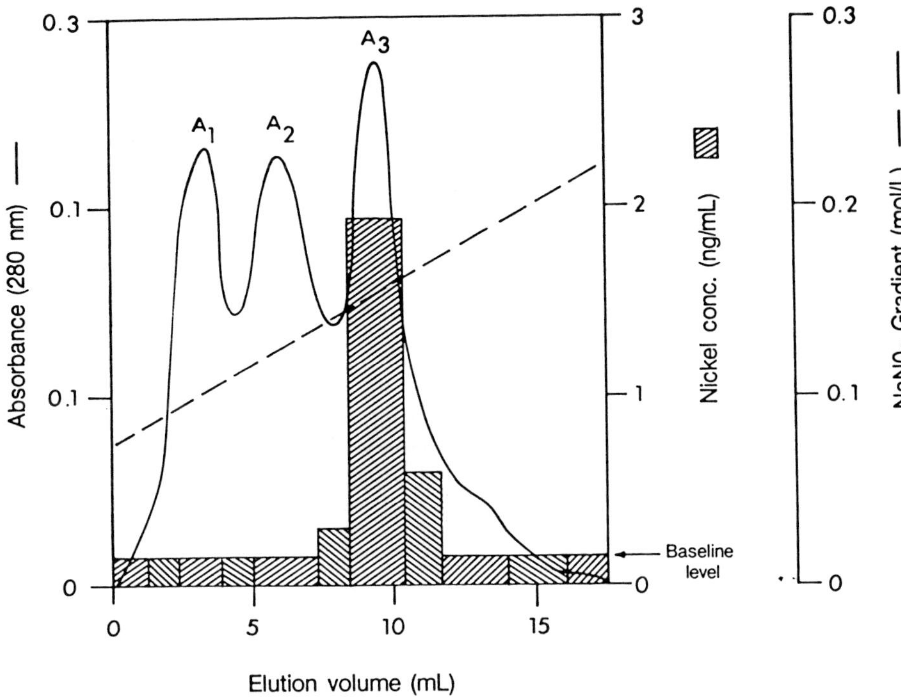

FIGURE 4. Chromatographic profiles of Ni and A_{280} nm in effluent from an ion-exchange column of "Mono-Q", with elution in tris buffer containing a linear gradient of sodium nitrate (0.075 to 0.27 mol per L). The starting material was peak "A" obtained by gel-filtration chromatography of human serum (see figure 1). The A_{280nm} plot has been corrected for background absorbance of the sodium nitrate gradient. The chromatographic profile shows a single nickel-containing peak ("A_3").

Zinc containing proteins.

Thereafter we applied our new system to investigation of zinc-containing protein in human serum.

Figre 5 showing the basic knowledge of this field established by A. F. Parisi, et al. (4) , R. I. Henkin and E. L. Giroux, et al (5). during 1970 to 1975.

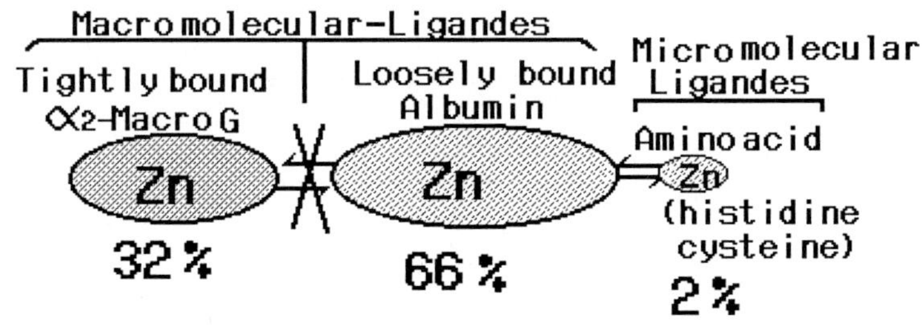

Figure 5. Binding of serum zinc.
Reproduced from Henkin (5)

According to them, zinc is unexceptionally bound to some ligands in human blood, as illustrared in this figure. Approximately 66 % of plasma zinc is combined to albumin, 32 % to alpha2-M, and 2 % to amino acids such as histidine and cyctein. The zinc bound to albumin is in equilibrium with the zinc bound to amino acid. Thus, about 1 to 2 % of circulating zinc is easily movable between albumin and aminoacids. Zinc is, however, unexchanges between alpha2-M and albumin, since the association constant is very high between alpha2-M and zinc, that association constant is grater than 10^{10}. It has been acsepted that only liver tissue can incorporate zinc into alpha2-M and also metabolizes them (4, 5).

Materials and methods.

Figure 6 is a diagram of LC-AAS system, which we newly designed to analyze zinc-containing protein in blood plasma or serum. As you see the left inside of the figure, the first step of this system is a column chromatography. The column we chose are HR-5/20 from Pharmacia for general screening test and HR-10/30 for preparative work for zinc binding alpha2-M. They are filled with Superose-6. A 100 microliter loop injector is connected between eluent-pump and the column.

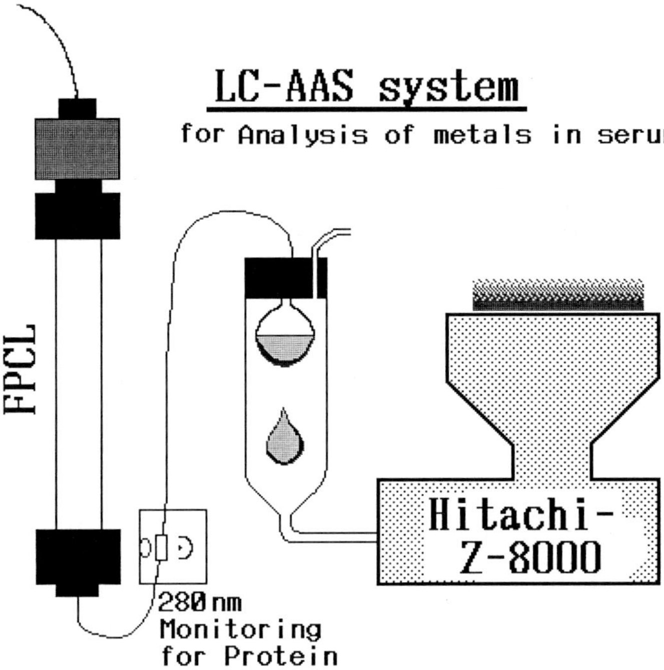

Figure 6.

The second step of the system is a flame type of atomic absorption spectrophotometer for zinc detection. A drip infusion type of injector connects in between the column and the AAS. This injector is newly designed by us. Each drop carries about 70 microliter quit reproducibly, and the elute drops in every 20 seconds when set the eluent flow rate at 200 mocrolite per minute.

Figure 7 is a picture showing a representative of analytical pattern of normal human serum applied to HR-10/30, a preparative column. The first peak corresponds to alpha2-M, and the second to albumin.

Figure 8 is a representative pattern of normal serum applide to a smaller column ,HR-5/20 for genelal screening.

Figure 9 is the result of an experiment of additive zinc. It was a repetition of an experiment exactly same as figure 8 except zinc was added to the sample before injection. Surprisingly, almost all additive zinc has appeared on the alpha 2-macroglbulin region, as you can see here.

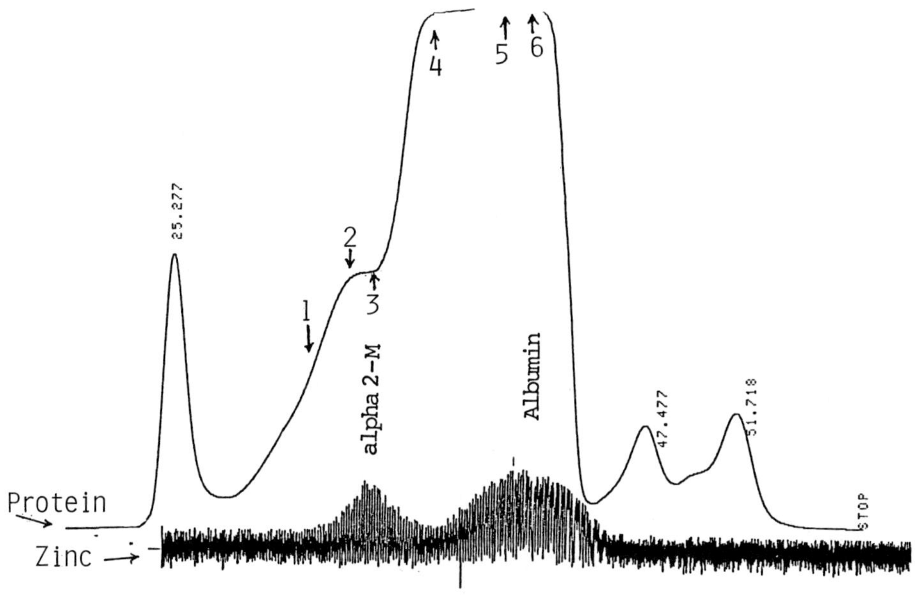

Figure 7. A typical chromatographic profiles of Zinc and Proteins in effluent from gel-filtration column of " Superose 6, HR-10/30 "

We could obtain further purified solution of alpha2-M and albumin combined to zinc with our preparative LC-AAS system just mentioned above. Such sample have led us to some new findings about biding condition of zinc and nickel to the proteins, as follows:

1. Both zinc and nickel bound to alpha 2-macroglobulin are easily exchangable at least in vitro.
2. Maximum zinc binding capacity of alpha 2-macroglobulin is 700 to 1000 microgram of zinc/gram of protein, and that of albumin was 40 to 50 microgram.
3. Zinc normally occupies approximately one third of the binding capacity of alpha 2-macroglobulin in vivo.

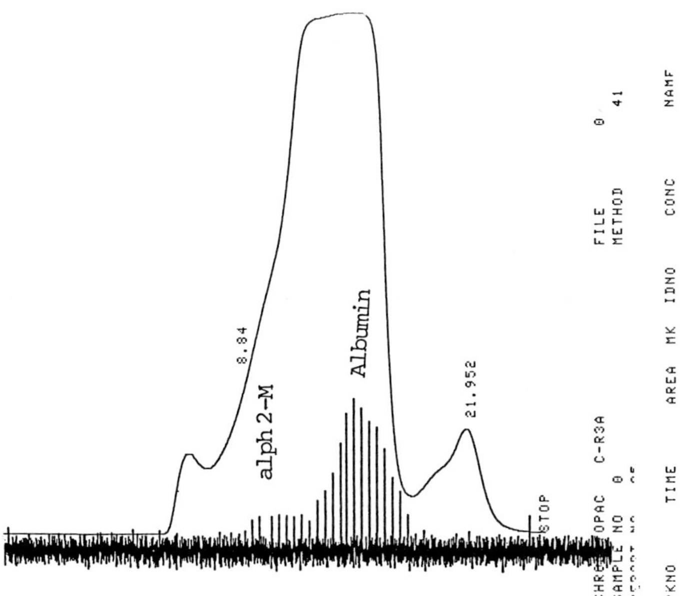

Figure 8. A typical chromatographic profiles of Zinc and Proteins in effluent from gel-filtration column of " Superose 6, HR-5/20 "

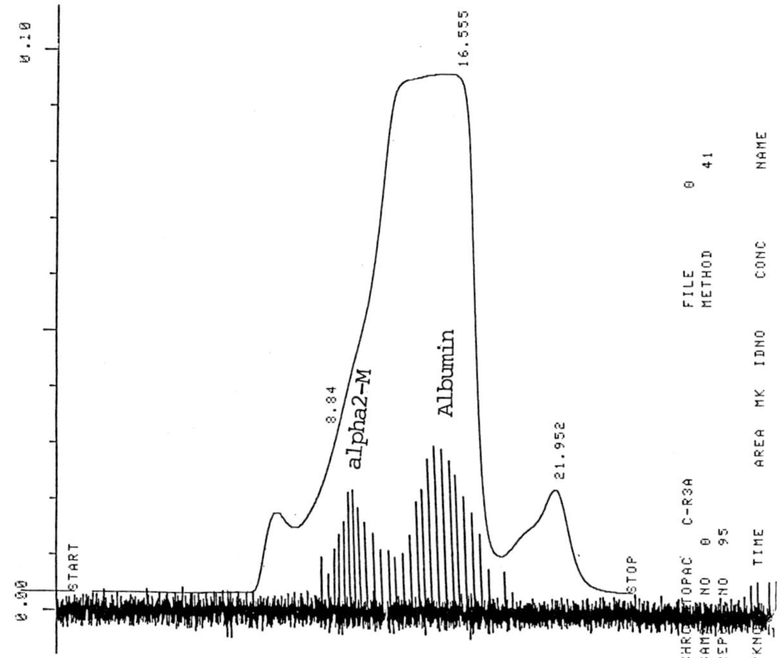

Figure 9. A typical chromatographic profiles of Zinc and Proteins in effluent from gel-filtration column of " Superose 6, HR-5/20 " (Zinc was added to serum just before sample injection)

References

1. Nomoto, S., McNeely, M. D., and Sunderman, F. W., Jr. : Isoration of a nickel alpha2-macroglobulin from rabbit serum. Biochemistry 10: 1647-1651, 1971.
2. Sunderman, F. W., Jr., Decsy, M. I., Nomoto, S. and Nechay, M. W. : Isoration of a nickel alpha2-macroglobulin from human and rabbit serum. Fed. Proc. 30: 1274(Abstr. 1294), 1973.
3. Nomoto, S., Decsy, M. I., Murphy, J. R., and Sunderman, F. W., Jr. Isoration of 63Ni-labelled nickeloplasmin from rabbit serum. Miochem. Med. 8:171-181, 1973.
4. Parisi, A. F. and Vallee, B. L. : Isolation of a zinc alpha2-macroglobulin from human serum. Biochemistry, 9: 2421-2426, 1970.
5. Henkin, R. I. : Metal-albumin-amino acid interactions. Chemical and physiological interactions. Adv. Exp. Med. Biol. 48: 299-328, 1970.

Simultaneous determinations of essential trace metals in biological fluids and their significance

Kazuo Nomiyama and Hiroko Nomiyama

Department of Environmental Health, Jichi Medical School,
Tochigi-Ken 329-04, Japan

Abstract - From the toxicological viewpoint, we discuss the importance of determining multiple trace elements in the diagnosis of health effects of heavy metals by citing two episodes: lead-induced zinc-deficiency acrodermatitis and the reduction of cadmium induced health effects by copper supplementation. Based on these two episodes, the following aspects were discussed: 1) the necessity to determine multiple trace elements, 2) tissue metal shifts (interaction), 3) the early diagnosis of the health effects of heavy metals, 4) how to avoid mis-diagnosis (renal molybdenum in renal dysfunctions), 5) the pitfalls of biological monitoring, 6) the difficulty in discriminating between essential and toxic metals, and 7) the appropriate methods for determining trace elements in biological specimens.

INTRODUCTION

We shall discuss the importance of careful assessment of data for an excess or deficient state in a particular metal and the rationale for our recommendation that multiple trace elements should be determined when assessing pathological status of a disease.

1 LEAD-INDUCED ZINC DEFICIENCY ACRODERMATITIS (ref. 1)

Seven male rabbits each weighing 3 kg at the start of the experiment were intravenously given lead acetate 3 times a week at a dose level of 2 mg/kg through an ear vein. Body weight and health effects were determined at specific intervals. Two rabbits suffered from acrodermatitis in the 7th week of the experiment. The acrodermatitis deteriorated into broken skin, visible muscle and finally fragile tissue that started to bleed even by softly touching the animal area, , as shown Fig. 1a. Another 2 rabbits suffered from mild acrodermatitis (Fig. 1b) in the 8th week, and an additional 2 rabbits developed acrodermatitis by the 10th and 17th week, respectively. In total, 6 rabbits out of 7 suffered from acrodermatitis; the prevalence of acrodermatitis was 87 %.

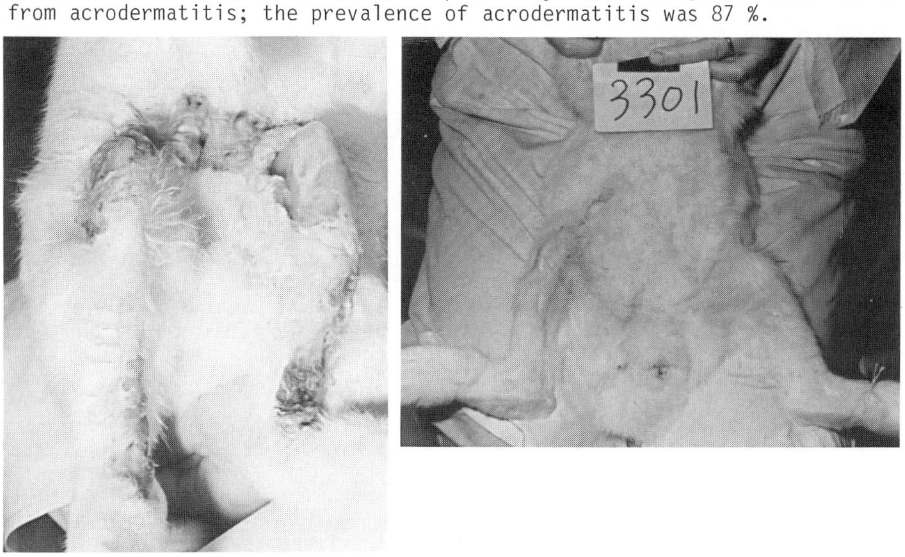

Fig. 1 Lead-induced zinc-deficiency acrodermatitis
Right and left photographs represent severe and mild cases respectively (cited from ref. 1).

Food intake was not decreased in rabbits given lead. As seen in Fig. 2, plasma alkaline phosphatase and zinc levels decreased significantly in the 2nd week. The normal alkaline phosphatase level in the rabbits is between 6 and 10 U/l. Acrodermatitis appeared when plasma alkaline phosphatase decreased to below 3 U/l and became aggravated when plasma alkaline phosphatase decreased to below 2 U/l.

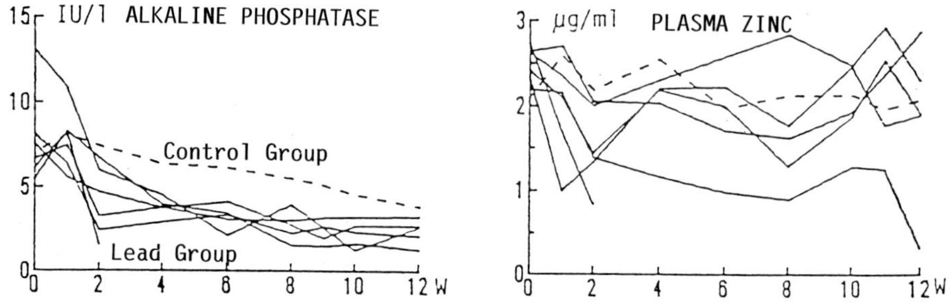

Fig. 2 Plasma alkaline phosphatase and zinc in rabbits given iv lead (cited from ref. 1).

The rabbits suffering from serious acrodermatitis were given oral zinc sulfate at the dose of 50 mg, daily, regardless of continued lead exposure. Oral intake of zinc hardly improved plasma alkaline phosphatase, but improved the level of plasma zinc. Even serious acrodermatitis was relieved by oral administrations of zinc. Hair appeared again after 4-5 weeks of zinc treatment. Mild acrodermatitis was completely healed by oral administration of zinc.

The above clinical signs and symptoms suggest that lead-induced acrodermatitis is a symptom of zinc deficiency. Because it is very difficult to induce acrodermatitis by feeding rabbits with a zinc deficient diet, why is it so easy to induce serious acrodermatitis by lead exposure ? The following is an explanation for this phenomenon: lead in the liver binds with and inactivates hepatic delta-aminolevulinate dehydratase. Lead disturbs heme synthesis and induces anemia. To rescue delta-aminolevulinate dehydratase synthesis, zinc comes to the liver from zinc stock organs such as the hair and skin. Furthermore, experimental lead administration induces diarrhea in our rabbits. The diarrhea may disturb the intestinal absorption of zinc, which results in an acceleration of zinc deficiency at the zinc stock organ, skin, and finally leads to zinc-deficient acrodermatitis.

Cadmium and mercury also induce zinc-deficient acrodermatitis. The rabbits were given pelleted food containing cadmium at a dose level of 300 ppm over a period of 20 weeks. The acrodermatitis in this case was not as serious as the lead-induced one.

Lead or cadmium-induced zinc-deficient acrodermatitis may warn us of the following: 1) not to simply assess the excess or deficiency of metals by biological monitoring, and 2) a state of tissue metal imbalance can cause ill health.

2 CADMIUM HEALTH EFFECTS AND COPPER DEFICIENCY (ref. 2)

Twenty six male rabbits, each weighing 2.6 kg at the start of the experiment, were given subcutaneous injections of cadmium chloride at a dose level of 0.5 mg/kg over a period of 21 weeks. Another 2 rabbits served as the control animals. Body weights were measured every week, and blood and urine specimens were subjected to assess health effects of cadmium every other week. Animals were autopsied at an certain interval, and their levels of renal cadmium, copper and zinc were determined.

As shown in Fig. 3, renal cadmium increased with the dose of cadmium. Renal zinc and copper increased with the dose as well. Renal copper, however, reached a maximum in the 4th week and then decreased thereafter. The rate of increase in renal cadmium began to slow down after the 4th week, and cadmium reached its maximum of 425 ug/g in the 14th week and then decreased thereafter. On the other hand, renal dysfunctions such as proteinuria, glycosuria, aminoaciduria and enzymuria became apparent after the 9th week.

The above data suggest that the mechanism of cadmium intoxication is related to the decrease in renal copper and suggest that copper supplementation prevents cadmium intoxication.

In another experiment, 33 male rabbits were divided into 3 groups (ref. 3): rabbits of the first group were given subcutaneous injections of cadmium chloride at a dose level of 0.5 mg/kg everyday, rabbits of the second group were administered cadmium chloride and intravenous injections of copper acetate at a dose of 50 μg/kg, once a week; and rabbits of

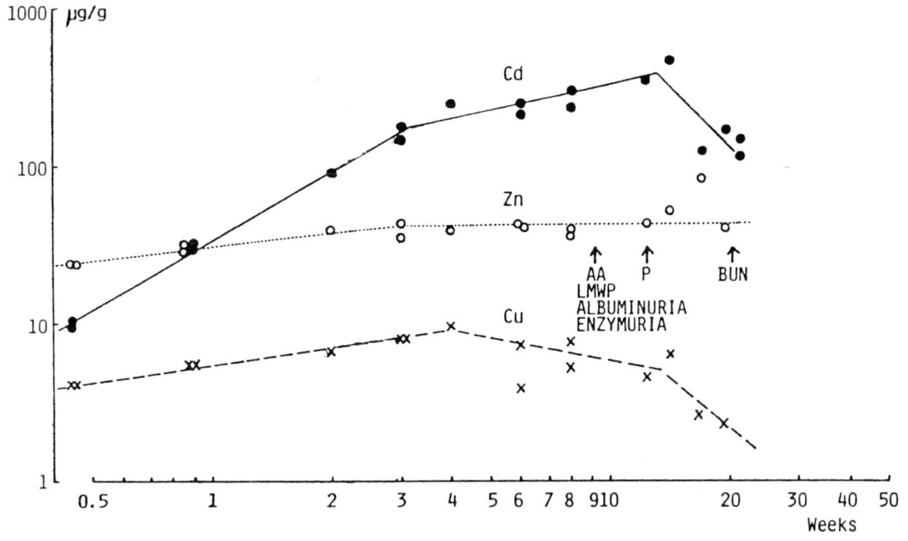

Fig. 3 Cadmium health effects and renal cadmium, zinc and copper in rabbits given sc cadmium at a dose level of 0.5 mgCd/kg over a period of 21 weeks (ref. 2). Mark P, LMWP or AA represent for proteinuria, low-molecular-weight proteinuria or aminoaciduria was detected in rabbits exposed to cadmium.

the last group served the as control animals.

As seen in Fig. 4, cadmium-induced body weight loss was moderated by copper supplementation. Compared to the non-supplemented group, the appearance of cadmium-induced proteinuria, glycosuria and aminoaciduria were delayed by 1-6 weeks in the supplemented group. Although copper supplementation could not completely prevent cadmium intoxication, but it relieved cadmium intoxication at least.

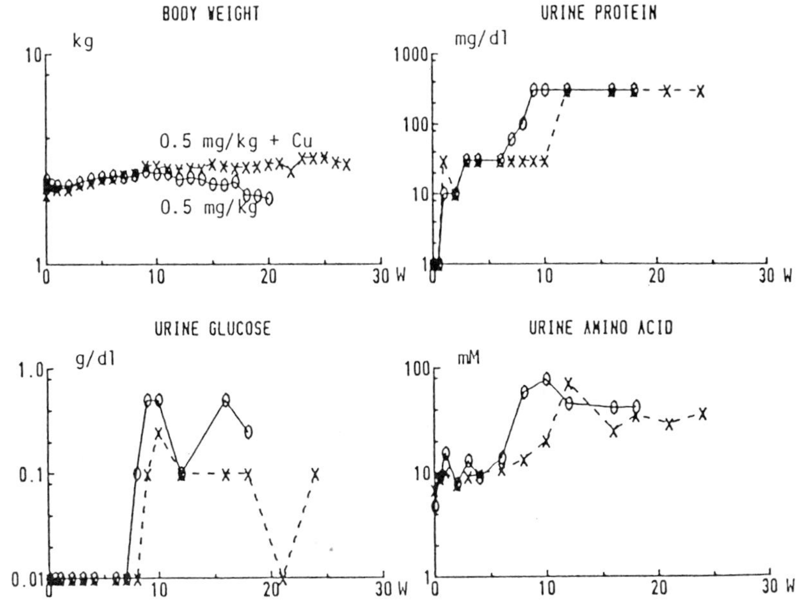

Fig. 4 Alleviating effects of iv copper on cadmium health effects in rabbits (cited from ref. 3).
Open circle and cross represent the mean of the cadmium group and the cadmium with copper supplementation group, respectively.

The above data may indicate that cadmium health effects are associated with a cadmium-induced imbalance of tissue metals.

3 BIOLOGICAL MONITORING OF CADMIUM EXPOSURE AND ITS HEALTH EFFECTS BY URINE COPPER DETERMINATION

Some areas of Japan have been contaminated with cadmium, and health effects among the residents of cadmium-polluted areas have been studied under the sponsorship of the Japanese Environmental Agency. As seen in Table 1, urine copper was found to have a much closer relationship to cadmium health effects than urine cadmium (ref. 4). At first, we could not imagine why urine copper was a better monitoring parameter for cadmium health effects.

Table 1 Correlation between urine cadmium, copper, zinc and lead and renal effects in residents of 5 cadmium-polluted areas in Japan (data were cited from ref. 4).

	Urine Cd	Urine Cu	Urine Zn	Urine Pb
Urine protein		**, *		
glucose				**
amino acids				
β_2-microglobulin		**, *		
retinol-binding protein		**		
lysosome		**		*

Marks ** and * represent statistically significant correlation at 1 and 5 % level, in one cadmium-polluted area out of 5.

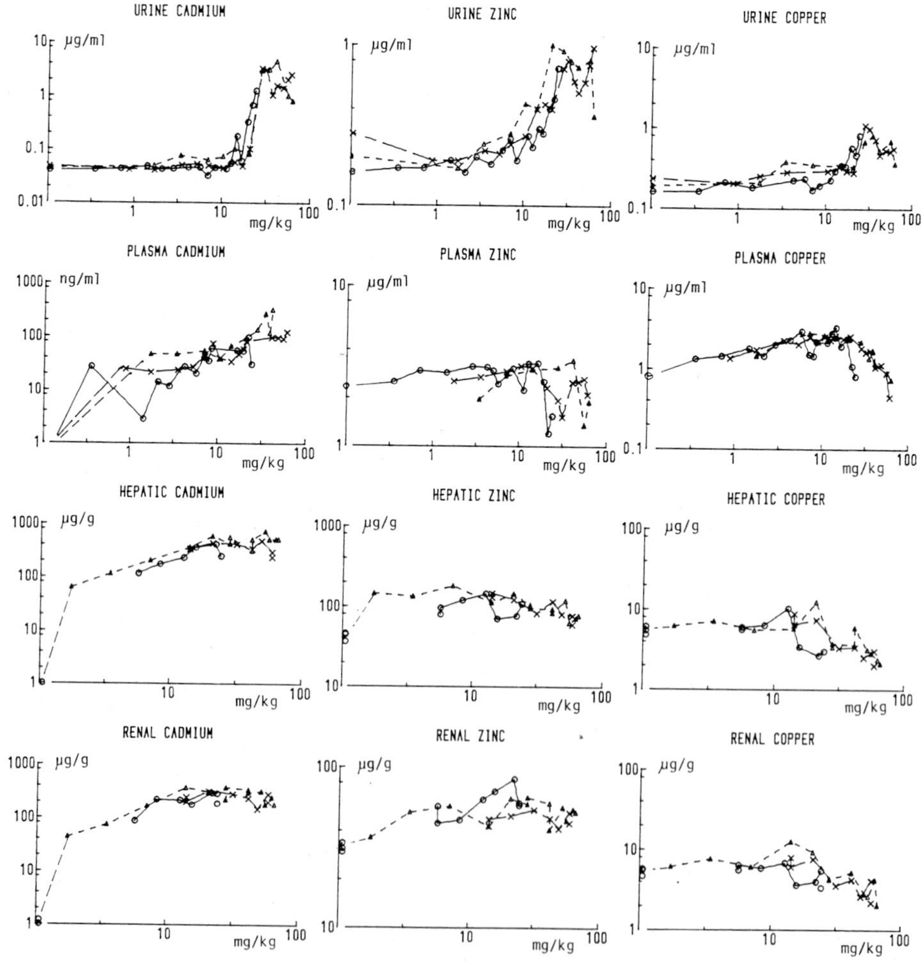

Fig. 5 Plasma, urine, hepatic and renal metals (cadmium, zinc and copper) in rabbits given sc cadmium at a dose level of 0.1, 0.25 or 0.5 mgCd/kg, daily, over a period of 34 weeks (cited from ref. 5).

We carried out an experiment on rabbits to elucidate the mechanism (ref. 5). Thirty-three male rabbits were given cadmium chloride subcutaneously at a dose level of 0, 0.1, 0.25 or 0.5 mg/kg, everyday, over a period of 34 weeks. As seen in Fig. 5, regardless of the cadmium dose level, hepatic and renal copper increased with the dose of cadmium, and then decreased. Plasma copper increased to 3 times the normal level at a total cadmium dose of 14 mg/kg, and then it decreased to half of the normal level at a total cadmium dose of 60 mg/kg. Urine copper, on the other hand, suddenly increased at a total cadmium dose of 20 mg/kg, when hepatic, renal and plasma copper began to decrease.

Cadmium exposure elevated hepatic, renal and plasma copper. However, excess cadmium, which accumulated in the liver and renal cortex, may decrease the production of copper-binding proteins such as metallothionein and ceruloplasmin, and thus the liver and the kidneys hardly retain any copper. This may result in increasing copper excretion into the urine. Therefore, an increase in urine copper level may be a very early sign of renal or hepatic dysfunctions preceding proteinuria, glycosuria, aminoaciduria, or elevations in the level of plasma enzymes such as aspartate aminotransferase, alanine aminotransferase and lactic dyhydrogenase. Therefore urine copper was found to be an excellent parameter for monitoring cadmium exposure and cadmium health effects.

4 COMPREHENSIVE APPRAISAL OF ELEMENT DETERMINATION

The above data indicate that it is not wise to simply conclude that high plasma or urine copper indicates an excess intake of copper.

We have discussed copper, a "miracle metal". However, copper is not the only metal that is shifted by cadmium. Listed in Table 2 are 16 tissue metals in the liver and the kidneys of rabbits and monkeys exposed to cadmium, lead, chromium or copper for a long period of time (refs. 6-9). Heavy metal exposures induced shifts in various tissue metals. The mechanism of tissue metal shift is not yet fully elucidated, but may be clarified in the near future.

Table 2 Tissue Metal Shift in Chronic Metal Intoxication (data cited from 6, 7, 8 and 9)

Metal	Cadmium		Lead		Chromium		Copper	
Animal	Rabbits		Rabbits		Monkeys		Monkeys	
Route	sc		iv		or		or	
Period	34 Weeks		18 Weeks		40 Months		40 Months	
Tissue	Kidneys	Liver	Kidneys	Liver	Kidneys	Liver	Kidneys	Liver
Cd	↑↑,↓	↑↑,↓	-	-	-	-	-	-
Cu	⇡,↓	-,↓↓	↑	↑	-	-		
Zn	⇡	↑↑,↓	↑	-	↑	-	↑	-
Pb	↑↑,↓,-	↑↑,↓	↑	↑	↑	-	↑	-
Cr	-	⇣,-	-	-	↑↑	↑↑	↓	-
Ca	↑↑	↑↑	↑	-	↑↑	↑	⇡	-
Mg	⇣	⇣	↑	-	↑↑	-	↑	↑
Mn	↓↓	↑	↑	-				
Fe	⇣	↓↓	-	-	↑↑	↑	↑↑	↑
Co	⇣	⇡,⇣	-	↑	-	-	↑↑	-
Ni	↑	↑↑,-	-	-	↑	-	↑↑	-
Mo	-	⇣	-	-	-	-	-	-
Ti			-	-	-	-	-	-

CONCLUSION

Finally, we propose that it is worthwhile to determine more elements when attempting to elucidate the mechanisms of various diseases. Dr. Tanaka has recommended the determination of molybdenum in the study of Wilson's disease (ref. 10). It is quite wise to determine antagonistic elements of copper such as molybdenum and zinc. Multi-elemental analyses may give us more informations which will help us to fully understand the pathological status of a disease.

ACKNOWLEDG

This work was partl
Japanese Ministry o

REFERENCES

1. K. Nomiyama, H.
219 (1986).
2. K. Nomiyama and
New York (1982).
3. K. Nomiyama and
(1983).
4. I. Shigematsu an
5. K. Nomiyama and
(1983).
6. K. Nomiyama and
7. K. Nomiyama, H.
(1988).
8. K. Nomiyama, H.
9. K. Nomiyama and
(1985).
10. Y. Tanaka, 3rd

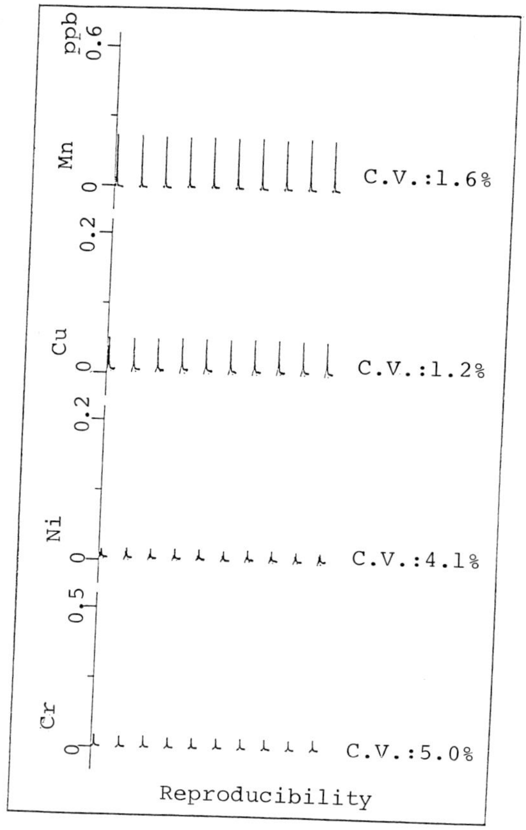

Fig. 7. Reproducibility on analysis of Mn, Cu, Ni and Cr in serum

REFERENCE

1) J. V. Sullivan and A. Walsh, Appl. Opt., 7, 1271(1968).
2) A. T. Zander, T. C. O'Haver and P. N. Keliber, Anal. Chem., 48,1166(1976).
3) B. V. L'vov, Atomic Absorption Spectrochemical Analysis, P. 193, Adam Hilger, (1970).
4) M. Hashimoto, H. Yamada, K. Ohishi and K. Yasuda,Anal. Sciences, 2 109(1986).
5) H. Koizumi and K. Yasuda, Spectrochim, Acta. 31B, 523(1976).
6) B. V. L'vov, Spectrochim. Acta, 33B, 153(1978).
7) C. L. Chakrabarti, C. C. Wan and W. C. Li, Ibid., 35B, 93(1980).
8) I. Atsuya, K. Ito and M. Otomo, Anal. Chim. Acta, 147, 185(1983).

Production of a transgenic mouse model for human dominantly inherited disease

Ken-ichi Yamamura, Shoji Wakasugi, Takeaki Inomoto**,
Tomohisa Iwanaga*, Shigehiro Yi*, Shuichiro Maeda**,
Makoto Naito*, Kiyoshi Takahashi* and Kazunori Shimada*

Institute for Medical Genetics, *Department of Pathology, and
**Department of Biochemistry, Kumamoto University Medical School
Kuhonji 4-24-1, Kumamoto 862, Japan

Abstract - Familial amyloidotic polyneuropathy is an autosomal dominant disorder, characterized by the extracellular deposition of fibrillar amyloid protein and by prominent peripheral nerve involvement. We have produced transgenic mice by microinjecting the human mutant transthyretin gene. Amyloid deposition had begun at 6 months of age and was observed mainly in the mucosa of intestinal tract. Although the clinical symptoms have not developed yet, it is possible to establish an animal model for human dominantly inherited disease by an introduction of mutant gene into mouse germ line.

INTRODUCTION

Amyloidosis comprises a heterogenous group of diseases of diverse etiology characterized by the extracellular deposition of a number of fibrillar proteins which may be distinguished from each other biochemically and immunohistologically. One type of systemic amyloidosis may occur in association with familial amyloidotic polyneuropathy (FAP). FAP is an autosomal dominant disorder, characterized by the extracellular deposition of fibrillar amyloid protein and by prominent peripheral nerve involvement (ref. 1). This protein is mainly composed of transthyretin (TTR) with a substitution of methionine for valine at position 30 in the FAP type I, as reported in Japan, Sweden and Portugal (ref. 2). This amino acid substitution is thought to lead to amyloid deposition. The human TTR gene has been cloned and well characterized at the molecular level (ref. 3-5). All the FAP patients so far examined carry one mutant gene (ref. 6, 7). Thus it is clear that the main cause of this disease is the presence of mutant TTR. However in patients with FAP, the age at onset varies from 20 to 60 years even among the same family members. These data suggest involvement of factor(s) other than the single nucleotide mutation the TTR gene. To elucidate this factor(s) and to examine the pathological process of amyloid deposition, we have produced transgenic mice by microinjecting the cloned human mutant TTR gene into fertilized eggs of C57BL/6 mice.

PRODUCTION OF TRANSGENIC MOUSE LINE

We choose the inbred strain of mouse, C57BL/6 (B6), as recipient for DNA microinjection, because amyloid deposition itself can be influenced by genetic background. In order to produce large quantities of variant TTR in transgenic mice, we prepared two constructs. One is the 7.6-kilobase (kb) HindIII-EcoRI fragment containing about 600-base pair (bp) upstream region and entire human mutant TTR gene in which the promoter region of the mouse metallothionein-I gene was ligated to the structural gene of human mutant TTR gene (MT-hTTR30). About 200 copies of each construct (0.6-hTTR30 and MT-hTTR30) were microinjected into fertilized mouse eggs and we obtained 9 and 5 transgenic mice, respectively.

TISSUE- AND STAGE- SPECIFIC EXPRESSION

It has been shown that the TTR gene is expressed not only in liver but also in other tissues including brain and yolk sac (ref. 8, 9). In our transgenic mice 0.6-hTTR gene is expressed in liver and yolk sac, and also in brain but at very low level. Costa et al. (ref. 10) recently showed that the enhancer-like element is located between 1.6 to 2.15 kb upstream region of TTR gene and that the level of TTR gene and that the level of TTR gene expression decreased to one-tenth in the absence of this enhancer element. In our transgenic mice the level of human TTR mRNA was exactly one-tenth of that of mouse endogenous TTR mRNA. All these results suggest that both the promoter region (up to 600 bp upstream region) and the enhancer element will be required for the efficient expression of TTR gene in liver and brain. To analyze the developmental regulation, RNAs were extracted from liver and yolk sac of fetuses of 13, 15, and 17 days' gestation. In the liver human TTR mRNA was detected as early as 13 days' gestation and the level of

mRNA increased gradually during development and reached maximum at 17 days' gestation. On the other hand, the level of human TTR mRNA in yolk sac did not vary appreciably during the period of 13-17 days of gestation. Although the level of expression of human TTR gene is low, the pattern of expression during development is exactly the same as that of endogenous mouse TTR gene (ref. 11).
These results clearly suggest that the expression of mutant TTR gene in FAP patients is regulated normally and that the late onset of this disease is not due to the dysregulation of mutant TTR gene. In contrast to the 0.6-hTTR30 gene, the MT-hTTR30 gene is expressed in various tissues including liver, heart, brain, and kidney.

SERUM LEVELS AND FORMATION OF HYBRID TETRAMER

Serum levels of human TTR in each transgenic mouse was analyzed by Western blot assay and were ranged from 0.2 to 3.0 mg/dl and 1.0 to 4.8 mg/dl in 0.6-hTTR30 and MT-hTTR30 transgenic line, respectively. As the TTR molecule is composed of four identical subunits, it is possible that human TTR are associated with mouse endogenous TTR to form hybrid tetramers if the human TTR gene is expressed in liver or brain. This possibility was confirmed by the Ouchterlony test.

AMYLOID DEPOSITION IN TRANSGENIC MICE

The presence of amyloid substance in each tissue was examined using pathological criteria, that is, the ability to bind Congo red and to give an apple-green birefringence under polarized light, and its fibrillar ultrastructure. In the MT-hTTR30 line amyloid starts to deposit mainly in the mucosa of small intestine at around 6 months of age. At 12 month-old, amyloid deposition appeared more remarkably, in the same tissues and in addition was present around the blood vessels in the submucosa of the esophagus, colon, rectum and anus and in about 10% of the renal glomeruli. However, there were no amyloid deposits in peripheral nervous tissues, choroid plexus and heart, areas where amyloid deposition is commonly observed at the time of autopsy on FAP patients.
The components of amyloid deposit were examined by the peroxidase-antiperoxidase (PAP) method. These amyloid substances were stained with anti-human TTR and anti-mouse amyloid P-component antisera. These results clearly demonstrated that the variant TTR was deposited as amyloid fibrils.
Recent technical advances in the manipulation of mouse embryos have facilitated direct approaches for acquiring a mouse model in which the molecular defect is exactly the same as that seen in human. We produced transgenic mice in which amyloid was deposited under the same mechanism as in human. Although the peripheral polyneuropathy has not developed in these transgenic mice, these transgenic mice could be used to devise methods of altering progression of amyloid deposition.

ACKNOWLEDGEMENTS

We are grateful to Ms. R. Kitamura for her assistance in the preparation of this manuscript. This work was supported by a grant from the Ministry of Education, Science and Culture, Japan.

REFERENCES

1. C. Andrade, Brain, 75, 408-427 (1952).
2. S. Tawara, M. Nakazato, K. Kanagawa, H. Matsuo and S. Araki, Biochem. Biophys. Res. Commun., 116, 880-888 (1983).
3. T. Tsuzuki, S. Mita, S. Maeda, S. Araki and K. Shimada, J. Biol. Chem., 260, 12224-12227 (1985).
4. H. Sasaki, N. Yoshioka, Y. Takagi and Y. Sakaki, Gene, 37, 191-197 (1985).
5. S. Maeda, S. Mita, S. Araki and K. Shimada, Mol. Biol. Med. 3, 329-338 (1986).
6. M. Ide, S. Mita, S. Ikegawa, S. Maeda, K. Shimada and S. Araki, Mol. Cell. Biol., 6, 4697-4708 (1986).
7. S. Mita, S. Maeda, M. Ide, T. Tsuzuki, K. Shimada and S. Araki, Neurology, 36, 298-301 (1986).
8. P.M. Dickson, P.D. Aldred, T. Marley, T. Guo-Fen, G.J. Howlett and G. Schreiber, Biochem. Biophys. Res. Commun., 127, 890-895 (1985).
9. D.R. Soprano, K.J. Soprano and D.S. Goodman, Proc. Natl. Acad. Sci. USA, 83, 7330-7334 (1986).
10. R.H. Costa, E. Lai and J.E. Darnell, Jr., Mol. Cell. Biol., 6, 4697-4708 (1986).
11. K. Yamamura, S. Wakasugi, S. Maeda, T. Inomoto, T. Iwanaga, M. Uehira, K. Araki, J. Miyazaki and K. Shimada, Dev. Genet., 8, 195-205 (1987).

Clinical application of restriction fragment length polymorphisms (RFLPs)

Yusuke Nakamura

Howard Hughes Medical Institute, University of Utah, Salt Lake City, Utah

Abstract - DNA technology based on RFLPs (Restriction Fragment Length Polymorphisms) has brought a new system to the fields of medicine and forensic science, especially for the study of genetic diseases and for identification of individuals for forensic purposes. Linkage analysis based on segregation of RFLPs in affected families has already determined the chromosomal localization of genes that harbor mutations responsible for many genetic diseases, and highly polymorphic VNTR (Variable Number of Tandem Repeat) markers are now being used to increase the efficiency of such studies.

INTRODUCTION

Segregation studies based on RFLPs (Restriction Fragment Length Polymorphisms), normal variations in DNA at many sites in the human genome, often allow us to distinguish whether a chromosome is of maternal or paternal origin. When that is possible, we can follow the inheritance of a gene that is known only by a phenotype that is segregating in a family, if the phenotype co-segregates with a polymorphic "marker" locus. Co-segregation, or "linkage", depends on physical proximity on a chromosome between the marker and the unknown gene. Genetic linkage analysis using this powerful property of normal polymorphism has been contributing to research on human genetic diseases and has led to chromosomal localization of dozens of genes that harbor mutations responsible for inherited disorders, such as Duchenne muscular dystrophy (1), cystic fibrosis (2-4), polycystic kidney disease (5), familial adenomatous polyposis (6,7), and multiple endocrine neoplasia types 1 and 2A (8-10). The gene that is defective in Duchenne muscular dystrophy has been isolated, and the product of this gene is undergoing intensive investigation (11, 12). Isolation and characterization of other genes that have been localized by linkage analysis will occur before long, and when the molecular basis of defects in such genes is understood, new therapies can be devised.

Polymorphic loci usually consist of only two possible alleles, generated by a substitution of one nucleotide for another in human genomic DNA, at a site recognized for cleavage by a bacterial endonuclease ("restriction enzyme"). However, another type of RFLP, known as a VNTR (Variable Number of Tandem Repeat), is generated by variation from one individual to another in the number of tandemly repeated sequences at a particular locus (13). Because the number of different alleles possible in the population can be large at such a locus, VNTRs are very informative in a linkage study. VNTRs are also helpful in forensic studies because of their highly polymorphic nature, and they are being used in clinical settings to monitor recipients of bone marrow transplants.

RFLPs (SITE POLYMORPHISMS AND VNTRs)

When we digest genomic DNA with restriction enzymes, the sizes of the fragments at some loci are sometimes different among the tested population due to base substitution at the recognition site. Fig. 1 shows schematically the pattern of a site polymorphism on a Southern blot. Because thymine (T) has been substituted for cytosine (C) as the second nucleotide in the recognition sequence for the enzyme TaqI, chromosome B yields a 4-kilobase-size band upon hybridization with a DNA probe that is specific for this locus, and chromosome A yields a 2-kb band on the electrophoretic gel. If the individual is a heterozygote at the locus detected by the probe (as in lane 2 of Fig. 1), we can distinguish two homologs of the same chromosome. In this case, the locus serves as a recognizable "marker" for a specific point in the human genome.

However, the theoretical maximum heterozygosity within the population that is provided by a site-polymorphic RFLP "marker" locus is 50%. This means that we will be able to get segregation information from this marker in fewer than 50% of tested individuals; more than 50% of the population will be uninformative for linkage studies at that particular locus.

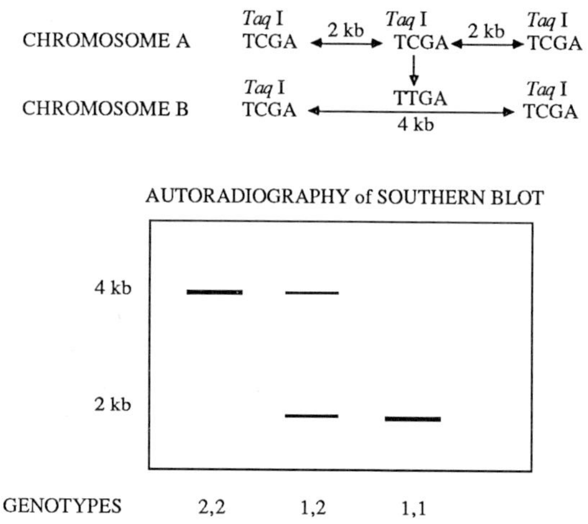

Fig. 1. The typical autoradiographic pattern and the mechanism of a site polymorphism at a DNA marker locus. Because allele 2 (on chromosome B) is missing one copy of the correct recognition sequence for cleavage by TaqI, it is longer (heavier) than allele 1 and does not travel as fast on the electrophoretic gel as allele 1. Genomic DNA has been denatured to the single-stranded form and transferred to a membrane ("Southern blot") after electrophoresis; when the probe, a single-stranded segment of DNA specific for this locus, is radiolabeled and hybridized to the membrane, autoradiography reveals the allele pattern at the locus. Under stringent conditions no other loci will be labeled.

To increase the informativeness of DNA markers and increase the efficiency of linkage studies we have isolated within the past three years more than 200 VNTRs, the type of RFLP illustrated in Fig. 2. Each vertical lane again represents the alleles at one locus (YNH24, on chromosome 2) from one of 15 unrelated individuals. Nineteen different alleles are visible in this small population sample.

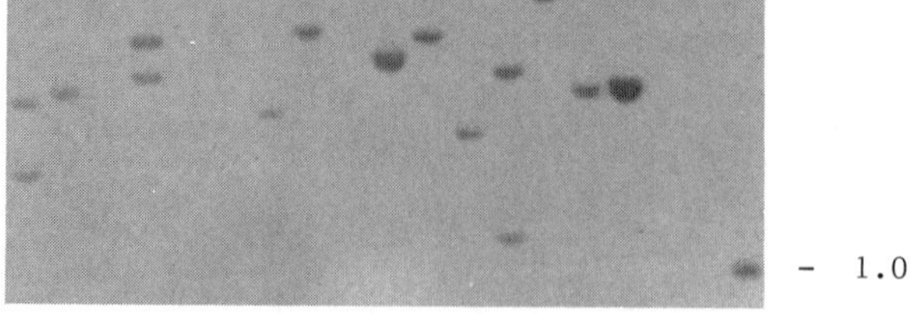

Fig. 2. Autoradiograph of DNA from a random population sample, digested with the restriction enzyme MspI and hybridized to a probe for locus YNH24. M, lane for molecular size markers (in kilobases).

The first VNTR marker - pAW101 (D14S1), later mapped on chromosome 14 - was reported by Wyman and White in 1980 (14,15). VNTR sequences were subsequently found in a 5' flanking region of the insulin gene (16), a 3' flanking region of the H-ras gene (17), an intron of the myoglobin gene, and a region near the pseudogene of zetaglobin (18). These observations suggested the existence of many VNTR loci in the human genome. In 1985, Jeffreys et al.

reported a "minisatellite" sequence that showed a hypervariable "fingerprinting" pattern on Southern blots (19). This evidence supported the idea that there are many VNTR loci and provided a hint as to how to isolate such loci efficiently, because VNTR loci seem to have some sequence similarity to each other. To test this possibility for selecting VNTR loci, we used the oligonucleotides shown in Table 1 for screening human genomic cosmid libraries at relatively lower stringency. Several hundred cosmid clones that hybridized with each oligonucleotide were isolated and tested for polymorphisms with nine enzymes (MspI, TaqI, RsaI, BglII, PstI, PvuII, HindIII, EcoRI and BamHI).

TABLE 1. DNA sequences and hybridization conditions for oligonucleotide probes.

Probe	Sequences	Temp. (°C) of: Hybridization	Washing
Zeta-globin	TGGGGCACAGG$^{T}_{C}$TGTGAG	42	48
Insulin	ACAGGGGTGTGGGG	30	37
Myoglobin-1	GGAGGTGGGCAGGAAG	37	44
Myoglobin-2	GGAGGCTGGAGGAG	37	42
HBV-1	GGAGTTGGGGGAGGAG	37	44
HBV-2	GGACTGGGAGGAGTTGGGGG	50	60
HBV-3	GGTGAAGCA$^{G}_{C}$AGGTG	37	42
HBV-4	GAGAGGGGTGTAGAG	37	42
HBV-5	GGTGTAGAGAGGGGT	37	42
YNZ22	CTCTGGGTGTCGTGC	37	42
Core	18 nucleotides including GNNGTGGG	45-55	50-60

TABLE 2. Summary of screening for VNTR polymorphism.

Probe	Positive clones per genome *	Clones tested for polymorphism	VNTR polymorphism	Percent **	Site polymorphism ***
Zeta-globin	180	57	12	21	20 (6)
Insulin	220	20	4	20	8 (1)
Myoglobin-1	150	65	8	12	19 (8)
Myoglobin-2	18	18	8	44	8 (2)
HBV-1	200	75	13	17	38 (13)
HBV-2	40	15	2	13	10 (3)
HBV DR 1	50	26	6	23	6 (2)
HBV DR 2 and 3	150	58	15	26	40 (19)
YNZ22	38	38	9	24	25 (11)
GNNGTGGG (18mer)		102	34	30	40 (20)
Totals		474	111	23	214(85)

* We screened one genomic equivalent (almost 75,000 colonies) to two genomic equivalents for each probe. The number of positive clones per genome means the number per 75,000 colonies. ** The proportion of VNTR DNA markers among the tested cosmids. *** The number of cosmids that showed site polymorphisms with two or more restriction enzymes is shown in parentheses.

Table 2 summarizes the results of the screening procedure (13,20). Nearly 30% of the clones tested showed the VNTR type of polymorphism. When we screened the clones randomly, we obtained VNTR loci from only 3% of the tested clones. Prescreening with oligonucleotides that have been identified as sequences common to VNTR markers is therefore an efficient approach, enriching the harvest of VNTR loci approximately 10-fold. Furthermore, as the insert size of cosmid clones is as large as 35-45 kb, we also had a better chance of identifying a site polymorphism with one or more enzymes (13).

RECOMBINATION FREQUENCY AND THE DISTANCE BETWEEN DNA MARKERS

For the construction of a genetic linkage map that will be useful in detecting the location of a genetic defect segregating in a family, we need to estimate the distance between DNA markers. Such estimates derive from the frequency of recombination events between pairs of markers. During meiosis, the homologous chromosomes line up in paris; crossing-over of segments of DNA occurs between the homologs, and this exchange of material (recombination) produces chimeric chromosomes, a patchwork of DNA segments derived from each parent (Fig. 3). During one meiosis, an estimated 30 recombination events occur throughout the genome. From this phenomenon and the estimated size of the human genome (3×10^9 base pairs), we can calculate roughly that a 1% frequency of recombination between two markers reflects an average of 1,000 kb, or 1 million nucleotide base pairs, of physical distance on a chromosome.

Our analysis of genotypic data for several DNA markers in a large number of 3-generation families, using a sophisticated computer program (21), has produced genetic linkage maps for several human chromosomes; chromosome 17 is shown in Fig. 4 (22). This linkage map covers 218 centimorgans (cM) in males and 279 cM in females, and covers the chromosome from the telomeric region of the short arm to the telomeric region of the long arm. If the gene associated with any genetic disease lies within the mapped region of this chromosome, it will be linked in affected families with one or more of the markers if a sufficient number of meiosis are available for analysis. So far, genetic linkage maps of human chromosomes 1 (ref. 23),

5 (ref. 7), 6p (ref. 24), 9 (ref. 25), 10 (refs. 26,27), 11p (ref. 28), 12 (ref. 29), 13 (ref. 30), 14q32 (ref. 31), 15 (ref. 32), 17 (ref. 22), 18 (ref. 33), and 19 (ref. 34) have been published from our laboratory at the University of Utah, and other groups have published similar maps (35).

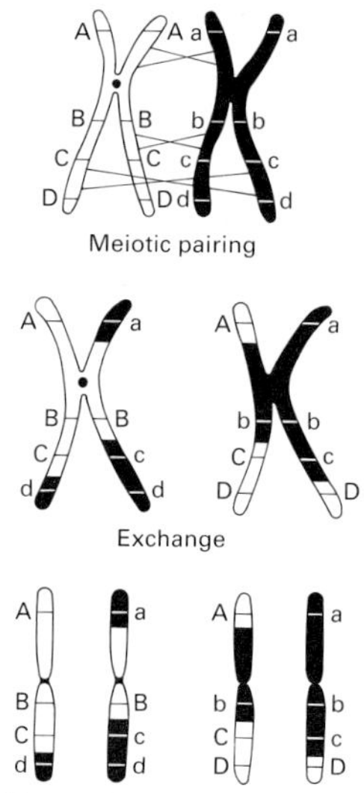

Fig. 3. The segmental nature of inherited chromosomes. A single meiosis produces four recombinant chromosomes; each of them contains a different mosaic of segments, here illustrated in black and white, derived from both parental homologues. An offspring will inherit only one of the four from this parent and an equally random mosaic on the homologous chromosome from the other parent, making him genetically different from any sibling except a monozygotic twin.

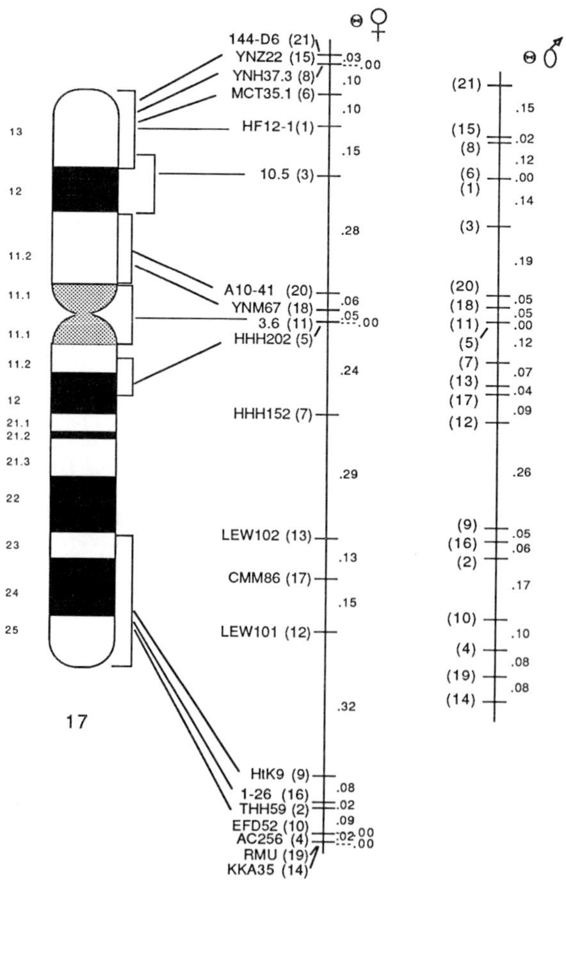

Fig. 4. Sex-specific genetic maps of human chromosome 17, with physical localizations of selected markers, derived from cytogenetic methods, indicated on the ideogram. θ = percent recombination, expressed as a fraction. Two genetic maps are necessary for this chromosome, because significant differences in the frequency of crossingover appear to occur in some intervals between loci, as a function of whether the meiosis are in males or in females. This phenomenon has not yet been fully explained. The order of the loci on the map will not vary with sex, however. (From ref. 22, reprinted by permission. (c) 1988, Academic Press, Ltd.)

LOCALIZATION OF GENETIC DISEASE LOCI BY LINKAGE ANALYSIS

Figure 5 shows typical patterns of cosegregation between DNA markers and genetic diseases. Among the diseases showing an autosomal dominant mode of inheritance (Fig. 5-a), more than a dozen have been localized to chromosomes by linkage analysis, e.g. familial adenomatous polyposis (FAP) (6,7), multiple endocrine neoplasia (MEN) types 1 and 2A (8-10), polycystic kidney disease (5), Huntington's disease, and neurofibromatosis types 1 and 2 (36-39). Figure 5-b shows the autosomal recessive pattern of inheritance associated with two other diseases that have been mapped by linkage analysis, cystic fibrosis (2-4) and Wilson's disease (40). Figure 5-c illustrates the inheritance pattern of an X-linked recessive gene, such as is found for the numerous diseases including Duchenne and Becker muscular dystrophies (1,41) and Wiscott-Aldrich syndrome (42), that have now been localized on the X chromosome. In Fig. 5-d, the Southern blot indicates coinheritance of the phenotype of FAP, an autosomal dominant condition, with a particular allele of the DNA marker YN5.48 (43).

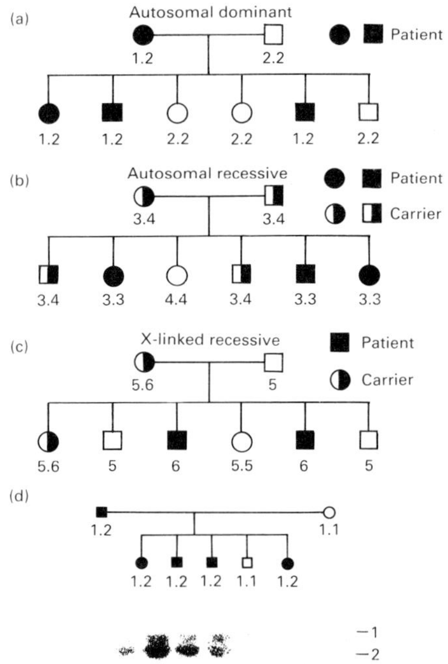

Fig. 5. Patterns of inheritance. Round symbols indicate female members of each family, squares males. (a): the disease gene cosegregates with allele 1 of the marker, and all members of this family who have this allele will be affected with the disease. (b): a family member carrying one allele 3 at the marker locus will not be affected with the disease, but may pass the defective gene to an offspring who will be affected if his or her other parent also transmits the defect. (c): only males are likely to be affected by an X-linked defect, because their sisters will have inherited another X chromosome (from their fathers) whose normal function will substitute for the mother's defective allele. In the family shown here, the defective allele, which cosegregates with marker allele 6, can be transmitted by one of the daughters to her offspring although she herself will not be affected. (d): FAP, an autosomal dominant defect, appears in all the children in this family except the son who inherited marker allele 1, linked to the normal gene at the FAP locus in this family, from both parents.

Having accumulated a large set of linkage data between genotypes at DNA marker loci in the region in normal families and phenotypes in families segregating the disease, we can now define the location of the FAP locus within a 10-cM segment on the long arm of chromosome 5, between YN5.64 and MC5.61 in Fig. 6 (43).

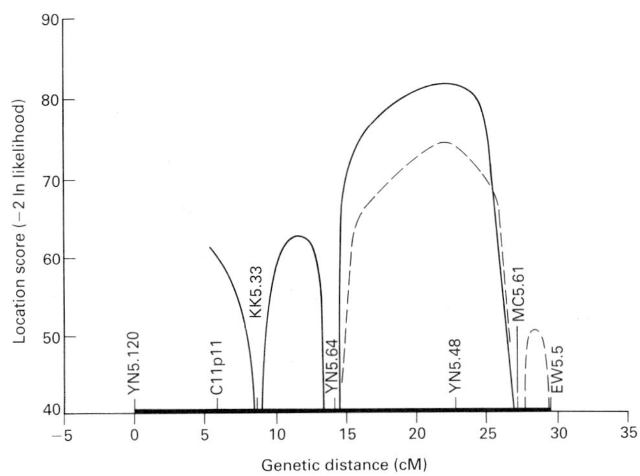

Fig. 6. Location score (26) for the FAP gene on the map of closely-linked markers on chromosome 5p. The solid line indicates location score with respect to the subset of loci C11p11, KK5.33, YN5.64, and YN5.48; the dashed line indicates location score with respect to the subset YN5.64, YN5.48, MC5.61 and EW5.5. Both curves indicate that the most likely location of FAP is very close to the YN5.48 locus. (From ref. 43, reprinted by permission. (c) 1988 American Society of Human Genetics.)

Finding the chromosomal location of the gene associated with a genetic disease is the first step toward isolation of the gene itself; linkage analysis can define and narrow the target region. The regions containing many of the genes listed above have been narrowed to the 1 - 10 cM (1,000 - 10,000 kb) range. These genes will be isolated within a few years, and their function will become clear.

Application of highly polymorphic markers to individual identification

As the VNTR markers have a large number of different alleles represented in the population, they can distinguish even siblings from each other. For example, the two markers in Fig. 7 (pYNH24 and pMLJ14) distinguish seven brothers and sisters.

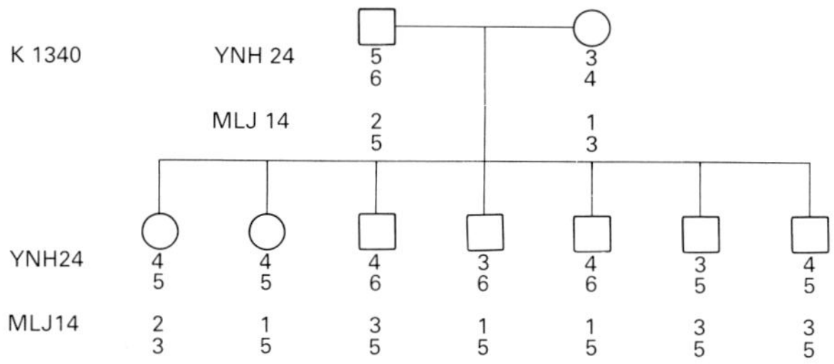

Fig. 7. Genotypes of two highly polymorphic VNTR markers in one family.

Each of the seven siblings has a different genotype when the two VNTR loci are combined. This result illustrates the potential power of VNTR markers for monitoring bone marrow transplantation to distinguish the donor and recipient lymphocytes. Of course, this technique is also available for paternity testing or other forensic purposes, and intensive investigation of its reliability for these applications is underway.

Technology with respect to polymorphic DNA markers has been expanding very rapidly, and prenatal or presymptomatic diagnosis for some genetic diseases is already routine. Diagnostic and forensic applications carry certain ethical burdens. However, I believe that DNA technology will often give answers that are faster and more precise than conventional methods.

REFERENCES

1. J.M. Murray, K.E. Davies, P.S. Harper, L. Meredith, C.R. Mueller and R. Williamson, Nature 300, 69-71 (1982).
2. R. White, S. Woodward, M. Leppert, P. O'Connell, Y. Nakamura, M. Hoff, J. Herbst, J.-M. Lalouel, M. Dean and G.V. Woude, Nature, 318, 382-384 (1985).
3. B.J. Wainwright, P. Scambler, J. Schmidtke, E.A. Watson, H.-Y. Law, M. Farrall, H.J. Cooke, H. Eiberg and R. Williamson, Nature, 318, 384-385 (1985).
4. L.-C. Tsui, M. Buchwald, D. Barker, J. Braman, R. Knowlton, et al., Science, 230, 1054-1057 (1985).
5. S.T. Reeders, M.H. Breuning, K.E. Davies, R.D. Nicolls, A.P. Jarman, D.R. Higgs, P.L. Pearson and D.J. Weatherall, Nature, 317, 542-544 (1985).
6. W.F. Bodmer, C.J. Bailey, J. Bodmer, H.J.R. Bussey, A. Ellis, P. Gorman, F.C. Lucibello, V.A. Murday, S.H. Rider, P. Scambler, D. Sheer, E. Solomon and N.K. Spurr, Nature, 328, 614-616 (1987).
7. M. Leppert, M. Dobbs, P. Scambler, P. O'Connell, Y. Nakamura, D. Stauffer, S. Woodward, R. Burt, J. Hughes, E. Gardner, M. Lathrop, J. Wasmuth, J.-M. Lalouel and R. White, Science, 238, 1411-1413 (1987).
8. C.P.G. Mathew, K.S. Chin, D.F. Easton, K. Thorpe, C. Carter, G.I. Liou, S.-F. Fong, C.D.B. Bridges, H. Haak, A.C. Nieuwenhuizen Krusenman, S. Schifter, H.H. Hansen, H. Telenius, M. Telenius-Berg and B.A.J. Ponder, Nature, 328, 527-528 (1987).
9. N.E. Simpson, K.K. Kidd, P.J. GOodfellow, H. McDermid, S. Myers, J.R. Kidd, C.E. Jackson, A.M.V. Duncan, L.A. Farrer, K. Brasch, C. Castiglione, M. Genel, J. Gertner, C.R. Greenberg, J.F. Gusella, J.J.A. Holden and B.N. White, Nature, 328, 528-530 (1987).
10. C. Larsson, B. Skogseid, K. Oberg, Y. Nakamura and M. Nordensjold, Nature, 332, 85-87 (1988).
11. E.P. Hoffman, R.H. Brown and L.M. Kunkel, Cell, 51, 919-928 (1987).

12. C. Webster, L. Silberstein, A.P. Hays and H.M. Blau, Cell, 52, 503-513 (1988).
13. Y. Nakamura, M. Leppert, P. O'Connell, R. Wolff, T. Holm, M. Culver, C. Martin, E. Fujimoto, M. Hoff, E. Kumlin and R. White, Science, 235, 1616-1622 (1987).
14. A.R. Wyman and R. White, Proc. Natl. Acad. Sci. USA, 77, 6754-6758 (1980).
15. T.A. Donlon and R.E. Magenis, Cytogenet. Cell Genet., 37, 453-454 (1984).
16. G.I. Bell, M.J. Selby and W.J. Rutter, Nature, 295, 31-35 (1982).
17. D.J. Capon, E.Y. Chen, A.D. Levinson, P.H. Seeberg and D.V. Goeddel, Nature, 302, 33-37 (1983).
18. S.E.Y. Goodbourn, D.R. Higgs, J.B. Clegg and D.J. Weatherall, Proc. Natl. Acad. Sci. USA, 80, 5022-5026 (1983).
19. A.J. Jeffreys, V. Wilson and S.L. Thein, Nature, 314, 67-73 (1985).
20. Y. Nakamura, M. Carlson, K. Krapcho, M. Kanamori and R. White, Am. J. Hum. Genet., 43, in press.
21. G.M. Lathrop, J.-M. Lalouel, C. Julier and J. Ott, Am. J. Hum. Genet., 37, 482-498 (1985).
22. Y. Nakamura, M. Lathrop, P. O'Connell, M. Leppert, D. Barker, E. Wright, M. Skolnick, S. Kondoleon, M. Litt, J.-M. Lalouel and R. White, Genomics, 2, 302-309 (1988).
23. P. O'Connell, G.M. Lathrop, Y. Nakamura, M. Leppert, R.H. Ardinger, J.L. Murray, J.-M. Lalouel and R. White, Genomics, in press.
24. R. Leach, R. Demars, S. Hasstedt and R. White, Proc. Natl. Acad. Sci USA, 83, 3909-3913 (1986).
25. M. Lathrop, Y. Nakamura, P. O'Connell, M. Leppert, S. Woodward, J.-M. Lalouel, and R. White, Genomics, in press.
26. M. Lathrop, Y. Nakamura, P. Cartwright, P. O'Connell, M. Leppert, C. Jones, H. Tateishi, T. Bragg, J.-M. Lalouel, and R. White, Genomics, 2, 157-164 (1988).
27. Y. Nakamura, M. Lathrop, T. Bragg, M. Leppert, P. O'Connell, C. Jones, J.-M. Lalouel, and R. White, Genomics, in press.
28. R. White, M. Leppert, T. Bishop, D. Barker, J. Berkowitz, C. Brown, P. Callahan, T. Holm, and L. Jerominski, Nature, 313, 101-105 (1985).
29. P. O'Connell, G.M. Lathrop, M. Law, M. Leppert, Y. Nakamura, M. Hoff, E. Kumlin, W. Thomas, T. Elsner, L. Ballard, P. Goodman, E. Azen, J. Sadler, G. Cai, J.-M. Lalouel, and R. White, Genomics, 1, 93-102 (1987).
30. M. Leppert, W. Cavenee, P. Callahan, T. Holm, P. O'Connell, K. Thompson, G.M. Lathrop, J.-M. Lalouel and R. White, Am. J. Hum. Genet., 39, 425-437 (1986).
31. Y. Nakamura, M. Lathrop, P. O'Connell, M. Leppert, J.-M. Lalouel, and R. White, Genomics, in press.
32. Y. Nakamura, M. Lathrop, P. O'Connell, M. Leppert, J.-M. Lalouel and R. White, Genomics, in press.
33. P. O'Connell, G.M. Lathrop, M. Leppert, Y. Nakamura, U. Muller, J.-M. Lalouel and R. White, Genomics, in press.
34. Y. Nakamura, M. Lathrop, P. O'Connell, M. Leppert, J.-M. Lalouel, and R. White, Genomics, 3, 67-71 (1988).
35. H. Donis-Keller and 32 other authors, Cell, 51, 319-337 (1987).
36. D. Barker, E. Wright, K. Nguyen, L. Cannon, P. Fain, D. Goldger, D.T. Bishop, J. Carey, B. Baty, J. Kivlin, H. Willard, J.S. Waye, G. Greig, L. Leinwand, Y. Nakamura, P. O'Connell, M. Leppert, J.-M. Lalouel, R. White and M. Skolnick, Science, 236, 1100-1102 (1987).
37. R. White, Y. Nakamura, P. O'Connell, M. Leppert, J.-M. Lalouel, D. Barker, D. Goldgar, M. Skolnick, J. Carey, C.E. Wallis, C.P. Slater, C. Mathew and B. Ponder, Genomics, 1, 364-367 (1987).
38. G. Rouleau, W. Wertelecki, J. Haines, W. Hobbs, J. Trofatter, B. Seizinger, R. Martuza, D. Superneau, P.M. Conneally, and J. Gusella, Nature, 329, 246-248 (1987).
39. J.F. Gusella, N.S. Wexler, P.M. Conneally, S.L. Naylor, M.A. Anderson, R.E. Tanzi, P.C. Watkins, K. Ottina, M.R. Wallace, A.Y. Sakaguchi, A.B. Young, I. Shoulson, E. Bonilla, and J.B. Martin, Nature, 306, 234-238 (1984).
40. M. Frydman, B. Bonne-Tamir, L.A. Farrer, P.M. Conneally, A. Magazanik, S. Ashbel and Z. Goldwitch, Proc. Acad. Sci. USA, 82, 1819-1821 (1985).
41. S. Fadda, M. Mochi, L. Roncuzzi, D. Sangiorgi, D. Sbarra, M. Zatz and G. Romeo, Hum. Genet., 71, 33-36 (1985).
42. M. Peacocke and K.A. Siminovitch, Proc. Natl. Acad. Sci. USA, 84, 3430-3433 (1987).
43. Y. Nakamura, M. Lathrop, M. Leppert, M. Dobbs, J. Wasmuth, E. Kumlin, E. Fujimoto, M. Carlson, K. Krapcho, T. Sears, J.-M. Lalouel, and R. White, Am. J. Hum. Genet., in press.

1. Development of rapid identification kits

Attempts at development of simple identification kits have been made for more than 10 years. While various problems have been discussed, this method has settled in among the laboratory tests for application. As shown in Table 2, methods for Enterobacteriaceae have been developed rather early, followed by similar attempts for gram-positive organisms such as Staphylococcus, Streptococcus, gram-negative bacteria such as Neisseria gonorrhoeae, N. meningitidis and Branhamella, gram-negative rods such as Pseudomonas, anaerobic bacteria, yeast-like fungus, and acid-fast bacteria. Although some problems have prevented the identification of all bacteria by this method, further developments of a new technique are expected.

TABLE 2. Commercially available kits for identification of isolates

Family Enterobacteriaceae	N.gonorrhoeae & N.meningitidis
API 20E [Asuka]	Minitek [BBL]
Micro ID [Ono]	Phadebacto test [Shionogi]
ID test EB 20 [Nissui]	Anaerobes
Biotest No.1 [Eiken]	API [Asuka]
Enterotube II [Roche]	Minitek [BBL]
Pile tube No.1 [Eiken]	RaPID ANA system [Amuco]
Nonfermenting bacteria	Anaerobe-Tek System [Flow Lab.]
API 20E [Asuka]	Acid-fast bacteria
Oxiferm [Roche]	Acid-fast bacteria differentiation set[Kyokuto]
Pile tube No.2 [Eiken]	Yeasts
Minitek-BBL system [BBL]	API oxanogram [Asuka]
YY system [BBL]	Minitek Yeast [BBL]
Streptococci	Germtest [Asuka]
API strep 20 [Asuka]	Candida Check [Dai-Iatron]
API strep [Asuka]	Mycotube [Roche]
Phadebacto test [Shionogi]	
Slidex strepto kit [Synthetic]	
Strep ID [Tomoe]	
Staphylococci	
API Staph [Asuka]	
ID test SP-18 [Nissui]	
Phadebacto test [Shionogi]	
Staph Slide test [Synthetic]	
PS Latex [Eiken]	

2. Automated instruments

Generally, automations are considered to be difficult for the bacteriological tests. However, automations of bacteriological tests are in progress, and instruments such as Autobac, MS-2, AMS, AutoScan, Sceptor, Cobas Bact, Bactec and MIC 2000 are commercially available. By using Autobac, MS-2, AMS and Cobas Bact, the susceptibility test and screening test for bacteriuria are possible, along with the identification test. Bactec is used for the examination of bacteria in blood, which proved to be useful for the rapid diagnosis of septicemia. By utilizing a computer, the process of identification has become more complex, and the number of items for examination is increased as it is requested.

3. Immunological methods for antigen detection

The detection of antigen weighs greater in the rapid diagnosis of infectious diseases, especially in virus examination. Methods shown in Table 3 are well known.

TABLE 3. Methods for detection of microorganisms

Organisms	Methods								Nucleic acid	
	LA	CoA	FA	EIA-ELISA	RIA	IP	PAP	ABI	HD	REA
Staphylococcus sp.	●									
Streptococcus sp.	●	●								
Streptococcus group A	●		●	●						
group B	●	●								
Streptococcus pneumoniae	●	●								
Neisseria sp.	●	●	●	●						
Escherichia coli									●	
Salmonella sp.	●			●						
Vibrio cholerae		●								
Pseudomonas sp.			●							
Haemophilus sp.	●	●								
Bordetella pertussis				●						
Campylobacter sp.	●								●	
Mycobacterium sp.									●	
Bacteroides fragilis			●							
Legionella pneumophila			●							●
Candida albicans	●									
Cryptococcus neoformans	●									
Aspergillus			●							

TABLE 3. Methods for detection of microorganisms (continued)

Organisms	Methods									
	LA	CoA	FA	EIA-ELISA	RIA	IP	PAP	ABI	Nucleic acid HD	Nucleic acid REA
Hepatitis Bc antigen				●						
Be antigen				●	●					
Bs antigen	●			●	●				●	
Herpes simplex virus	●		●	●		●	●	●	●	●
Varicella zoster virus			●						●	
Cytomegalovirus			●	●		●			●	●
Epstein-Barr virus									●	
Adenovirus			●	●					●	●
Influenza virus type A			●	●						
type B			●	●						
Respiratory syncytial virus			●	●				●		
Rotavirus	●		●	●						●
Human immunodeficiency virus				●						
Yellow fever virus					●					
Mycoplasma pneumoniae			●			●				
Chlamydia trachomatis			●	●		●			●	
psittaci			●							
Treponema pallidum			●							

LA:Latex agglutination, CoA:Coagglutination, FA:Fluorescent antibody test, EIA:Enzyme immunoassay, ELISA:Enzyme-linked immunosorbent assay, RIA:Radio-immunoassay, IP:Immunoperoxidase test, PAP:Peroxidase-antiperoxidase test, ABI:Avidin-biotin immunoassay, HD:Hybridization, REA:Restriction enzyme analysis

They include latex agglutination test (LA), fluorescent antibody test (FA) and enzyme immunoassay (EIA) which are used for laboratory tests.

1) Latex agglutination test (LA)

LA is extensively utilized for detecting general bacteria, fungi and viruses. It is especially used in the detection of viruses, as the isolation of organisms is generally difficult and time-consuming. Therefore, the utility of a simple method for antigen detection is very high.

2) Fluorescent antibody test (FA) or Immunofluorescence test (IF)

As a rapid method for detection of antigen, FA is generally applied to detection of general bacteria, fungi, rickettsia and viruses. FA is also used for detecting antibody in syphilis or EB virus infections. Recently, high specific methods using monoclonal antibody have been applied to general microbiological laboratory test. The test results of Chlamydia trachomatis, herpes simplex virus (HSV) and respiratory syncytial (RS) virus are acceptable.

3) Enzyme immunoassay (EIA) or Enzyme-linked immunosorbent assay (ELISA)

As the sensitivity of EIA is high, the test can be performed within a short time. As the method of laboratory diagnosis, EIA is applied to detection of hepatitis virus, HSV, rota-virus, cytomegalovirus, RS virus, C.trachomatis, and bacteria such as Neisseria, Group A Streptococcus and Campylobacter. The antigens can be detected in clinical specimens containing a large amount of virus, for instance, the serum from patients with type B hepatitis and the feces from infants with diarrhea due to rotavirus.

4) Counter immunoelectrophoresis (CIE)

CIE has been first applied to detection of hepatitis type B (HB) virus, then to H.influenzae type b, Group B Streptococcus, N.meningitidis (group A, C and D) and S.pneumoniae. The kits are commercially available.

5) Coagglutination test (CoA)

This method utilizes the binding of protein A from the cell wall of Staphylococcus aureus to Fc portion of immunoglobulin. CoA has been applied to detection of N.gonorrhoeae, S. pneumoniae, Streptococcus pyogenes group A and B, H.influenzae and N.meningitidis (A, B, C, YW135). The kit is commercially available under the name of Phadebact [Pharmacia].

6) Passive hemagglutination test (PHA)

This method is widely used as an antibody test for syphilis, mycoplasma infection, toxoplas-mosis and viral diseases.

7) Reversed passive hemagglutination test (RPHA)

This method is applied to detection of HB virus and rotavirus. The detection of rotavirus in feces has become possible by using RPHA. The globulin fraction obtained by the purifi-cation of antiserum which is raised against each antigens is adsorbed onto the surface of fixed sheep red blood cells. The sensitized blood cells are then mixed with specimens. In the presence of antigen, reaction with the sensitized blood cells takes place to cause agglutination.

These are the outline of the immunoserological methods for antigen detection. These methods above mentioned are now readily applicable to daily use by utilizing commercially available kits.

4. Metabolic products or toxin measurement

Recently, gaschromatography has been used for measuring microquantities of the chemical markers characterizing microorganism, and for analyzing the metabolic products and cellular constituents to help identifying anaerobic bacteria.

5. Application of flow cytometry
Attempts are also made to introduce a new method of flow cytometry. The utility of this method is summarized in Table 4.

TABLE 4. Applications of flow cytometry to bacterial infection diagnosis

Analysis of cell mass and nucleic acid during the cell growth cycle
Analysis of antimicrobial action on bacteria
Antibiotic receptors
DNA synthesis
Double fluorescence staining for DNA base composition
Chromomycin A3(C) ⟶ GC
Hoechst 33258 ⟶ AT
Immunofluorescence staining of bacteria using specific monoclonal antibody

6. Rapid and simple tissue-culture method for isolation of viruses
The isolation of viruses generally takes a long time. And the technique is complicated. Microplate method developed by Numazaki et al. [National Sendai Hospital] utilizes a microplate on which attempts are made to isolate virus from 4 kinds of cells. The isolation of various respiratory viruses has thus become possible in a hospital clinical laboratory. Rapid and direct isolation of the causative virus is significant.
7. Nucleic acid hybridization method
Hybridization technique using DNA and RNA probes has been applied to the detection and identification of viral genomes in clinical specimens. It is also being used for general bacteria such as Campylobacter, Mycoplasma and Legionella. These subjects will be discussed in detail by the next author.
8. Application of these methods to detection of causative agents
The major diseases and the causative organisms to which these methods are applied are listed next.
1) Application to detection of bacteria
a) Streptococcus pyogenes group A infection
LA and CoA are used for attempting to classify the groups directly from the colony. The commercially available kits have been used in daily tests.
b) Bacterial meningitis
For the purpose of direct detection of meningococcus antigen in cerebrospinal fluid, the following methods are used. (1)CIE, (2)EIA or ELISA, (3)CoA, (4)LA.
With CIE, it is possible to detect Group A, C and D meningococcus, but not other Groups. EIA is useful for the antigen detection of Group A meningococcus, Type b influenza bacillus and Pneumococcus. By using these methods combined with Gram staining, the rate of detection is higher than that obtained by using CIE alone by 20-30%. CoA can be performed with commercially available kit of reagents [Pharmacia]. CoA has a higher sensitivity than CIE, but not all of the meningococcal antigens can be detected by CoA.
c) Syphilis
LA has been applied to measurement of antibody in various other infections. In syphilis, the serum test for syphilis is carried out by using Treponema pallidum (TP) antigen adsorbed onto latex particles. No false-positive result is noted, in excellent agreement with the result of TPHA.
d) Gonococcal infection
As a method based on an immunologic reaction, EIA has been developed. Gonozyme [Abbott] is the name of the commercially available kit.
e) Legionellosis
In legionellosis, simultaneously with the isolation of bacteria and measurement of serum antibody titer, IF is used for demonstration of bacteria in specimens. By using IF, causative agent, Legionella, is demonstrated in sputum, pleural effusion, lung biopsy specimen and lung tissue specimen.
f) Mycotic infection
For the diagnosis of mycotic infections, the isolation and identification of fungus along with histopathological examination are important. Especially in deep-seated fungal infection, the direct demonstration of fungus is not always easy, thus necessitating serological methods for diagnosis. Antibody can be detected by the serological methods, but the antigen tests are more important.
(1)Candidiasis:LA and double antibody sandwich EIA are used. The former is used more frequently. In cases of fungal infection, antibody detection is carried out using a serological test. The detection of antigen is attempted next if the test is negative.
(2)Aspergillosis:The main serological test is directed to the antibody. In many of the patients with mycotic infection such as aspergillosis, the antibody production is reduced, thus the antigen detection becomes necessary. The application of CIE, ELISA and radioimmunoassay (RIA) has been reported.
(3)Cryptococcosis:For the detection of polysaccharide antigen in the capsule of Cryptococcus, LA is widely used. ELISA, complement fixation test (CF) and CIE are also used.
g) Clostridium difficile infection
For the detection of C.difficile toxin in feces, the method for the demonstration of

cytotoxin (D-2 toxin, toxin B) using cultured cells, Ouchterlony method, CIE and ELISA (especially useful for the detection of D-1 toxin, toxin A) are used. LA has been also developed by Ueno et al. for laboratory application. The reagents of LA used for detection of enterotoxin consist of immunoglobulin fraction which is specific to D-1 toxin (toxin A) purified from high titer anti-toxin serum. This was obtained by the immunization of rabbit with toxoid prepared from purified D-1 toxin (toxin A) of C.difficile. It was adsorbed onto latex particle to produce agglutination specific to D-1 toxin. The lower limit of detection of D-1 toxin with latex photoimmunoassay (LPIA) was 10 ng/ml. The highest level of 750 ng/ml was obtained from healthy subjects (mostly less than 10-60 ng/ml) and 804-8280 ng/ml (mostly higher than 1000 ng/ml) from patients with enteritis and diarrhea induced by antibiotics. By using the slide-glass method, it is possible to make the diagnosis in 3 minutes in the presence of more than 500 ng/ml toxin in feces.

h) Rickettsiasis

In rickettsiasis, the test for antibody is first carried out by using IF, EIA and microagglutination mehtod. CF and Weil-Felix reaction are further used as supplemental tests. For the diagnosis of tsutsugamushi desaese, immunoperoxidase method (IP) has been developed which is an excellent method. Especially in the measurement of IgM and IgG antibody titer with IF and IP, the causative organism can be predicted with reasonable certainty. In the detection of antigen, on the other hand, the isolation and identification of rickettsia are carried out along with the demonstration of rickettsial antigen.

i) C.trachomatis infection

IF and EIA have been used.

(1)IF:MicroTrak kit [Syva] is commercially available along with the product of Orion. Monoclonal antibody used in the kit reacts with all 15 serotypes of C.trachomatis but does not react with C.psittaci.

(2)EIA:A 5 hr-EIA, Chlamydiazyme [Abbott], was compared with cell culture (HeLa 229) for detection of chlamydial antigen in 300 urethral specimens from male patients with non-gonococcal urethritis (Table 5). Although Chlamydiazyme failed to detect chlamydial antigen in 3 of 100 specimens which were positive in cell culture, the antigen was detected in 15 of 200 culture-negative specimens by Chlamydiazyme. Thus, Chlamydiazyme is a rapid, sensitive and specific method for diagnosis of chlamydial infection in urogenital tract (ref. 4).

2) Application to detection of viruses

Virus isolation, electron microscopy (EM), IF and EIA have been used for detection of virus or viral antigen. Selections are made from these methods for each virus for clinical laboratory tests. LA is also used for detection of antigen and antibody. In virological studies, antibody tests have been used widely with great significance. The demonstration of antigen or pathogenic organism has ever greater diagnostic significance as a direct proof of the presence of pathogenic organism. The methods for detection of antigens using immunologic techniques are important from the viewpoint of rapidity and simplification.

a) Rotavirus infection

In infections due to rotavirus, measurement of antibody titer is carried out with CF and immune adherence hemagglutination (IAHA), but these are indirect methods for demonstration of recent rotavirus infection. They are more frequently used for seroepidemiologic studies than diagnosis of desease. For the diagnosis the antigen detection method such as RPHA, ELISA, LA, EM and polyacrylamide gel electophoresis (PAGE) are used.

b) HSV infection

The detection of HSV antigen has also been attempted by IF using type-specific monoclonal antibodies [MicroTrak, Syva](Table 6). The direct microscopic examination is used to detect directly HSV-infected cells in clinical specimens. The combined use of the direct examination and cell culture followed by IF is recommended for enhanced detection of HSV (ref. 5).

TABLE 5. Comparison of Chlamydiazyme with culture method for detection of C.trachomatis in urethral specimens

Methods		Chlamydiazyme* (+)	Chlamydiazyme* (-)
Culture method	(+)	97	3
	(-)	15	185

*Sensitivity 97/100(97%)
Specificity 185/200(93%)

TABLE 6. Comparison of direct examination with culture method using IF staining for detection of HSV in clinical specimens

Methods		Direct examination* (+)	Direct examination* (-)
Culture method	(+)	67	11
	(-)	0	25

*Sensitivity 67/78(86%)
Specificity 25/25(100%)

SUMMARY

In tests for microorganisms, the direct detection of pathogenic organism is important for general bacteria. The isolation and identification may be carried out routinely. The isolation and culture of virus, rickettsia and chlamydia are so difficult that such methods cannot be widely practiced. Methods for direct detection of pathogenic organisms or antigens become very significant. Including general bacteria which may be cultured, it generally takes a long time for microorganism testing than in other clinical examinations, and the need for rapid testing is greater. The tests for various important microorganisms are becoming more useful clinically through the progress of rapid diagnosis and development of new techniques. Major examples of these were explained along with their applications. Rapid methods for diagnosis have made progress not only in the immunological field but also in other fields. An overall approach is required to establish significant methods for diagnosis of infectious diseases.

REFERENCES

1. L.R. McCarthy, Rapid Detection and Identification of Infectious Agents, p. 165, Academic Press, London (1985).
2. M. Nakamura, Igaku no ayumi, 146, 84-86 (1988).
3. M. Nakamura, J. Med. Technol., 29, 1643-1651 (1985).
4. M. Nakamura and S. Nishida, Jap. J. Clin. Pathol., 34, 1293-1299 (1986).
5. S. Nishida and M. Nakamura, Jap. J. Clin. Pathol., 36, 101-106 (1988).

New assays for the diagnosis of viral infections

Robert H. Yolken

Johns Hopkins University School of Medicine

Abstract - The advent of antiviral chemotherapy has led to an increased need for the accurate diagnosis of viral infections. The fastidious nature of viruses which infect the gastrointestinal and respiratory tracts has prevented the widespread application of cultivation techniques for the detection of these agents. For this reason, we and others have developed a number of techniques for the direct detection of viruses in human body fluids. Some of these techniques involve the recognition of defined viral antigens by means of solid phase immunoassay methods. While there are a number of different labels which can be utilized for the quantitation of antigens in immunoassay systems, molecules which possess enzymatic activity have proven to be the most useful for the practical detection of viral antigens. These assays have the advantage that they are relatively inexpensive and simple to perform. In addition, acceptable levels of sensitivity and specificity can be obtained if high affinity immunoreagents are utilized and if adequate control reactions are performed. However, the use of immunoassays requires the identification of a immunogenic viral proteins which can be used as a marker of viral infection. Since some pathogenic human viruses do not have recognizable antigens which are shared by all infecting species, non-immunological methods for viral diagnosis have also been devised. The recent development of simplified methods for the extraction of nucleic acids from virions, the labelling of probes with non-isotopic markers, and the hybridization of probe and target nucleic acid in liquid phase may result in the development of practical assays for viral detection. Furthermore, the utilization of methods for the amplification of target nucleic acids may allow for the attainment of high degrees of assay sensitivity.

The effective management of patients with viral infections depends to a great extent upon the accurate diagnosis of the infection. In addition, viral diagnosis allows for the monitoring of disease frequency in high risk populations and for the efficient distribution of health care resources (ref. 1). Unlike most pathogenic bacteria, viruses are obligate intracellular parasites and require living cells for propagation. The high cost of constructing tissue culture facilities and the expertise required for the maintenance of a sterile environment has, in the past, limited the availability of viral diagnostic testing to centralized laboratories. This limitation has precluded the wide-scale application of viral diagnostic techniques to clinical medicine.

Recently, however, a number of techniques have been devised which allow for the performance of viral diagnosis without the need to isolate virus in in vitro systems. Many of these techniques utilize immunoassay formats which make use of specific interactions between viral antigens and labelled antibodies. While there are many formats which can make use of labelled immunoreactants, most assays for the detection of viral antigens in clinical specimens have made use of a solid phase format in which immunoglobulins are directly linked to the marker molecule (ref. 2). In such formats, an unlabelled anti-viral antibody is immobilized onto the surface of a solid phase. Numerous solid phases can be utilized including the wells of microtiter plates, plastic beads, nylon filters and latex particles. The solid phase antibody is then reacted with the clinical sample. If the sample contains the virus to which the antibody is directed, a portion of the viral protein will bind to the solid phase surface. Extraneous material is removed by means of washing steps which are generally performed with a buffer-containing detergent solution. The washing step is important since it allows the subsequent reactions to be performed under controlled conditions without interference from extraneous materials which might be present in human body fluids. Following this washing step, the immobilized antigen is again reacted with specific anti-viral immunoglobulin. This immunoglobulin can be directly labelled with the marker, in which case the assay is generally referred to as a "direct" immunoassay. Alternately, unlabelled immunoglobulin can be utilized, in which case the binding is quantitated by another reaction in which the unlabelled immunoglobulin is reacted with a second labelled molecule. In such "indirect" immunoassay formats the second reactant can be a labelled molecule capable of recognizing immunoglobulin, such as an anti-species immunoglobulin antibody or a bacterial protein capable of recognizing immunoglobulins of defined species (e.g. Staphylococcal Protein A, Streptococcal Protein G).

A number of labels have been devised which can be coupled to anti-viral immunoglobulins with little, if any, alteration in the ability of the immunoglobulin to couple with viral antigen. Initially, many assays made use of radioactive isotopes as ^{125}I as immunoglobulin markers. Radioactive isotopes have the advantages that they can be efficiently coupled to immunoglobulins and can be measured in low concentrations using equipment available in most laboratories (ref. 3). In fact, immunoassays using radioactive isotopes, generally known as radioimmunoassays or RIAs, have been extremely valuable for the diagnosis of viral antigens, such as hepatitis B, which are evaluated in large numbers in clinical laboratories (ref. 4). However, there are a number of problems associated with the use of RIAs for the detection of viral antigens. Most importantly, the potential biohazard and disposal problems inherent in the use of radioisotopes and the need for instrumentation for assay quantitation make it difficult to utilize RIAs outside of central laboratories. Even in central laboratories, the safety and disposal requirements of radioisotopes impede the use of this form of assay when alternative diagnostic systems are available. Also, the inherent instability of radioisotopes makes it difficult to standardize reagents so that the same activity can be achieved over an extended period of time. Finally, the absolute requirement for instrumentation for the measurement of the radio-labelled immunoglobulin precludes the use of RIAs in situations, such as small clinics, physicians' offices and field sites, in which instruments are difficult to purchase and maintain.

For these reasons there has been a great deal of interest in the development of assays for the detection of viruses which utilize non-isotopic markers. The substitution of non-isotopic markers for radioisotopes allows for the retention of many of the advantages inherent in solid phase radioimmunoassays while avoiding the limitations inherent in the use of radioisotopes.

There are many non-isotopic markers which can be utilized of for the detection of anti-viral immunoglobulin in solid phase systems. Perhaps the most widely used are molecules which possess enzymatic activity (ref. 5). In such cases the reactions are quantitated by the measurement of the amount of product generated following addition of the appropriate enzyme substrate. Enzymes have a number of advantages as reagents for diagnostic immunoassays. These include the fact that enzyme substrate reactions utilizing colorigenic products can be evaluated qualitatively by means of visual inspection or measured quantitatively with simple instrumentation. Also, many enzymes are relatively stable, allowing for assay standardization over extended periods of time. Also, the use of enzyme-substrate systems poses little biohazard risks. Furthermore, assays which utilize enzymatic markers can take advantage of the sensitivity inherent in the fact that single molecules of enzyme can catalyze the reaction of multiple molecules of substrates within a finite period of time. The magnification of the enzyme substrate system can be further enhanced by the use of cycling systems which make use of multiple enzymatic reactions (ref. 6 and 7). However, it should be noted in this regard that the ultimate limitations of the sensitivity of solid phase immunoassays lie in the interactions of the viral antigens with the labelled antibodies rather than in the degree of enzymatic magnification achieved by the enzyme substrate reactions. However, even in cases in which enzymatic magnification does not lead to an increase in ultimate sensitivity, the time required for the attainment of optimal sensitivity can often be diminished substantially. This improvement in speed of performance can be very important in clinical situations in which a rapid result is necessary for clinical decision making and for disease control.

While enzymes offer a number of advantages as markers for viral diagnostic assays, there are a number of problems associated with the co-valent linkage of immunoglobulins to macromolecular enzymes. Such linkage reactions can be difficult to perform in a controlled, reproducible fashion. In addition, immunoglobulins coupled with macromolecules such as enzymes can display suboptimal degrees of antigen-binding kinetics. For these reasons, alternate means for the labelling of immunoglobulin molecules have been devised (ref. 8). For example, immunoglobulins can be labelled with low molecular weight markers and allowed to react with solid phase antigens. Following the completion of the antigen-antibody reaction binding is quantitated by a subsequent reaction with an enzyme-linked marker. While a number of markers can be used for this purpose, the system which has attained the most widespread usage utilizes the vitamin biotin as the immunoglobulin marker. This molecule can be coupled to immunoglobulins by means of a number of chemical reactions which yield enzyme-biotin conjugates with high degrees of antigen-reactivity (ref. 9). The biotin-labelled immunoglobulins are quantitated by reaction with enzyme-labelled avidin, a protein derived from egg white or bacteria with a very high affinity for biotin anb biotin-substituted macromolecules. Alternately, avidin can be reacted with biotin-substituted enzyme to form a biotin-avidin-enzyme complex which is capable of binding to biotin-labelled immunoglobulin. This system combines the advantages of enzyme labelled assays while avoiding some of the problems inherent in the linkage of immunoglobulins with enzymatic molecules. Immunoglobulins can also be labelled with molecules that emit fluorescent, chemiluminescent, or other types of non-isotopic energy. Reactions using such labels can be quantitated without the need for the performance of enzymatic reactions. However, since these systems do not take advantage of enzymatic magnification, they generally require specialized instrumentation for accurate quantitation of low levels of activity.

The above discussion relates to the use of antigen-antibody interactions for the diagnosis of infectious diseases. Recently, systems have been devised for the diagnosis of infectious diseases by the detection of viral DNA or RNA by means of nucleic acid hybridization reactions (ref. 10). The use of hybridization reactions offers a number of advantages for infectious disease diagnosis. These advantages include the inherent sensitivity of nucleotide base-pairing reactions, the defined nature and stability of nucleic acid probes and the ability to test for multiple pathogens under similar conditions. The development of methods fór magnifying the amount of nucleic acids present in a specimen by means of repeated reactions with DNA polymerase or other enzymes allow for the potential measurement of very small amounts of nucleic acids which might be present in a sample (ref. 11). Furthermore, the development of non-isotopic methods for the labelling of nucleic acids allows for the performance of the hybridization reactions without the need for radioactive isotopes, thus avoiding the problems inherent in radioactivity-based assays which are discussed above (ref. 12). However, there are still some problems inherent in the application of hybridization techniques for the practical diagnosis of viral infections. Most importantly, the detection of viral nucleic acids requires that the nucleic acids be extracted from viral surface and nucleocapsid proteins. While this extraction can be accomplished readily in research laboratories, the need for toxic solvents such as phenol and chloroform limits the usefullness of these procedures in clinical laboratories. Furthermore, the specificity of hybridization binding under reaction conditions likely to be encountered in clinical laboratories has not been documented. This is of particular concern since studies have documented non-specific reactions when viral nucleic acid is analyzed in the presence of an excess of irrelevant nucleic acid as might occur in the testing of crude clinical samples. Despite these problems, it is likely that nucleic acid hybridization reactions will come to play a role in the diagnostic armamentarium of the clinical virologist. The nature and extent of this role will be determined, to a great extent, by the finding of practical solutions to these and other problems related to the current protocols for the performance of the hybridization reactions.

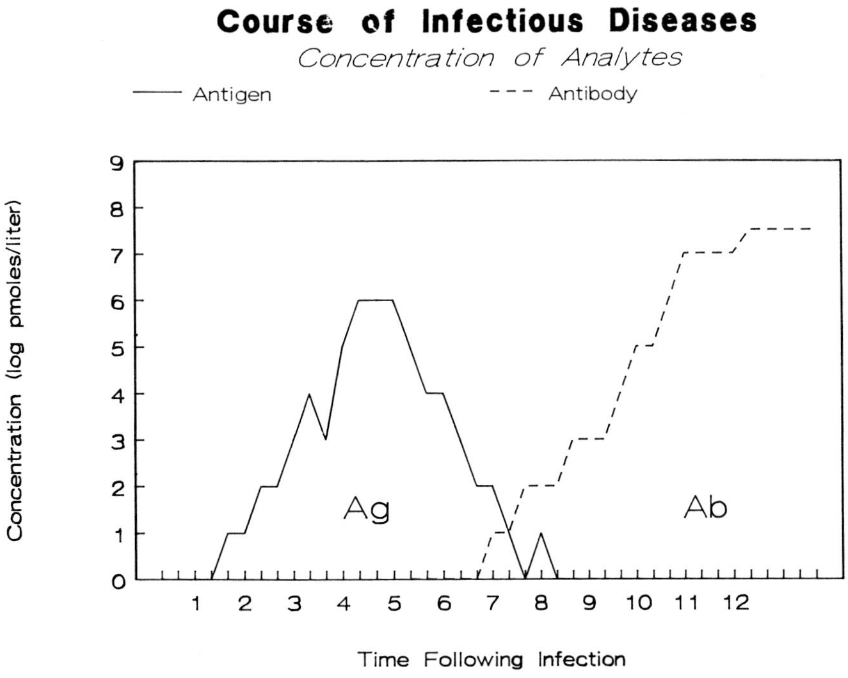

Figure 1: Idealized time course of human infection. See text for detailed description.

One of the most critical areas concerning the usage of assays for the diagnosis of viral infections concerns the question of whether a given assay system has sufficient sensitivity to allow for disease diagnosis. This question is a difficult one to address since the concentrations of virus particles, antigens, nucleic acids and antibodies which are present in the infected body fluid vary during the course of infection. A hypothetical course of a viral infection is presented in figure 1. As can be seen, the initial concentration of virus is quite low due to the fact that the infection is initiated by single or small numbers of organisms. As viral replication occurs, the concentration of virus and detectable viral products increases. However, it should be noted that the increase is not totally regular due to the fact that host factors are functioning at variable levels to inhibit viral replication. In most cases, these host factors will eventually result in a diminution of viral replication with a subsequent decrease in the level of viral products. Due to the kinetic nature of these interactions, this decline will not be regular and transient elevations of detectable viral products can be expected to occur. Finally, the development of an effective host response will be manifested by the attainment of detectable levels of anti-viral antibodies and measurable anti-viral cellular immunity.

This course of infection has a number of implications in terms of assay systems for the diagnosis of viral infections. First of all, it can be seen that it will be easiest to detect viruses and viral products at the height of infection when the concentrations are at their peak. Conversely, it will be difficult to detect any viral product very early in the course of infection, before replication has occurred, and later in the course when viral replication has been inhibited by the host immune response. This phenomenon explains why several different assay systems can be used to detect evidence of viral infection at the peak of replication while few are sufficiently sensitive to allow for detection very early or late in the course of the infection. Assays which display greater degrees of sensitivity will allow for the attainment of an accurate viral diagnosis for relatively greater portions of the overall infectious process. After the host response has been established, few, if any techniques will allow for the direct identification of viral infections. However, serological methods will allow for the retrospective detection of the immune response. It should be noted in this regard that the concentration of antibodies generated in response to infection is generally greater than the maximum level of antigen generated during the course of infection. This fact explains why less sensitive methods can be used for the detection of viral antibodies provided that sufficient time has elapsed since the occurrence of the initial infection.

From the above discussion, it is clear that immunoassays and nucleic acid hybridization reactions will play an ever increasing role in the diagnosis of viral infections. Since a great deal of work is currently being applied to the development and evaluation of immunoassay systems, the optimal format for viral diagnosis remains to be conclusively determined. It is also likely that the nature of the diagnostic tests which will find clinical usage will depend, to a great extent, on the environment in which the testing is performed and the nature of the target viruses. The determination of the efficiency of the individual assays systems will rely on the performance of carefully controlled clinical studies as to the sensitivity and specificity of the systems under actual clinical conditions. The performance of these evaluations will serve to validate some existing tests and, at the same time, stimulate the development of new assay systems. The wide-scale application of practical assay systems for the efficient detection of viral infections should allow for the accurate diagnosis and effective clinical management of patients with viral infections, the control of epidemic diseases, and a worldwide diminution of the morbidity and mortality associated with viral infections.

REFERENCES

1. D Richman, N. Schmidt, S. Plotkin, R. Yolken, M. Chernesky, I. McIntosh and M. Mattheis, Journal of Infectious Diseases, 150, 941-951 (1984).

2. R. Yolken, Review of Infectious Diseases, 4, 35-68 (1982).

3. J.D. Rosenthal, K. Hayashi and A.L. Notkins, Applied Microbiology, 25, 567-573 (1973).

4. N.J. Schmidt, Antiviral Agents and Viral Diseases of Man, 2nd Edition, 179-206 (1984).

5. A. Voller and D. Bidwell, Manual of Clinical Laboratory Immunology (Rose, Friedman and Fahey), 3rd Edition, 99-109 (1986).

6. E. Ishikawa, M. Imagawa and S. Hashide, Immunoenzymatic Techniques (Avrameas, Druet, Masseyeff and Feldman), 219-232 (1983)

7. A. Johannsson, D.H. Ellis, D.L. Bates, A.M. Plumb and C.J. Stanley, Journal of Immunological Methods, 87, 7-11 (1986).

8. T.T. Ngo, International Journal of Biochemistry, 15, 583-590 (1983).

9. R.H. Yolken, R. Viscidi, F. Leister, C. Harris and S-B Wee, Manual of Clinical Laboratory Immunology (Rose, Friedman and Fahey) 3rd Edition, 573-581 (1986).

10. R.P. Viscidi and R.H. Yolken, Molecular and Cellular Probes, 1, 3-14 (1987).

11. R.K. Saiki, D.H. Gelfand, S. Stoffel, S.J. Scharf, R. Higuchi, G.T. Hort, K.B. Mullis, and H.A. Erlich, Science, 239, 487-489 (1988).

12. P.R. Langer, A.A. Waldrop and D.C. Ward, Proceedings of the National Academy of Sciences, USA, 78, 6633-6637 (1981).

Recent development of nucleic acid probes in clinical microbiology

Takayuki Ezaki and Eiko Yabuuchi

Department of Microbiology, Gifu University
School of Medicine, 40 Tsukasa-machi
Gifu, 500 Japan.

Abstract - Nonradioactive DNA-DNA hybridization method in microtiter wells was developped for the routine Single stranded DNAs from 30 reference strains of streptococci, 23 type strains of legionellae, and 37 strains of aerobic gram-negative nonfermenting rods were immobilized in microtiter wells. The microtiter plates thus fixed with reference DNAs were kept at a dried condition before use.

When an organism suspected of belonging to the above reference organism, the DNA was extracted from 1 to1.5 ml of overnight culture broth, within 30 min. The DNA was then immediately labelled with photobiotin within 15 min. The labelled DNA and reference DNAs immobilized in microtiter wells were hybridized for 2 hr. After washing the microplate, biotinylated DNAs in microtiter wells were quantitatively detected with an enzyme, streptavidin conjugated β-D-galactosidase and the substrate,4-methylumbellyferyl-β-D-galactopyranoside.

INTRODUCTION

Quantitative DNA-DNA hybridization is an important technique for the determining genetic relatedness among microorganisms. However, this method requires radioisotopes and involves complex procedures. Thus, the application is limited to research laboratories.

Forster et al.(1) have reported a simple DNA-labelling method which uses photobiotin instead of radioisotope. Since photobiotin bound DNA under visible light within a few minutes, labelling procedures became simple. Detection of photobiotinylated DNA was simplified by availability of commercial streptavidin conjugated β- D-galactosidase.

We selected a fluorogenic substrate, 4-methylumbellyferyl-β-D-galactopyranoside for the quantitative fluorometry. we can list up several advantages to carry out hybridization in microdilution wells. The most advantage of this method is the point to be applicable for the automated identification system .

PREPARATION OF REFERENCE DNA PLATE

Unlabeled single stranded DNAs were suspended in phosphate bufffered saline containing 0.1 M $MgCl_2$. Hundred microliter of each DNA solution was distributed into each microwell and immobilized by the method described before (2).

Table 1. DNA plate for streptococci

1	*S. pyogenes*	ATCC 12344
2	*S. agalactiae*	NCTC 8181
3	*S. equi*	NCTC 9682
4	*S. dysgalactiae*	ATCC 27541
5	*S. canis*	ATCC 43496
6	*S. porcinus*	NCTC 10228
7	*S. iniae*	ATCC 29178
8	*S. suis*	NCTC 10234
9	*S. bovis*	NCFB 597
10	*S. equinus*	ATCC 9821
11	*S. saccharolyticus*	NCFB 2594
12	*S. cecorum*	NCFB 2674
13	*S. pneumoniae*	NCTC 7465
14	*S. oralis*	NCTC 11427
15	*S. mitis*	NCTC 3165
16	*S. sanguis*	ATCC 10556
17	*S. salivarius*	ATCC 7073
18	*S. morbillorum*	ATCC 27824
19	*S. anginosus*	NCTC 10713
20	*S. mutans*	ATCC 25175
21	*S. ratus*	ATCC 19645
22	*S. ferus*	ATCC 33477
23	*S. sobrinus*	ATCC 33478
24	*S. cricetus*	ATCC 19642
25	*S. macacae*	NCTC 11558
26	*S. dwonei*	MFe 28
27	*S. uberis*	NCTC 3858
28	*S. acidominimus*	NCFB 2025
29	*G. hemolysans*	ATCC 10379
30	*A. viridans*	NCTC 8251

Table 2. DNA plate for nonfermenters

			GIFU
1	*Pseudomonas*	*aeruginosa*	274
2	*Pseudomonas*	*stutzeri*	404
3	*Pseudomonas*	*mendocina*	1953
4	*Pseudomonas*	*alcaligenes*	2492
5	*Pseudomonas*	*pseudoalcaligenes*	363
6	*Pseudomonas*	*cepacia*	645
7	*Pseudomonas*	*pickettii*	11738
8	*Pseudomonas*	*diminuta*	657
9	*Pseudomonas*	*vesicularis*	2388
10	*Pseudomonas*	*paucimobilis*	2395
11	*Xanthomonas*	*maltophilia*	2491
12	*Crysemonas*	*luteola*	11360
13	*Flavimonas*	*orizihabitans*	11359
14	*Shewanella*	*putrefaciens*	11744
15	*Pseudomonas*	*fluorescens*	11688
16	*Pseudomonas*	*putida*	1081
17	*Comamonas*	*terrigena*	11739
18	*Comamonas*	*acidovorans*	11501
19	*Comamonas*	*testosteroni*	11737
20	*Acinetobacter*	*calcoaceticus*	1888
21	*Acinetobacter*	*lwoffii*	1951
22	*Acinetobacter*	*baumanii*	11741
23	*Acinetobacter*	*haemolyticus*	11740
24	*Acinetobacter*	*johnsoni*	11743
25	*Acinetobacter*	*junii*	12492
26	*Flavobacterium*	*meningosepticum*	1203
27	*Flavobacterium*	*indologenes*	1347
28	*Flavobacterium*	*breve*	3159
29	*Flavobacterium*	*odoratum*	1357
30	*Flavobacterium*	*thalpophilum*	10877
31	*Sphingobacterium*	*multivorum*	2812
32	*Sphingobacterium*	*spiritivorum*	3101
33	*Sphingobacterium*	*mizutae*	2055
34	*Alcaligenes*	*faecalis*	1056
35	*Alcaligenes*	*xylosoxidans*	543
36	*Alcaligenes*	*denitrificans*	852
37	*Agrobacterium*	*radiobacter*	1950

The microplates immobilized reference DNAs were dried and kept at room temperature before use. Lists of bacterial strains immobilized were shown in Table 1 to Table 3.

SMALL-SCALE DNA PREPARATION FROM UNIDENTIFIED STRAINS

Organisms were firstly suspended in 2 ml of saline and the concentration was adjusted equivalent to McFarland turbidity standard No. 3. 1.5 ml of bacterial suspension was transferred to each Eppendorf tube and precipitated. Streptococci were then suspended in 5mM EDTA,pH 8.0 and lysed with achromopeptidase (2). Legionellae and nonfermenters were suspended in EDTA-saline, pH 8.3 and lysed with sodium dodecyl sulfate as described previously (3,4).

Table 3. DNA plate for legionellae

	Organism		ATCC
1	*Legionella*	*pneumophila*	33152
2	*Legionella*	*bozemanii*	33217
3	*Legionella*	*micdadei*	33218
4	*Legionella*	*dumoffii*	33279
5	*Legionella*	*gormanii*	33297
6	*Legionella*	*longbeachae*	33462
7	*Legionella*	*jordanis*	33623
8	*Legionella*	*oakridgensi*	33761
9	*Legionella*	*wadsworthii*	33877
10	*Legionella*	*feeleii*	35072
11	*Legionella*	*sainthelensi*	35248
12	*Legionella*	*macechernii*	35300
13	*Legionella*	*jamestowniensis*	35298
14	*Legionella*	*rublilucens*	35304
15	*Legionella*	*erythra*	35303
16	*Legionella*	*hackeliae*	35250
17	*Legionella*	*spiritensis*	35249
18	*Legionella*	*parisiensis*	35299
19	*Legionella*	*cherrii*	35252
20	*Legionella*	*steigerwaltii*	35302
21	*Legionella*	*santicrusis*	35301
22	*Legionella*	*anisa*	35292
23	*Legionella*	*islaelensis*	43119

After phenol-chloroform-isoamyl alchohol extraction to remove proteins, DNA containing water phase were precipitated with room-temperature ethanol.
Precipitated DNA were washed with a washing buffer (2) to remove RNA and proteins and precipitated with room-temperature ethanol. This crude DNA was enough for labelling and for hybridization.

PHOTOBIOTINYLATION OF DNA

DNAs thus prepared were labelled with photobiotin under a sunlamp for 15 min as described previously (3). After labelling, extraamount of free photobiotin were removed with 1-butanol.

HYBRIDIZATION AND DETECTION

Labelled DNAs were heat denatured and briefly sonicated.
Hybridization with reference DNAs were carried out for 2 hr in microtiter plate (3).
After hybridization, the microplate was washed and streptavidin-conjugated beta-D-galactosidase was bound to biotinylated DNAs and the enzyme activity of each well was determined after adding a fluorogenic substrate, 4-methylumbellyferyl β-D-galactopyranoside. By this hybridization method, all reference strains immobilized in microdilution wells were clearly diffrentiated.

PRACTICAL IDENTIFICATION OF UNKNOWN ORGANISMS

Clinical strains identified by this microplate-hybridization method. were examplified in Fig. 1.
All 27 legionellae strains isolated from human clinical specimens and envirinmental water could be speciated by this method although most strains (18 strains) were L. pneumophilla . Most strains of streptococci and nonfermenters could be identified by this method, however, some typical strains and also atypical strains failed to hybridize to any DNAs . Homology values of these unidentified strains to any reference strains were less than 60 % by quantitative hybridization. These results indicate that current taxonomy of streptococci and nonfermenters is still not satisfactory.
Johnson (5) suggested that a species should be genetically independent and that the homology values among established species and other species should less

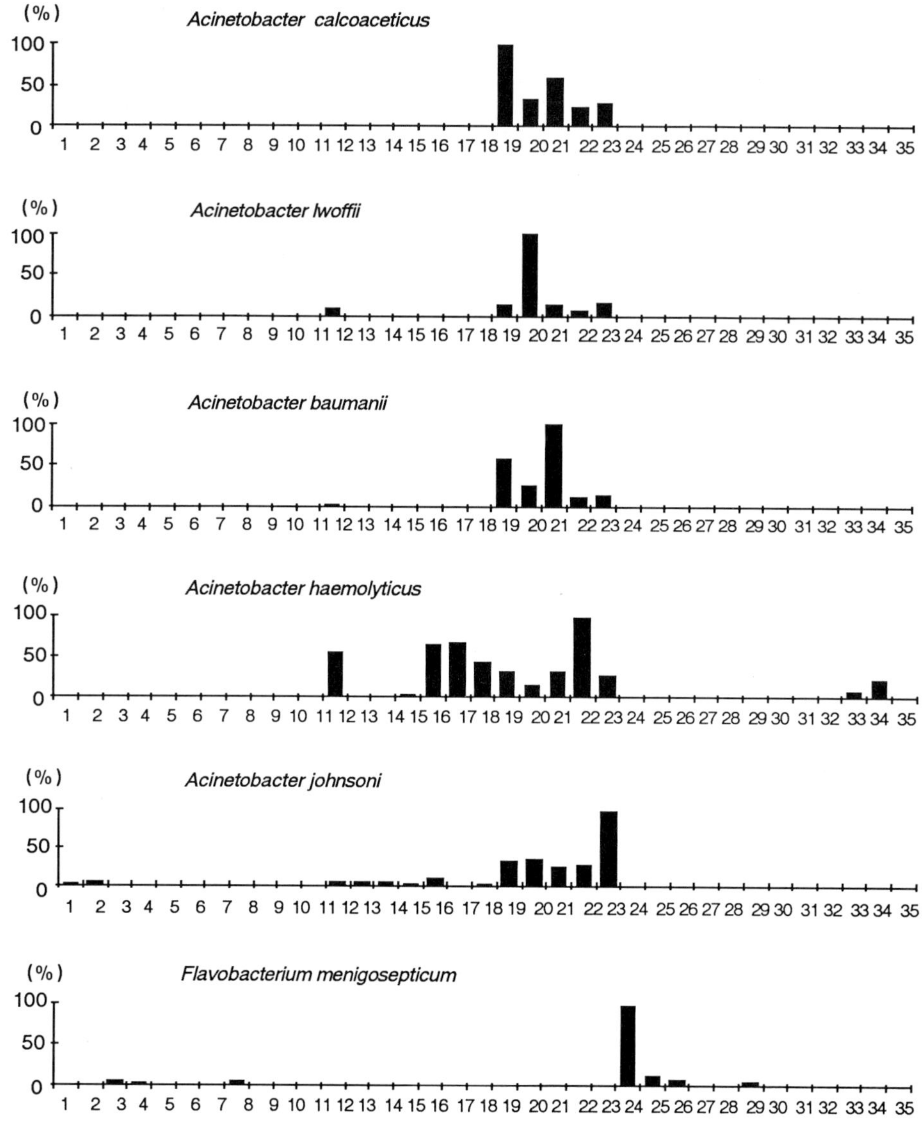

Fig. 1. Practical identification of nonfermenters by microplate hybridization method. Number of holizontal axis is corresponding to the organisms listed in Table 2. Vertical bar indicates relative homology value of each organism when the strongest fluorencence value is calculated as 100 %.

than 60% under optimal condition. However, in medical microbiology, there are many cases in which two genetically closely related species are allowed to exist as independent species only because one species is pathogenic in human and the other is not. We expect that such pathogenic and nonpathogenic organisms should be included in a single species and call the pathogenic strain as "pathovars " . Development of specific DNA probes corresponding to the pathogenic factors are expected for the identification of pathogenic strains .

If bacterial taxonomy is rearranged by Johnson's criteria , our microplate-hybridization method will be an important and decisive tequnique to identify organisms in clinical microbiology.

REFERENCES

1. A. E. Forster, J. L. M cInnes, D. C. Skingle and R. H. Symons. Nucleic Acids Research, 3,745-761 (1985).

2. T. Ezaki, Y. Hashimoto, N. Takeuchi, H. Yammoto, S. L. Liu, H. Miura, K. Matsui, and E. Yabuuchi. J. Clin. Microbiol. 26, 1708-1713 (1988).

3. T. Ezaki, N. Takeuchi, S. L. Liu , A. Kai, H. Yamamoto, and E. Yabuuchi. Microbiol. Immunol. 32, 141-150 (1988).

4. T. Ezaki, S. Dejsirilert, H. Yamamoto, N. Takeuchi, S. L. Liu and E. Yabuuchi . J. Gen. Appl. Microbiol. 34, 191-199 (1988).

5. J. L. Johnson. In Krieg and J. G. Holt (ed) Bergey's Manual of Systematic Bacteriology . Vol 1. William & Wilkins, Baltimore / London. p8-11. (1984).

Molecular diagnosis of rotavirus infection

Osamu Nakagomi and Toyoko Nakagomi

Departments of Laboratory Medicine and of Microbiology, Akita University School of Medicine, Akita 010, Japan

Abstract - Recent advances in molecular biology have captured the attention of clinical microbiologists seeking for new assays which allow in-depth characterization of clinical isolates at molecular level. This paper reviews application of molecular probe technology to the diagnosis and characterization of rotaviruses, the single most important etiologic agent of acute diarrhea worldwide. RNA-RNA hybridization assay not only can predict serotypes but reveals the presence of "genogroups" among rotavirus isolates which may provide a clue to understand transmission and evolution of rotaviruses.

INTRODUCTION

Recent advances in molecular biology suggest that application of techniques originally developed for the analyses of nucleic acids to the diagnosis and characterization of infectious diseases are increasingly practical. Such techniques include: (1) Analysis of nucleic acids by molecular weight, i.e., electrophoresis with or without restriction endonuclease digestion, (2) Analysis by sequence homology, i.e., nucleic acid hybridization, (3) Determination of amino acid sequence deduced from nucleotide sequence, i.e., DNA or RNA sequencing. Improvement and refinement of these techniques not only provide us of alternative detection methods of infectious agents but allow us in-depth characterization of each clinical isolate at molecular level, making it possible to identify the offending microorganism at "strain" level. Sharing such information between clinical microbiologists and clinicians taking care of individual patients will eventually lead to the prevention of disease transmission within hospitals.

Of enteric viral infections, rotavirus has been the major target of extensive research including efforts to develop vaccines against severe diarrheal illness of children under two years of age (ref. 1). This is because a number of studies performed to date clearly indicate that rotavirus is the single most important etiological agent of acute gastroenteritis of the children in both developed and developing regions of the world. In addition to the clinical importance of the disease caused by rotavirus, rotavirus provides materials suitable for the development and evaluation of new assays for virus detection and characterization since a large number of virus particles are excreated in fecal specimens at the acute phase of the disease.

This paper reviews the application of molecular probe technology to the diagnosis and characterization of rotavirus infection. Since detection of viruses or other microorganmisms by molecular probe technology are reviewed elsewhere (ref.2-4, and a few preceding papers in this book), we will focus our attention on further genetic characterization of rotavirus isolates by RNA-RNA hybridization assay and nucleotide sequencing.

ROTAVIRUS

Rotavirus, a member of the family Reoviridae, is a non-enveloped double shelled virus which contains eleven segments of double-stranded (ds) RNA genome. The largest gene segment, approximately 3,300 bp, is referred to as gene 1 and the smallest one, approximately 680 bp, is designated gene 11. Estimated molecular weight of the 11 gene segments is 11 to 14 million daltons and the number of nucleotide base pairs was calculated to be 18,300 bp (ref. 1). Each gene segment encodes one viral protein except gene 8 or 9 (depending on strains) which codes for two outer-capsid glycoproteins [VP7(1) and VP7(2)] that are synthesized by the start of translation in a bicistronic mRNA at two distinct in-frame initiation sites (ref. 5). VP7 at which virus-neutralizing antibodies are directed is a cell attachment protein (ref. 6) and rotavirus serotype is primarily determined by the antigenic specificity of this protein. VP3, hemagglutinin, is also the target of virus-neutralizing antibodies and has been reported to be involved in the process of virus entry into the cell (ref. 7, 8). VP6, the product of the gene 6, bears either subgroup I or II determinant as well as the determinant common to all group A rotaviruses. Immunologic assays, such as enzyme-linked immunosorbent assay, are believed to react mostly with these antigenic determinants. Rotavirus particles contain an endogenous RNA-dependent RNA polymerase. The polymerase is activated by conversion of infectious double-shelled particles into single-shelled particles with chelating agents. This endogenous polymerase synthesizes large amounts of single-stranded (ss) RNA transcripts representing each template RNA genome segment. The RNA probes prepared in this way have been used for hybridization studies (ref. 9-11).

FORMATS FOR HYBRIDIZATON REACTIONS

Two major formats for hybridization reactions i.e., in solution and on a solid support, have successfully applied for rotavirus characterization (ref.9-18). To carry out hybridization in solution, dsRNA from rotavirus strains are denatured, mixed with the radiolabeled probe prepared from a reference strain, and then incubated for at least 16 h at various temperatures (for example, at 65 C for high stringency hybridization and at 52 C for low stringency hybridization). The resulting hybrids are separated on a polyacrylamide gel and are subjected to autoradiography. This assay allows the side-by-side comparison of homology between dsRNA from a given strain and the probes prepared from multiple reference strains. However, the heterologous hybrids do not necessarily comigrate on a gel with the homologous hybrids (hybrid molecules formed by reannealing the radiolabeled transcript and the separated minus strands of the same gene). It is, therefore, not always possible to identify the genes which show homology with those of the reference strain.

The other format which utilizes solid-phase support is often referred to as Northern blot hybridization. To do this, dsRNA from various strains are separated on a polyacrylamide gel, denatured in situ, and then transferred to a filter membrane such as Nylon or DBM paper. Hybridization is allowed to occur between denatured dsRNA fixed on a filter membrane and the radiolabled probe prepared from a reference strain. Since dsRNA fixed on a membrane retains the original electrophoretic mobility on a polyacrylamide gel, identification of each of the 11 gene segments after hybridization is possible. In addition, it is convenient to examine sequence homology between many isolates and a given single probe simultaneously, but not multiple probes. A low stringency condition used in this assay is 52 C in the absence of formamide and a high stringency condition is 52 C in the presence of 50% formamide. The former condition is reported to detect up to 34% of base mismatches and the latter condition is reported to detect up to 8% base mismatches (ref. 17).

As to types of probes used in these hybridization studies, transcript probes (ref. 9-15), random primed cDNA probes (ref. 16-18) and cloned cDNA probes (ref. 19-21) have been reported. Transcript probes can be made easily with the endogenous RNA-dependent RNA polymerase, if purified single-shelled particles are available. In addition, ssRNA transcripts prepared in this way faithfully represent each of the 11 genomic RNA segments. Random primed cDNA probes can also be prepared with ease and may be less labor-intensive. However, the cDNA reverse transcription of the genome segments is not equimolar; therefore, the absolute differences in the intensities of hybridization signals observed on the blots cannot be precisely correlated with degrees of sequence homology (ref. 4). Finally, cloned cDNA probes are recently available with the successful cloning of increasing number of rotavirus genes. The use of cDNA clones has obvious advantage over the others, such as feasibility of preparing large amount of probes and possible feasibility of using gene-specific probes if such clones are available.

IDENTIFICATION OF ROTAVIRUS SEROTYPE BY RNA-RNA HYBRIDIZATION

Four distinct serotypes of human rotavirus have been identified by several techniques, including plaque-reduction neutralization assay (ref. 22), enzyme-linked immunosorbent assay with serotype-specific monoclonal antibodies (ref. 23-25), and solid-phase immune electron microscopy (ref. 26). Recently it was shown that RNA-RNA hybridization using single human rotavirus gene substitution reassortants as probes can provide an alternative method for identifying the serotype of stool rotaviruses (ref. 15) These reassortants contained only the VP7 gene of their human rotavirus parent (representing serotypes 1, 2, 3, or 4), and the remaining 10 genes were derived from their bovine rotavirus strain UK parent. The rationales for this assay are as follows: (1) A high degree of homology is observed among the VP7 genes of a same serotype but not among the corresponding genes from different serotypes. (2) The probe made from the bovine rotaviru s UK strain does not hybridize to the corresponding genes of human rotaviruses. It is, therefore, possible to predict the serotype of a given strain, if dsRNA extracted from that stool specimen is hybridized to each of the probes made from single human rotavirus VP7 gene substitution reassortants representing serotypes 1 through 4. If, for example, a hybrid band is formed between a given strain and the serotype 3 probe, it is indicated that this strain belongs to serotype 3. Actually, genomic RNAs extracted directly from stool specimens of children with rotavirus diarrhea formed a hybrid specifically with the VP7 gene of only one of the four reassortant probes, indicating that they belonged to that particular serotype.. Then, what is the advantages of this assay over ELISA with serotype-specific monoclonal antibodies? Application of these ELISA to the epidemiological studies has revealed the presence of rotavirus strains that escape the recognition by the panels of serotype-specific monoclonal antibodies. These viruses could represent either new serotypes or naturally occurring antigenic variants. Coulson (ref. 27) has described the existence of serotype 1 rotaviruses with various reactivity patterns with three different serotype 1-specific momoclonal antibodies and has proposed that these variants be designated monotypes. Serotyping by RNA-RNA hybridization can circumvent such problems encountered by certain monoclonal antibodies, although the hybridization assay is not as practical as serotyping ELISA. In addition, this method should help identify new serotypes, since viruses exhibiting a new VP7 antigen should fail to hybridize to any of the four reassortant rotavirus probes.

PREDICTION OF HUMAN ROTAVIRUS SEROTYPE BY NUCLEOTIDE SEQUENCE ANALYSIS OF THE VP7 GENE

Studies on serotyping based on the sequence relatedness of the VP7 genes have recently been extended by direct sequence analysis of the VP7 gene transcripts with synthetic oligonucleotide primers (ref. 28). Two regions, nucleotides 307 through 351 and 670 through 711, corresponding to amino acids 87 through 101 and 288 through 221, respectively, of the VP7 gene was chosen to be sequenced, since each of these two regions codes for a discrete cluster of amino acids in VP7 which are conserved within a serotype but are divergent among serotypes. The ssRNA transcripts were prepared from rotaviruses partially purified either directly from stool material or after a few passages in tissue culture. Dideoxynucleotide sequencing of rotavirus RNA was performed with two synthetic oligonucleotides, 5'CCATTGGATTACACAAC-CATTC3' and 5'GCTACGTTTTCTCTTGGTCC3', targetted to nucleotides downstream from each of the two divergent regions. The nucleotide and amino acid sequences for each field strain in the two divergent regions are compared with the sequences of reference strains representing human rotavirus serotypes 1 through 4. The serotype of each field strain could be predicted by identifying the reference strain to which the sequence of the two divergent regions of that field strain showed the greatest identity. The predicted serotype from the sequence analysis correlated in each of 35 cases with the serotype determined by plaque reduction neutralization assay or ELISA with serotype-specific monoclonal antibodies. It is, therefore, possible to predict the serotype of a rotavirus isolate by direct sequence analysis of its VP7 gene. Although sequence analysis may not be a practical method for routine typing in most diagnostic laboratories, comparison of the sequences with the reference strains will reveal at the molecular level whether the strain is a variant or a new serotype.

IDENTIFICATION OF ROTAVIRUS GENOGROUP BY RNA-RNA HYBRIDIZATION

We have reviewed the application of molecular probe technology to such fields of rotavirus diagnosis and characterization that can be approached by other methods. In this section, we will discuss molecular characterization of rotavirus genes which is possible only by RNA-RNA hybridization and propose "genogroup" classification based on the sequence relatedness among rotavirus strains.

RNA-RNA hybridization studies, using ssRNA transcripts as probes, have revealed two major human rotavirus families; one includes strains related to the prototype strain Wa (serotype 1, subgoup II) family, and the other includes strains related to the prototype strain DS-1 (serotype 2, subgroup I) family (ref. 9-11). Interestingly, these two families correspond to two distinct electropherotypes of viral RNA, i.e., "long" patterns (faster-moving 10th and 11th gene segments) and "short" pattens (slower-moving 10th and 11th gene segments). Furthermore, until recently, short and long patterns were believed to be associated with subgroup I or II specificity, respectively (ref. 29-32).

Eariler, in 1982, we isolated a novel rotavirus strain designated AU-1 from a child with acute gastroenteritis. The AU-1 strain was interesting in that it possessed a long RNA pattern yet belonged to subgroup I (ref. 33). Genetic studies utilizing RNA-RNA hybridization in solution at high stringency revealed that the AU-1 strain did not belong to either the Wa or the DS-1 family (ref. 14). Since animal rotaviruses have long RNA patterns and the majority belong to subgroup I, it was concluded that the AU-1 strain might be an animal rotavirus that had infected a human.

Recently, a few groups of investigators including ourselves have reported the presence of human rotaviruses similar to the AU-1 strain in that they have long RNA patterns yet belong to subgroup I (ref. 34-36). Although only one of such strains (the AU228 strain isolated by us) has been subjected to RNA-RNA hybridization, it appears that these strains belong to the AU-1 group of rotaviruses (Fig. 1). We, therefore, predict the presence of the third group of human rotavirus families. Since the presence of "family" within a "genus" (Rotavirus) does not conform to the taxonomic hierarchy, we propose that the grouping of rotavirus strins based on the genetic relatedness be designated "genogroup" (Fig. 2).

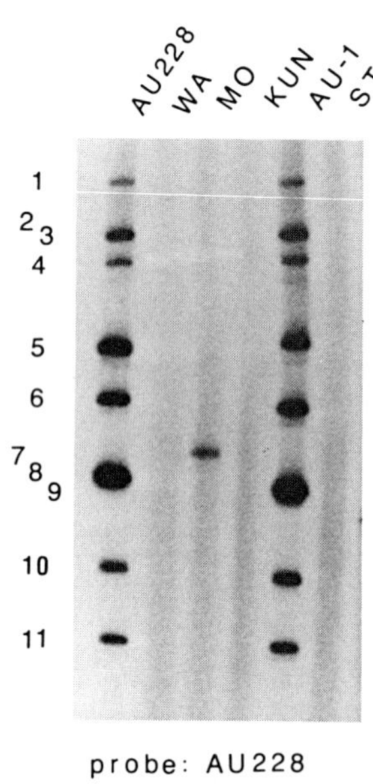

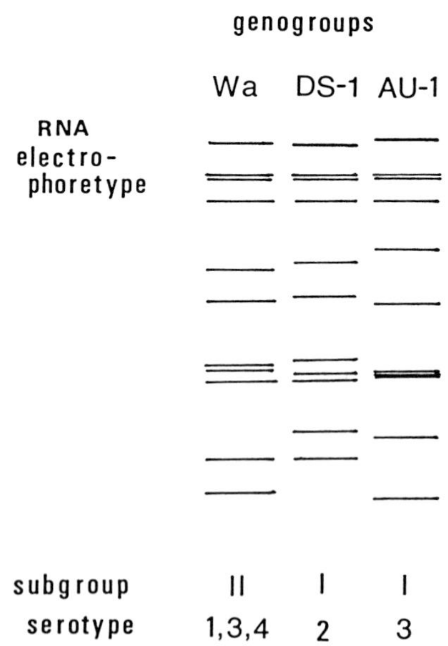

Fig. 1 (left). A hybridization pattern obtained between the AU228 probe and human rotavirus prototypes, Wa (serotype 1), MO (serotype 3), KUN (serotype 2), AU-1 (serotype 3) and ST3 (serotype 4).
Fig. 2 (right). Rotavirus genogroups and their relation to electrophoretypes, subgroups and serotypes.

To examine whether genogroups occur within rotavirus strains recovered from the same animal species other than humans, the probe prepared from the bovine rotavirus NCDV was hybridized to the genomic RNAs from bovine rotavirus strains which represent three distinct bovine rotavirus serotypes. All of these strains have high degree of homology with the NCDV strains (our unpublished observation). Furthermore, any of the three bovine serotypes did not show significant homology with four human rotavirus serotypes (our unpublished observation). These result indicate that bovine rotavirus belong to a single genogroup which is distinct from human genogroups.

Identification of genogroups of rotavirus isolates and quest for animal rotavirus strains that share genogroup with novel human rotavirus such as the AU-1 strain will provide a clue to find the evidence of interspecies transmission of animal rotavirus to humans and to understand genetic evolution of rotaviruses in nature.

CONCLUSION

Rapid detection of fastidious microorganisms with high sensitivity and specificity is definitely of vital importance in clinical microbiology and for this goal the molecular probe technology is expected to give a great impact. The importance of in-depth characterization of clinical isolates, however, should not be underestimated. The improvement and refinement of gene technology for application in clinical microbiology make possible the genetic characterization of the clinical isolates which used to be possible only at advanced research laboratories. Hopefully, in the near future, such techniques will be incorporated into the workflow of most of the clinical laboratories. Accumulation of knowledge obtained through such technology will provide a new perspective for the control and prevention of infectious diseases in humans.

REFERENCES

1. A.Z. Kapikian and R.M. Chanock, Virology, p.863-906, Raven Press, New York (1985).
2. R.H. Yolken, Mol. Cell. Probes 2, 87-96 (1988).
3. F.C. Tenover, Clin. Microbiol. Rev. 1, 82-101 (1988).
4. M.K. Estes and T. Tanaka, DNA Probes for Infectious Diseases, CRC Press, in press.
5. W.K. Chan, M.E. Penaranda, S.E. Crawford and M.K. Estes, Virology, 151, 243-252 (1986).
6. M. Sabara, J.E. Gilchrist, G.R. Hudson and L.A. Babiuk, J. Virol. 53, 58-66 (1985).
7. K.T. Kaljot, R.D. Shaw, D.H. Rubin and H.B. Greenberg, J. Virol. 62, 1136-1144 (1988).
8. N. Fukuhara, O. Yoshie, S. Kitaoka and t. Konno, J. Virol. 62, 2209-2218 (1988).
9. J. Flores, J. Myslinski, A.R. Kalica, H.B. Greenberg, R.G. Wyatt, A.Z. Kapikian and R.M. Chanock, J. Virol. 43, 1032-1037 (1982).
10. J. Flores, Y. Hoshino, E. Boeggeman, R. Purcell, R.M. Chanock and A.Z. Kapikian, Arch. Virol. 87, 273-285 (1986).
11. J. Flores, I. Perez-Schael, E. Boeggeman, L. White, M. Perez, R. Purcell, Y. Hoshino, K. Midthun, R.M. Chanock and A.Z. Kapikian, J. Med. Virol. 17, 135-143 (1985).
12. J. Flores, K. Midthun, Y. Hoshino, K. Green, M. Gorziglia, A.Z. Kapikian and R.M. Chanock, J. Virol. 60, 972-979 (1986).
13. K. Midthun, J. Valdesuso, Y. Hoshino, J. Flores, A.Z. Kapikian and R.M. Chanock, J. Clin. Microbiol. 25, 295-300 (1987).
14. O. Nakagomi, T. Nakagomi, Y. Hoshino, J. Flores and A.Z. Kapikian, J. Clin. Microbiol. 25, 1159-1164 (1987).
15. K. Midthun, J. Flores, K. Taniguchi, S. Urasawa, A.Z. Kapikian and R.M. Chanock, J. Clin. Microbiol. 25, 1269-1274 (1987).
16. J.E. Street, M.C. Croxon, W.F. Chadderton and A.R. Bellamy, J. Virol. 43, 369-378 (1982).
17. B.A. Schroeder, J.E. Street, J. Kalmakoff and A.R. Bellamy, J. Virol. 43, 379-385 (1982).
18. T. Tanaka, M.E. Conner, D.Y. Graham and M.K. Estes, Arch. Virol. 98, 253-265 (1988).
19. S. Pedley and M.A. McCrae, J. Virol. Meth. 9, 173-181 (1984).
20. D.H. Dimitrov, D.Y. Graham and M.K. Estes, J. Infect. Dis. 152, 293-300

(1985).
21. M. Lin, M. Imai, A.R. Bellamy, N. Ikegami, Y. Furuichi, D. Summers, D.L. Nuss and R. Deibel, J. Virol., 55, 509-512 (1985).
22. R.G. Wyatt, H.D. James, Jr., A.L. Pittman, Y. Hoshino, H.B. Greenberg, A.R. Kalica, J. Flores and A.Z. Kapikian, J. Clin. Microbiol. 18, 310-317 (1983).
23. B.S. Coulson, L.E. Unicomb, G.A. Pitson and R.F. Bishop, J. Clin. Microbiol. 25, 509-515 (1987).
24. R. Heath, C. Birch and I. Gust, J. Gen. Virol. 67, 2455-2466, 1986.
25. K. Taniguchi, T. Urasawa, Y. Morita, H.B. Greenberg and S. Urasawa, J. Infect. Dis. 155, 1159-1166 (1987).
26. G. Gerna, N. Passarani, A. Sarasini and M. Battglia, J. Infect. Dis. 152, 1143-1151 (1985).
27. B.S. Coulson, Virology, 159, 209-216 (1987).
28. K.Y. Green, J.F. Sears, K. Taniguchi, K. Midthun, Y. Hoshino, M. Gorziglia, K. Nishikawa, S. Urasawa, A.Z. Kapikian, R.M. Chanock and J. Flores, J. Virol. 62, 1819-1823 (1988).
29. A. Kalica, H.B. Greenberg, R.T. Espejo, J. Flores, R.G. Wyatt, A.Z. Kapikian and R.M. Chanock, Infect. Immun. 33, 958-961 (1981).
30. T. Kutsuzawa, T. Konno, H. Suzuki, T. Ebina and N. Ishida, Microbiol. Immunol. 26, 271-273 (1982).
31. L. Svensson, I. Uhnoo, M. Grandien and G. Wadell, J. Med. Virol. 18, 101-111 (1986).
32. L. White, I. Perez, M. Perez, B. Urbina, H. Greenberg, A. Kapikian and J. Flores, J. Clin. Microbiol. 19, 516-520 (1984).
33. O.Nakagomi, T. Nakagomi, H. Oyamada and T. Suto, J. Med. Virol. 17, 29-34 (1985).
34. A.D. Steele and J.J. Alexander, J. Med. Virol. 24, 321-327 (1988).
35. Y. Aboudy, I. Shif, I. Zilberstein and T. Gotlieb-Stematsky, J. Med. Virol, 25, 351-359 (1988).
36. T. Nakagomi, K. Katsushima and O. Nakagomi, Ann. Inst. Pasteur/Virol. 139, 295-300.

Technological trends of the modern hemostasis laboratory

Jeanine M. Walenga, Ph.D.

Department of Pathology, Loyola University Medical Center, Maywood, IL 60153, USA

Abstract - Current health trends point to increasing illnesses and deaths due to atherosclerosis, myocardial infarction, pulmonary embolism, venous thrombosis and other vascular disorders. These disorders are either from a direct cause or as a consequence of another disease state, eg. cancer, immune disorders. The evaluation of the hemostatic system has thus grown from a focus on hypocoagulation of blood to additionally encompass hyper(pro)coagulation, thrombolysis, cellular and vascular involvement with more target-specific therapeutic and prophylactic treatments. To fill these medical needs, the type and number of assays performed for patient work-ups has expanded to include global screening assays, whole blood analysis, and specific assays of factors, activators, inhibitors and cellular release products from the coagulation system, the fibrinolytic system, platelets and endothelium. Drug monitoring is also becoming more specialized. Incorporation of new technical developments which have made these assays feasible are synthetic substrates, ELISA and RIA. These methods allow for more biochemically defined systems and thus a more sensitive and specific analytical approach than provided by the earlier techniques. The commonly used coagulant and electrophoretic techniques will, however, remain in the lab. To accommodate the new techniques, many single detector instruments for both old and new assay techniques are rapidly becoming available in both manual and automated modes. Physicians's office testing, STAT analysis, panel profiling of disease states and individual instruments with multiple probes to perform coagulant, amidolytic and ELISA assays have also become available. The future hemostasis laboratory will be greatly expanded over the clotting laboratory of the past with highly specific and sensitive automated assays of all components of the hemostatic system.

INTRODUCTION

Thrombotic disorders, whether directly acquired of associated with another disease, are a major health hazard. In 1985 the National Institutes of Health estimated that venous thromboembolism accounted for 300,000 hospitalizations and 50,000 deaths in the USA alone. An in-depth assessment of the individual parameters of coagulation, fibrinolysis, platelets, and endothelium may help alleviate many of these complications (ref. 1,2,3).

Different scientific disciplines have contributed to a clearer understanding of the hemostatic mechanisms (ref. 4,5). It is now accepted that the prothrombin time (PT) and APTT are valid screening assays, but a new molecular approach can provide more specific and sensitive, thorough evaluation of hemostasis. Technologies are now available for biochemical analysis of individual activators, inhibitors, and early physiological markers of activation in hemostatic systems (ref. 6). Application of these concepts will provide the clinical laboratory with the ability to clinically diagnose and therapeutically intervene and monitor thrombosis at a more effective level (ref. 7).

Although important to the evaluation of coagulation, early assay developments focused only on clotting, with no direct evaluation of fibrinolysis or the full role of platelets. Emphasis was placed on bleeding disorders, with no concern for hyper(pro)coagulability. From 1970 through the early 1980's an explosion in the area of biochemical and molecular evaluation of specific individual components of the hemostatic system (Table I) occurred. In fact, hemostasis is no longer regarded merely as an independent system of clotting but rather as a general host response that, when uncontrolled, may contribute to the pathophysiology of inflammatory reactions, heart disease and cancer.

In addition to the activation and inhibition enzymes, low molecular weight peptides and other substances such as prostaglandins that specifically define the initial stages of coagulant, fibrinolytic, or platelet activation or endothelial function were identified (ref. 8). Antithrombotic, fibrinolytic and antiplatelet therapies came into being which could now be effectively monitored by these newer techniques.

TABLE I

RELATED SYSTEMS OF HEMOSTASIS

Blood coagulation (activators and inhibitors)
Blood cellular elements
Fibrinolysis (activators and inhibitors)
Endothelium/sub-endothelium
Complement
Eicosanoids
Inorganic ions
Other (viscosity, fluid dynamics)

ASSAY TECHNIQUES FOR HEMOSTASIS

Coagulant
Synthetic substrate
Immunologic: RID, RIA, EIA, ELISA, EIP
Platelet function

Current methodology developments have combined biochemical, immunologic, and physical techniques with colorimetric, radiochemical, and physical endpoint detection (Table I). Adaptation of these new techniques to automated instrumentation has been proven to be feasible. Many newer tests are commercially available as manual kits adaptable to clinical chemistry instrumentation. A spectrophotometer is required for enzymatic assays, and a gamma or beta counter or microtiter plate system is required for immunologic assays. Centrifugal, solid-phase, flow analyzers, dry chemistry, kinetic analyzers and immunoanalytic instruments including flow cytometry currently have hemostatic applications (Table II).

TABLE II

INSTRUMENTATION FOR HEMOSTASTIC TESTING

TYPE	DETECTOR	APPLIED TECHNIQUES
Clot analyzers	Visible light, mechanical	Coagulant
Platelet analyzers	Microscopic, aggregometer, flow cytometry	Platelet function, antibody detection
Centrifugal analyzers	Visible light, nephelometric, fluorescent light	Synthetic substrate, coagulant, immunologic
Kinetic analyzers	Visible light	Synthetic substrate
Solid-phase analyzers	Visible or fluorescent light, refraction	Synthetic substrate, immunologic
Laser or rate nephelometers	Immunoprecipitation	Immunologic
Electrophoresis	-	Immunologic
Microtiter plate systems	Visible light	Enzyme immunoassay, synthetic substrate
Gamma or beta counters	Radioactivity	Radioimmunoassay
Multiprobe	Visible light or laser	Synthetic substrate, coagulant, immunologic

Most recently the developments in hemostatic testing have led to the concepts of multiprobe instruments capable of performing any one of the three basic laboratory technologies, reagent coated tubes for STAT analysis (eg., AT III), the use of microtiter plates for synthetic substrate microanalysis and the incorporation of dry chemistry for a "dip stick" approach to analysis.

DEVELOPMENT OF LABORATORY TECHNIQUES

Coagulant Techniques

The basic coagulation assays are clot-based methods that employ the coagulant enzyme cascade and a fibrin endpoint. The PT and APTT are global methods that provide a generalized approach. Thus these assays provide basic clinical information on the overall function of the coagulant system. The utility of these assays has been proven by their long years of continued use in both research and clinical laboratories. The coagulant technique has also been applied for the measurement of specific coagulant factors, recently including protein C. The PT, APTT and other coagulant assays can also be used for heparin and warfarin monitoring.

Clotting assays were originally performed in glass by a "tilt-tube" technique and visual clot endpoint detection. Although inherently error-prone and highly subjective, the tilt-tube technique could be consistently performed by trained technicians. One of the first instruments developed to replace the tilt-tube in the late 1950s was the BBL Fibrometer (Becton Dickinson and Co., Rutherford, NJ). This semiautomated clot timer employs an electromechanical detector of clot formation which, because of its versatility and reproducibility, has become the mainstay of many coagulation laboratories. In the 1970s, semiautomated and fully automated optical clot detectors were introduced. These instruments detect a change in light transmission upon fibrin polymerization and have been satisfactorily dedicated for PT and APTT analyses. Organon Teknika Corp. (Parsippany, NJ), Lancer, a division of Sherwood Medical Industries (St. Louis, MO), Medical Laboratory Automation, Inc. (Mt. Vernon, NY) and Ortho Diagnostic Systems, Inc. (Raritan, NJ), are established manufacturers of these instruments.

Other clot-based instruments employ the concept of viscoelastic changes in whole blood or plasma as coagulation/fibrinolysis occurs. The Thrombelastograph (Hellige GmbH, Freiburg im Briesgau, W. Germany) and the Sonoclot (Sienco, Inc., Morrison, CO) kinetically measure clot formation. The Hemachron (International Technidyne Corp., Metuchen, NJ) and the Hepcon (HemoTec, Inc., Englewood, CO) are used for monitoring heparin by a viscomagnetic detector and an optical detector, respectively.

The current trend in coagulation instrumentation is to incorporate automated steps to pipet plasma directly from blood collection tubes and to evaluate the coagulation of whole blood in both laboratory instrumentation and easy-to-operate in-home or physicians's office testing devices. Most recently, the concept of multiple probes within one instrument has been developed for detection of coagulant, chromogenic (color), and immunologic assay endpoints. These techniques and instruments will be described.

Synthetic Substrate Techniques

Since clot-based assays rely on an intact coagulation system and fibrin formation, these techniques often require multiple assay steps to ensure an accurate measure of individual proteins. Certain assays have been found to suffer from nonlinearity due to the presence of fibrin degradation products (FDPs) which caused false results.

Synthetic substrate technology may be used to measure procoagulants, activated coagulants, coagulant cofactors, and protease inhibitor activities (ref. 9). This technology has been most successfully applied to protease inhibitors because the prior techniques were tedious, nonspecific and qualitative. Commercially available kits for assays are available from Diagnostica Stago (Asnieres, France), Boehringer Mannheim Diagnostics Division (Mannheim, W. Germany) and KabiVitrum (Stockholm, Sweden). These assays are unaffected by FDPs, fibrinogen concentration or the activity of other procoagulants. In general, synthetic substrate assays include fewer variables, fewer sources of error, and less speculation as to the identification of the analyte.

The principle of action of synthetic substrates, illustrated in Fig. 1, is where a synthetic amino acid sequence is recognized by an enzyme as the natural active site where it cleaves the peptide bond. For example, the natural substrate of thrombin, fibrinogen, has the following amino acid sequence at its cleavage site: Phe-X_7-Val-Arg-Gly-Pro-Arg. An appropriate synthetic chromogenic substrate has the sequence CBz-Gly-Pro-Arg-pNA (Chromozym TH, Pentapharm, Basel, Switzerland). The tripeptide sequence is coupled at the carboxyl end to the optically active (405 nm), chemically stable, chromophore para-nitroaniline (pNA). The enzyme (in this case thrombin) cleaves the bond between the amino acid and the pNA, releasing the pNA tag. Fluorescent tags may be preferred over chromogenic tags for their higher level of sensitivity, particularly when enzyme concentrations are excessively low.

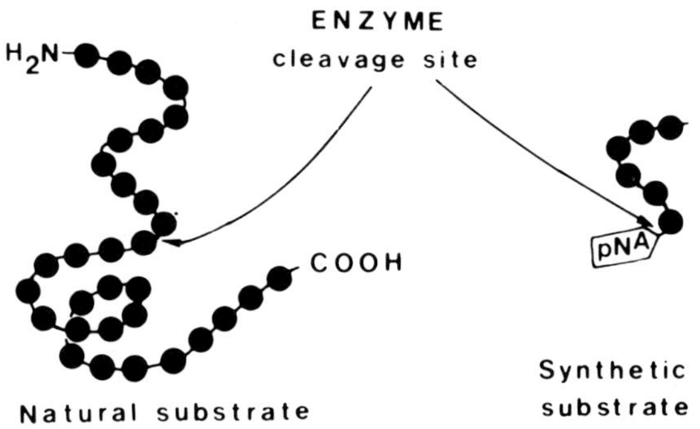

Fig. 1. The synthetic substrate mimics the enzymatic active site of the natural physiologic substrate, thereby providing a readily accessible reagent for sensitive and specific enzymatic analysis. The release of a chromophore, paranitroaniline (pNA), due to enzymatic cleavage produces a color that is easily quantitated (ref. 6).

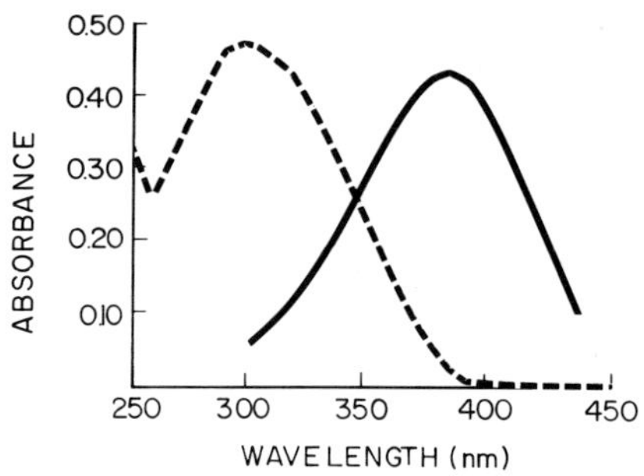

Fig. 2. Absorbance spectra of 0.25nM native substrate and free pNA. Because of the action of a serine protease on the substrate, the liberated pNA produces a shift in the peak absorbance compared to that of the native (coupled) substrate-pNA. Quantitation of free pNA is easily performed at 405nm, where no interference from the native substrate occurs.

Since the optical characteristics of the free tag are significantly different from those of the native substrate (Fig. 2), it is feasible to quantify enzymatic activity based on changes in optical density. These assays can be measured kinetically during the initial phases of the reaction or by an endpoint technique. In the latter technique, acetic acid is used to quench or stop the reaction after a specified time prior to measuring the reaction. The scheme below represents a general sequence of the biochemical reaction.

$$\underset{\text{(Achromogenic)}}{\text{Bz-CO-Phe-Val-Arg-pNA}} \xrightarrow{\text{Serine protease}} \underset{\text{(Chromogenic)}}{\text{Bz-CO-Phe-Val-Arg-OH + pNA}}$$

The schemes below illustrate the various general enzymatic reactions with synthetic substrates employed in the quantification of hemostatic parameters.

Proenzyme (indirect) assay: measures either proenzyme or activator activity level by measuring the generated enzyme.

1. Proenzyme $\xrightarrow{\text{Activator}}$ Enzyme
2. R-pNA $\xrightarrow{\text{Enzyme}}$ R-COOH + pNA

Enzyme (direct assay): directly quantitates the activity of an enzyme.

1. R-pNA $\xrightarrow{\text{Enzyme}}$ R-COOH + pNA

Inhibitor assay: quantitates the activity level of an endogenous inhibitor against exogenously added purified enzyme.

1. Enzyme + inhibitor ——— Enzyme-inhibitor complex + residual enzyme
2. R-pNA $\xrightarrow{\text{Residual enzyme}}$ R-COOH + pNA

Cofactor assay: quantitates the activity level of a cofactor normally present to enhance the rate of an enzymatic reaction.

1. Proenzyme $\xrightarrow{\text{Cofactor and activator}}$ Enzyme
2. R-pNA $\xrightarrow{\text{Enzyme}}$ R-COOH + pNA

Automated instrumentation designed for clinical chemistry testing can often be adapted to carry the synthetic substrate assays of hemostasis (Table II). More recently, dedicated instruments for hemostatic testing, application to microsystems (e.g., microtiter plate) and multiprobe instrumentation are under development.

The aca (E.I. DuPont de Nemours & Co., Inc., Wilmington, DE), originally designed for chemistry parameter analysis, has the capability of also performing plasminogen, AT III, fibrinogen, FDP and heparin determinations. This instrument uses individually assembled test packs for discrete sample analysis. These packs contain reagents in tablet form and are marked with a binary code that signals a microprocessor control. Under the direction of the microprocessor, the test pack is automatically filled with designated quantities of sample and diluent; the reaction proceeds according to design, and the results are determined photometrically.

The Hitachi 717 System (Boehringer Mannheim, Indianapolis, IN) is a selective, discrete multichannel kinetic analyzer that has been successfully adapted with many synthetic substrate assays for hemostatic testing. Due to its random access mode, STAT testing and assay flexibility are possible.

The FP-910 Coagulation Analyzer (Labsystems, Inc., Helsinki, Finland) is a unique, semi-automated, microprocessor controlled multiprobe instrument system. It is compatible with spectrophotometric, enzyme-linked immunosorbent assay and coagulant technologies. It simultaneously pipets or measures nine test samples in a cuvette block and measures them by vertical photometry. It is flexible, easy to use, economical, and compatible with commercial reagents for any assay and allows high throughput (150-200 tests/hr).

The concept of centrifugal analysis was to design an automated instrument, not based on continuous flow, in which analyses could be performed in parallel and computer interfaced. The basic concept is of a radial block of cuvettes rotating through a stationary light beam, in which absorbance readings are taken. A typical rotor contains twenty cuvettes and rotates at approximately 500 rpm, taking a reading every 100 ms. The major advantage to this system is the apparent simultaneous analysis of blank and test samples, allowing minimal electronic noise or signal shift between samples.

Individual cuvettes consist of at least two separate compartments divided by a dam separating reagents and test samples until centrifugal force causes them to mix. Mixing is completed in seconds, and data acquisition can begin just seconds after initiation of the reaction. The results may be photometric, fluorimetric, or turbidimetric and may be measured kinetically or by endpoint analysis. The Cobas Bio (Roche Inc., Nutley, NJ) and the Instrumentation Laboratory, Inc. (Lexington, MA) offer centrifugal analyzers.

The centrifugal analyzer has become a popular instrument for automated synthetic substrate assays. The most recent development in centrifugal analysis has been the ACL (Instrumentation Laboratory, Inc.). This instrument automatically performs both traditional clotting assays and synthetic substrate assays. Calibration and quality control programs are also automated and data can be stored in the instrument memory. The ACL is currently programmed for PT, APTT and fibrinogen (individual or simultaneous testing), as well as factor assays (individual or simultaneous profiling), heparin, AT III, plasminogen and α2-antiplasmin.

The concept of dry chemistry in which reagents are impregnated on a special paper has been introduced in clinical chemistry for analyte quantitation and therapeutic drug monitoring. Hemostatic testing has used a similar technique for the measurement of factor VIII:ag and several other parameters with the FIAX System (International Diagnostic Technology, Santa Clara, CA). This technique utilizes fluorescence to detect antigen-antibody complexes from a reaction on a test strip. Other "dipstick" and reagent coated tube systems which only require the addition of a diluted plasma sample (Coacute, KabiVitrum) for STAT analysis are currently under development.

<u>Immunologic Techniques</u>

Immunologic assays measure antigenically characterized protein without regard to the functionality of the protein. These immunoassays measure the concentration of proteins in nanogram per milliliter and picogram per milliliter ranges exceeding the sensitivity of synthetic substrate and coagulant techniques which measure in the milligram and microgram per milliliter ranges. Immunoassays are based on antigen-antibody reactions, in which the antigen is the substance to be analyzed (analyte) and the reactant is an antibody or immunoglobulin. Recent developments particularly in biotechnology have encouraged many developments of immunoassays in hemostasis (ref. 10).

Antibodies to the hemostatic proteins are produced either as polyclonal antibodies raised against human proteins in laboratory animals or as monoclonal antibodies raised in hybridoma culture. Monoclonal antibodies are more specific than polyclonal antibodies. A marker, or ligand, is covalently bound to the reagent antibody to provide a means of detection. Most antibodies are marked with radioactive ligands such as ^{125}I or enzymes such as peroxidase or alkaline phosphatase. In the latter, reagent enzymes react with reagent substrates to produce measurable color or fluorescence.

A recently advanced concept for the diagnosis of hemostatic disorders is measurement of molecular markers. Activation of, or imbalance in, any of the systems associated with hemostasis generates certain well-defined peptide cleavage products or cellular release products that have been termed molecular markers.

Based on their origin, these markers identify a specific pathway of activation. Because of the nature of their formation and their naturally low plasma concentrations, elevated levels of molecular markers indicate the initial stages of activity. Thus their measurement provides a reliable tool for identifying early underlying events leading to hemorrhagic or hypercoagulable disorders.

The assay for molecular markers quantitates the native substance and does not involve in vitro activation, generation or other manipulations prior to measurements, as was required in earlier methods such as the PT and APTT. This eliminates sources of error and possible nonphysiological interfering reactions. Because of the nature of molecular markers, special collection and handling procedures are required to maintain a physiologic sample for accurate quantitation.

Latex agglutination assays utilize latex particles coated with specific antibody which crosslink with soluble antigenic particles to create a visible precipitate. The limitations of this technique allow for identification of relatively large particles (50,000 daltons) at greater than 2 mg/ml. Most assays are performed manually; however, certain instruments have been adapted with this technique.

Nephelometric techniques employ a change in light scatter to quantitate the level of antigen-antibody complex formation. Original nephelometers measured the intensity of light scatter at a 90° angle to the incident light. To increase sensitivity, modifications were made including the measurement of only forward light scatter and incorporation of electronic devices to minimize background noise due to dust and other contaminants. The use of a polymeric buffer intensified light scatter by enhancing the insolubility of antigen-antibody complexes. The laser was a major development that created a more sensitive system with high-intensity monochromatic light sharply focused into one beam.

Immunodiffusion holds that the concentration of an antigen is directly proportional to the rate of precipitate produced as a result of its diffusion in an antiserum-containing agarose preparation. Current radial immunodiffusion (RID) methodology is based on the manual technique of Mancini in which a test sample, placed in a well cut into the agarose, diffuses radially from the well. The precipitate area is allowed to reach a maximal size; the square of the diameter of the ring is linearly proportional to the antigen concentration. This simple technique is reproducible but time consuming. Forty eight hours are required to obtain results.

The technique of electroimmunodiffusion (EID or EIP) is a powerful analytical tool. In the Laurell rocket technique, antigen migrates under an electric current through an antibody-containing medium, forming precipitate patterns in the shape of a rocket. Quantitation of antigen, which is proportional to the length of the rocket, can be achieved within 1 to 2 hours. Two dimensional electroimmunodiffusion provides more specific identification and characterization of antigens. In practice, one performs the first electrophoretic step as in the rocket assay, then rotates the agar containing antigen-antibody complexes 90° and performs a second electrophoretic step (second dimension) on the pre-electrophoretically separated antigens. Any antigen-antibody combination can be measured with this technique.

Radioimmunoassay (RIA) is based on either noncompetitive or competitive binding of radiolabeled and/or unlabeled (test sample) antigen to monospecific antibody. Quantitation can be done by several ways. In a noncompetitive binding assay, direct quantitation of antigen-antibody complexes is done. In a competitive binding assay the concentration of remaining free, unbound, radiolabeled antigen can be quantitated and related to the concentration of unlabeled test antigen through the use of standards. The amount of labeled protein bound to the antibody would be inversely proportional to the concentration of bound unlabeled test protein (Fig. 3). Radioimmunoassay is the most sensitive technique available for hemostatic testing; however, it requires special equipment (semiautomated and fully automated systems are available) and handling of isotopic material.

The technique of enzyme immunoassays (EIA) is similar to RIA except that the radionuclide marker is replaced by an enzyme. The final immunologic step is, therefore, followed by an indicator reaction to allow enzyme activity within the antigen-antibody complex to be photometrically determined. The "sandwich" technique is commonly used in ELISA (enzyme-linked immunosorbent assay) whereby antigens with multiple binding sites are used to bind together the reagent antibody and the labeled antibody (Fig. 3). Advantages of EIA over RIA are that reagents have a longer shelf-life, there are no regulations governing the handling of isotopes, and there is less expense. Numerous assays have recently been developed for EIA including tissue plasminogen activator, plasminogen activator inhibitor, d-dimer, fibrinopeptide A, thrombin-antithrombin complex, protein S and platelet factor 4. RIA methods are available also for the eicosanoids such as thromboxane and prostacyclin.

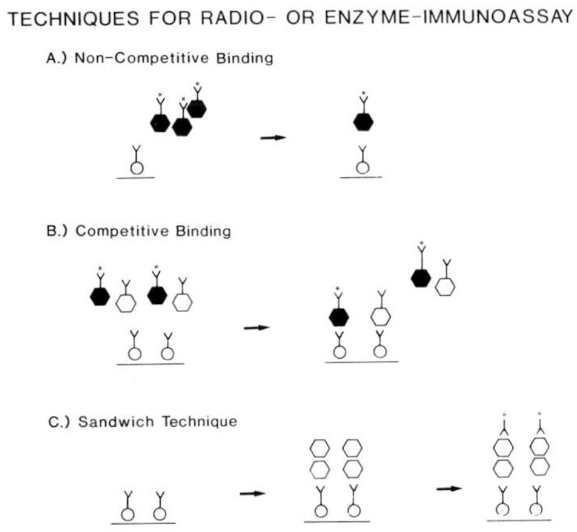

Fig. 3. Diagram of the basic principles of radio- or enzyme immunoassay. Antibody is bound to a solid surface. Added test unlabeled and/or labeled reagent antigen is added and labeled (*) antigen is then quantitated. The concentration of the bound, unlabeled test antigen is mathematically determined from the proportion of the total labeled antigen that was able to bind to the antibody. A.) Non-competitive binding, B.) Competitive binding and C.) Sandwich technique where * = radio or enzyme label.

Two distinct EIA methods are homogeneous and heterogeneous assays. The homogeneous test involves competitive binding between enzyme labeled antigen and unlabeled test antigen for a fixed number of antibody binding sites. The principle of quantitation is based on inhibition of the catalytic activity of the enzyme by the antigen-antibody complex. Because a separation step of reagents is not required, this system is referred to as a homogeneous test. This allows for ease of automation, yet it also allows for interference from plasma components.

The heterogeneous test principle, known by the term ELISA requires that the free reactant be separated from the solid-phase bound reactant after each reaction. Either competitive binding or more often noncompetitive binding ("sandwich technique") can be employed. The separation technique is usually a simple aspiration. However, some procedures may require centrifugation, sedimentation, double-antibody, or glass-bead separation. The ELISA principle involves either a competitive or noncompetitive binding system using an enzyme-linked antigen or antibody.

Several semiautomated and fully automated ELISA systems for microtiter plates are available with one or more of the following components: a wash/aspiration module, a pipettor/dilutor, and a reader. The microtiter plate allows up to 96 tests per run. Microsampling and low reagent consumption are positive features.

Fluoroimmunoassay (FIA) employs the same principle as ELISA, with the exception that a fluorophore is used in place of a chromophore. This may enhance the sensitivity of the reaction. Applications to microbeads and solid-phase dipsticks have been developed.

The FIAX Test System (International Diagnostic Technology, Inc., Santa Clara, CA) offers a dipstick technique. Reagents are contained on a StiQ sampler, upon which the reaction takes place and is read in a specially designed fluorometer. Currently applied coagulation parameters include α_1-antitrypsin ,α_2-macroglobulin, and the anaphylatoxins C3a, C4a and C5a. Other similar techniques are under development.

Flow cytometry and monoclonal antibodies have entered into the hemostasis laboratory for the evaluation of platelets. This technique has shown an importance for the detection of anti-platelet antibodies which lead to thrombocytopenia. It has also been used to determine structural variations on the platelet membrane surface.

SUMMARY

Hemostasis is a balance between complex interactions of directly opposing systems (coagulation and fibrinolysis) with seemingly unrelated systems on both the enzymatic (complement) and cellular (platelets, endothelium, leukocytes) levels. It should not be surprising that coagulation disorders often accompany many different disease states. Individual enzymes, inhibitors, cellular release products, and low molecular weight products of activation reactions (molecular markers) can now be measured in sensitive, specific assays that go far beyond the limits of the global PT and APTT. With this new perspective, pathologic hemostatic conditions can be identified during the early stages of disease (i.e., at subclinical stages before major pathologic complications are established), and more specifically targeted prophylactic as well as therapeutic intervention can be administered.

Technological advances in methodology and instrumentation have changed the scope of all clinical laboratories, but in particular the coagulation laboratory. The overall development has resulted from the influences of clinical chemistry, clinical immunology, pharmacology, biochemistry and biotechnology. Analytical instruments for use in hemostatic testing go beyond the clot-based readers and platelet aggregometers to a range of automated discrete chemistry analyzers, batch processors, microtiter systems and the newest multiprobe instruments designed to simultaneously measure different assay endpoints. Moreover, automation has the distinct advantages of operational simplicity, microsampling, low reagent consumption, cost-effectiveness and computer compatibility for fast and accurate data reduction. Instruments are designed for batch processing of single tests on multiple samples or multiple test panels on a single sample. Versatility ranges from instruments that only measure the final reaction solution, by endpoint or kinetic analysis, to instruments that automatically pipet reagents and sample, incubate and analyze the reaction.

These advances in methodology and instrumentation and other developments such as dry chemistry, flow cytometry, physicians office testing and disease panel profiling are providing the clinical hemostasis laboratory with tools to provide needed patient care against the risks associated with thrombosis and for monitoring of the new drug therapies.

REFERENCES

1. R. Bick, Disorders of Hemostasis and Thrombosis, Thieme Stratton, New York (1985).
2. O.D. Ratnoff, C.D. Forbes, Disorders of Hemostasis, Grune & Stratton, Orlando (1984).
3. M. Verstraete, J. Vermylen, Thrombosis, Pergamon Press, New York (1984).
4. D. Ogston, The Physiology of Hemostasis, Harvard University Press, Cambridge (1983).
5. A.R. Thompson, L.A. Harker, Manual of Hemostasis and Thrombosis, Davis, Philadelphia (1983).
6. J.M. Walenga, Hemostasis and Thrombosis in the Clinical Laboratory, p. 367, Lippincott, Philadelphia (1988).
7. J. Fareed (ed), Perspectives in Hemostasis, Pergamon Press, New York (1981).
8. R.W. Colman, J. Hirsh, V.J. Marder, E.W. Salzman (eds), Hemostasis and Thrombosis: Basic Principles and Clinical Practice, Lippincott, Philadelphia (1987).
9. H.C. Hemker, Handbook of Synthetic Substrates for the Coagulation and Fibrinolytic System, Martinus Nijhoff, The Hague (1983).
10. Z. Parvez, Immunoassays in Coagulation Testing, Springer-Verlag, New York (1984).

Automated fluorogenic prothrombin time method for the evaluation of hypercoagulability in human plasma

Hisao Kato, Kagehiro Uchida, Kentaro Takano and Takenori Yamaguchi

National Cardiovascular Center, Fujishiro-dai, Suita, Osaka 565, Japan

Highly sensitive automated methods for the evaluation of the extrinsic coagulation reactions in human plasma were developed by the combination of fluorogenic peptide substrate (Boc-Val-Pro-Arg-MCA) for thrombin and a centrifugal autoanalyzer (Cobas Bio). Fluorogenic prothrombin time (FPT) was measured by the reaction time to reach 0.1 relative fluorescence which was caused by the action of thrombin generated after the activation of 3 μl plasma with human placental tissue factor. FPT was expressed as per cent by dividing FPT of control plasma with FPT of patient's plasma. Factors X and VII contents in plasma were measured by the same method after mixing diluted plasma with each factor deficient plasma, tissue factor, calcium and the fluorogenic substrate. These fluorogenic methods were applied for the analysis of the hypercoagulability in plasmas from 31 patients with thrombotic and 28 with embolic infarctions. The average of FPT of the patient's plasmas which were collected within 48 hrs after onset was 156.1% in the former and 116.5% in the latter. The mean of the content of Factor VII in thrombotic infarction was significantly higher than that of embolic infarction (130.3% and 111.3%, respectively). There were no differences in the content of Factor X between two groups. These results indicate that these fluorogenic automated methods are highly sensitive to detect the hypercoagulability in cerebral thrombosis which is caused in part by the increase of Factor VII content in plasma.

Thrombosis is caused by complicated in vivo reactions which involve the damage or loss of endothelial cells, activation of platelets and leukocytes, activation of coagulation and fibrinolytic systems in plasma and alteration of their regulation systems. For the prognosis, diagnosis and therapy of the thrombotic diseases of cerebral and coronary arteries and lower limbs veins, the development of the highly sensitive method to detect the prethrombotic state is essential, together with the analysis of the prethrombotic state which precedes thrombus formation. In spite of the contribution of the hypercoagulability in plasma to the prethrombotic state, the conventional prothrombin time (PT) and activated partial thromboplastine time (APTT) methods and the chromogenic method recently developed, are not relevant to detect the hypercoagulability.

Blood coagulation proceeds by two pathways, that is, the intrinsic and extrinsic pathways, which are triggered by negatively-charged surfaces and tissue factor, respectively. Among the two pathways, it has been known that the extrinsic pathway is more important in in vivo reactions. In the present work, we intended to develop sensitive automated methods to estimate hypercoagulability in the extrinsic reactions, using fluorogenic peptide substrate for thrombin and a centrifugal autoanalyzer. Details for this work have been published (1).

FLUOROGENIC PROTHROMBIN TIME (FPT)

Three μl of human plasma was mixed with 300 μl of first reagent which contains human placental tissue factor(Thromborel S), calcium and phospholipid, using a centrifugal autoanalyzer, Cobas Bio. After 30 second, second reagent, 10 mM Boc-Val-Pro-Arg-methylcoumarylamide(MCA) was added and fluorescence readings at 60 second intervals were sent to a computer, NEC PC9801vm. Fluorescent intensity of amino methylcoumarin (AMC) increased sigmoidally after a lag time. Data were transformed into reaction times which were defined as the time elapsed to reach 0.1 relative fluorescence, using a program developed by us.

Figure 1 shows the increase of fluorescence intensity of normal and coagulation factors-deficient plasmas, which were measured by the FPT method. Thrombin activity was not significantly generated in Factor V-,

Factor VII- and Factor X-deficient plasmas and Warfarin-treated plasma. On the other hand, thrombin generation in other coagulation factors-deficient plasmas was the same as that of normal plasma or delayed to some extent.

Figure 2 shows the effect of the addition of the purified Factors VII, X and IX and prothrombin on the FPT of normal plasma and each factors-deficient plasmas. The addition of Factor X to control plasma or factor X-deficient plasma accelerated significantly their FPT. The addition of Factor VII moderately accelerated. The addition of prothrombin did not accelerate significantly FPT of normal plasma. The addition of Factor IX to normal plasma or Factor IX-deficient plasma did not accelerate their FPT. These results indicate that the FPT method is sensitive not only to the decrease of the concentration of Factors X and VII and prothrombin, but also sensitive to the increase of the concentration of Factor X and Factor VII in plasma.

When the FPT method was applied to plasmas from the patients with cardiovascular diseases, many plasmas gave shorter FPT than control plasma. Generally, PT has been expressed as per cent of control plasma by calculating from the standard curve, which was obtained by diluting the control plasma with buffer. Therefore, it is impossible to calculate PT which is shorter than control plasma. We divided FPT of control plasma with FPT of patient plasma and expressed as per cent for convenience. These per cent values of each plasma, which were thus calculated with different concentration of tissue factor, were approximately the same in spite of the different reaction times.

Figure 3 shows the comparison of the FPT of patient plasmas with PT of the same plasmas which were determined by conventional PT method, that is, clotting time method. The per cent values of patient plasmas from the two methods which were calculated by dividing clotting time or reaction time of control plasma with that of patient plasma, correlated with the coefficient of 0.90. However, 9 samples out of 84 samples gave more than 150 % in FPT, while they were between 100 and 130 %. This result indicates that the FPT method is sensitive not only to hypocoagulability, but also to hypercoagulability, while the conventional PT method is not relevant for the detection of hypercoagulability.

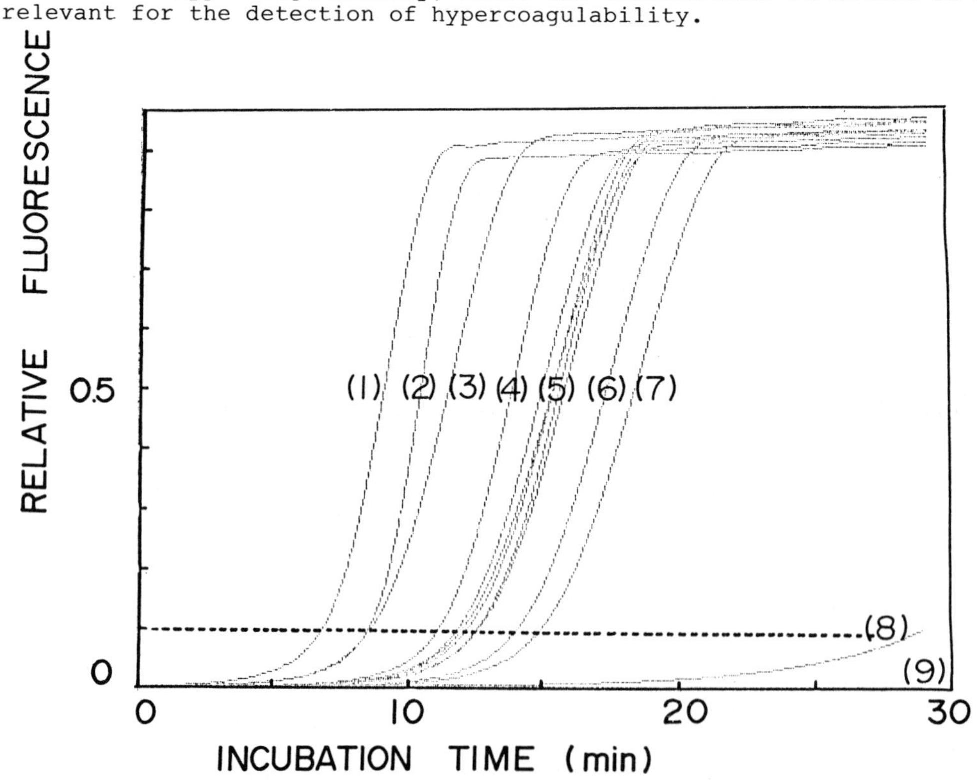

Fig. 1 FPT of coagulation factor deficient plasmas (1).
(1) protein C depleted plasma, (2) control plasma, (3) Factor XI deficient plasma, (4) prekallikrein deficient plasma, (5) fibrinogen, Factor VIII and HMW kininogen deficient plasmas, (6) Factor XII deficient plasma, (7) Factor IX deficient plasma, (8) Factor V deficient plasma and (9) Factor VII and Factor X deficient plasmas and Warfarin-treated plasma.

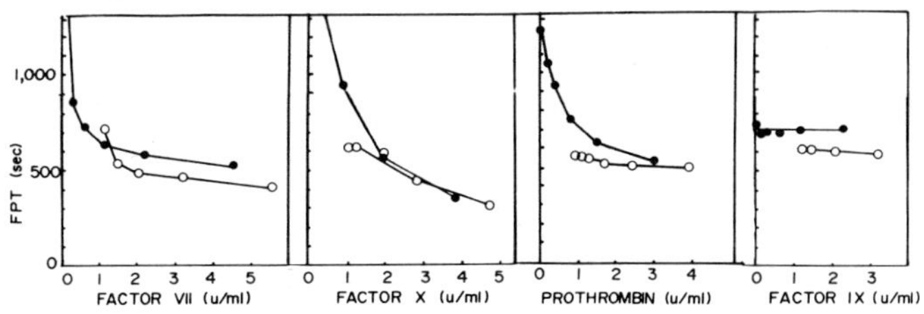

Fig. 2 Effect of the purified Factors VII, X and IX and prothrombin on FPT of control plasma and each factor-deficient plasmas (1).
The purified factor VII, Factor X, prothrombin or Factor IX was mixed with normal plasma (-o-) or each factor-deficient plasma (-●-) and their FPT's were calculated.

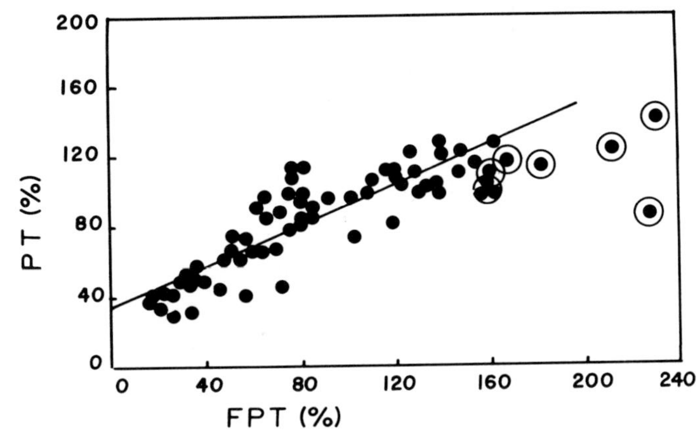

Fig. 3 Correlation of FPT with conventional PT(1).
Percentages of PT of patients which were calculated by dividing the clotting time of control plasma with that of patient plasma were compared with the percentages of FPT which were calculated by dividing reaction time of control plasma with that of patient plasma. The correlation of the samples (n=75) was calculated as follows; Y = 0.58 X + 34, r = 0.895
⦿; samples excluded for the calculation.

ESTIMATION OF CONCENTRATIONS OF FACTORS X AND VII IN PLASMA

The concentration of Factor X and Factor VII in plasma were measured by the same principle as FPT. Ten fold diluted plasma was mixed with Factor X deficient- or Factor VII deficient- plasma and then with the mixture of tissue factor, calcium and fluorogenic substrate. Fig. 4 (A) shows the generation of thrombin activity in the mixture of the serially diluted control plasma and Factor X deficient plasma.
From the data as shown in Fig. 4 (A), calibration curve for Factor X was obtained. Figure 4 (B) shows the calibration curves for Factor X and Factor VII. Ten fold diluted plasma was assumed to contain 100 % of Factor X or Factor VII. As shown in Fig. 4 (B), the concentrations of Factor X and Factor VII in plasma were measured from 10 % to 800 % by this method. The precision studies on these automated fluorogenic methods demonstrated that they can be used as the practical clinical method.

HYPERCOAGULABILITY IN CEREBROVASCULAR INFARCTIONS

Using these fluorogenic PT methods, we analyzed the coagulability of plasmas from the patients with cerebral infarctions, 27 cases of cerebral embolism and 35 cases of cerebral thorombosis. As shown in Table I, the averaged FPT of thrombotic patients was significantly shorter than that of embolic patients, 156.1 % in thrombosis and 116.5 % in embolism. Factor X contents were not different between embolism and thrombosis. On the other hand, Factor VII contents in thrombosis were significantly higher than that of embolic patients, 130.3 % in thrombosis and 100.9 % in embolism. These results indicate that thrombotic patients are in hypercoagulability, which is partly due to the increase of Factor VII content, while embolic patients are in normal or hypocoagulability.

In both cases, correlation between FPT and Factor VII content was very low, that is r =0.2. However, patients with either higher FPT or higher Factor VII content than 120 % or patients with both of them, were 11 cases in embolism (40.7 %), while 31 cases in thrombosis (91.2 %). These results indicate that FPT or Factor VII content or both of them are significantly higher in cerebral thrombosis, although no direct relation between them.

From these results, we speculate that patients with cerebral thrombosis were in prethrombotic state, which was caused by the increase of Factor VII content and other factors.

The fluorogenic PT methods described in this paper are supposed to be very promising as practical clinical method for the analysis of hypercoagulability in comparison with the conventional PT method and chromogenic PT method (2, 3). In FPT, hypercoagulability of many samples (25 samples) can be measured using small amounts of plasma (3 µl). Contents of Factors X and VII in plasma can also be measured using small amounts of deficient plasma (6 µl per sample). The application of FPT to

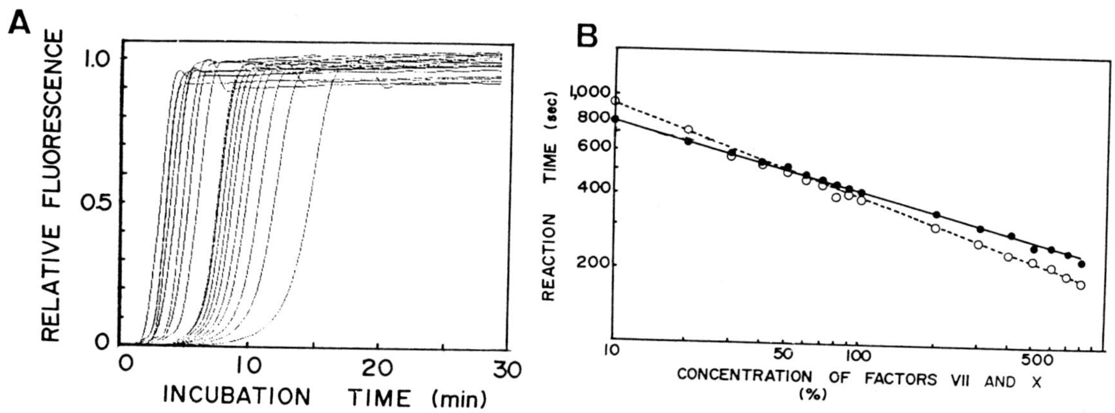

Fig. 4 Standard curves for the estimation of Factor X and Factor VII in plasma (1).
Control plasma was diluted with Tris-saline-BSA buffer and the concentration of each coagulation factors were measured using each coagulation factor deficient plasma. (A) Generation of thrombin activity in the mixture of diluted control plasma and Factor X deficient plasma. (B) Standard curves for Factors X and VII. Factor X;--○-- Factor VII;—●—

Table I FPT and concentrations of Factor X and Factor VII in plasmas from patients with thrombotic and embolic infarctions.

	Embolism	Thrombosis
FPT	116.5 + 45.4	156.1 + 45.2*
Factor X	106.0 + 31.8	111.3 + 35.2
Factor VII	100.9 + 38.6	130.3 + 42.3*

% ; Mean + S.D. * ; $p < 0.01$

the analysis of cerebrovascular infarction demonstrated that patients with thrombotic infarction are in hypercoagulable state which is partly caused by the increase of Factor VII content. Since the increase of Factor VII content in myocardial infarction has been reported (4-6), increase of Factor VII concentration in plasma might be a new risk factor in thrombotic diseases. However, the effects of other factors in plasma on hypercoagulability, for example, Factor Va, Factor Xa, tissue factor, Protein C, Protein S and protease inhibitors remain to be established.

REFERENCES

(1) Kato, H. and Uchida, K.: Automated fluorogenic methods for the evaluation of the extrinsic coagulation reactions in human plasma. Thrombosis Research 50, 77-90, 1988.
(2) Duncan, A., Bowie,, E. J. W., Owen, Jr., C. A. and Fass, D. N.: A clinical evaluation of automated chromogenic tests as substitutes for

conventional prothrombin time tests. Clin. Chem., 31, 853-855, 1985.
(3) Kolde, H. J. Chromo time system-A new generation of coagulation analyses. Behring Inst. Mitt., No. 78, 176-187, 1985.
(4) Meade, T. W. : Hypercoagulability and ischaemic diseases. Blood Reviews 1, 2-8, 1987.
(5) Hoffman, C., Shah, A., Sodums, M. and Hultin, M. B.: Factor VII activity state in coronary artery disease. J. Lab. Clin. Med. 111, 475-481, 1988.
(6) Carvalho de Sousa, J., Azevedo, J., Soria, C., Barros, F., Ribeiro, C., Parreira, F. and Caen, J. P.: Factor VII hyperactivity in acute myocardial thrombosis. A relation to the coagulation activation. Thrombosis Research 51, 165-173, 1988.

Rapid slide test for fibrin degradation products (FDP)

E. KITA

Department of Clinical Laboratory & Diagnostics, Nara Medical University, 840 Shijo, Kashihara, Nara 634, Japan

Recent elucidation of blood coagulation and fibrinolytic mechanisms allow us to detect many of molecular makers in hemostatic activation, when it takes place not in pathological but in physiological conditions. So, it is well established that FDP, degradation products both from fibrinogen and fibrin by the action of plasmin, might be heterogeneous.

However, still not a few clinical laboratories have detected FDP by only semi-quantitative aggulutination tests with anti-fibrinogen antibody in routine use. Quite often, quantitation of FDP in full detail may be requested in taking a share in decision making for clinical medical practices. For this instance, rapid, accurate and sensitive test for single sample is necessary.

Here, I would like to present a simple and rapid slide test for a part of FDP, from cross-linked fibrin. The original method is based on two-steps sandwich enzyme immunoassay (EIA) for FDP DD dimer.

Results in plasma and serum samples from pathological conditions, such as hematologic malignancies, DIC in various diseases, thrombosis with or without fibrinolytic agents and from normal volunteers under acute exposure to hypoxemia, which may alter fibrinolytic activities, and data in urine specimen would be presented.

Latex-particles, coated with anti-fibrinogen (fbg) antibody, has been used in many years as a maker of activated fibrinolysis. This method is very easy to handle with and reflect pretty well of fibrinolysis activation, but has some limitations (1,2), as the antibody may react not only with some of plasmin digested fbg metabolites (FgDP), but also with fbg itself, remaining in the sample. Also, it is not possible to identify fibrinolysis from fibrinogenolysis, due to the same reason.

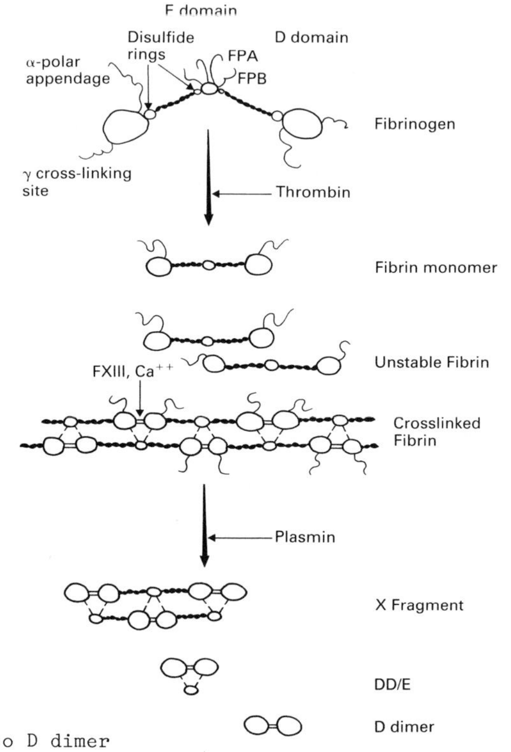

Figure 1 Fibrinogen to D dimer

Then, elucidation of detailed mechanism of blood coagulation and fibrinolysis, more specific and exact evaluation of fiblinolytic phenomenon is being demanded. As the laboratory tests, according to the development of biochemical, immunological and automational techniques, several kinds of different methods (3, 4) detecting fbg (FgDP) and fibrin degradation products(FDP)by the action of plasmin (plm), are now available in easy kit.

On the other hand, today, it is not sensible to abuse resources. So, we should carry out each hemostatic test, very carefully and effectively, without deterioration of quality of assessment. From this point of view, the slide-test for crosslinked fibrin delivatives (XDP) assay, which I will mention here, is an excellent specific, rapid and economic method.

Fbg is converted into fibron-monomer (FM) by the action of an enzyme, THROMBIN, releasing small peptides, called fibrinopeptide A and B (FPA and FPB), from alpha and beta chains, respectively. Then, FMs are polimelized by the FXIIIa (transglutaminase) and calcium ion (Ca^{++}), associating an E domein ina monomer with two DF domeins of neighbouring monomers. This results in the formation of a stable crosslinked fibrin network as the end-point of of blood coagulation.

Now, fibrinolytic mechanism (5) may play a role in hemostatics. Practically, the fibrinolysis may be going on at the same time as the activation of blood coagulation, still theoretically or for our convenience, always we are thinking it would be a succession of coagulation. In this mechanism, another major enzyme, PLASMIN (plm) interacts with crosslinked fibrin. Plm is generated from its precursor, plasminogen (plg) by the action of different types of plg-activators, such as tissue-plg activator (t-PA), Urokinase and Streptokinase. Degeneration of crosslinked fibrin leads to the characteristic production of dimetric units of d-d fragments, called D-dimer.

It is well known now, that the detection of D-dimer (6) would be the specific proof of actual fibrinolysis, which is different from the action of plm on fbg.

Terminology
FgDP: plasmic degradation of fibrinogen.
FDP : plasmic degradation of fibrinogen and/or fibrin not well identified.
XDP : plasmic degradation of crosslinked fibrin.

SIGNIFICANCE OF XDP ASSAY

Today, in most of the hemostatic laboratories, a large number of specimens belong to various kinds of thrombotic diseases, including DIC, cerebral and cardial infarcation, pulmonary embolism, and venous thrombosis. In diagnosis or monitoring of these diseases, the presence of elevated levels of XDP would be the most specific marker of ongoing fibrinolytic process (7). Sometimes, it is really necessary and useful to differentiate therapeutic fibrinolysis from unintended fibrinogenolysis in the course of thrombolytic therapy.

PRINCIPLE OF LATEX SLIDE TEST (RAPIDIA-D dimer, Fuji Rebio/MabCO)

The latex agglutination slide test (8) for XDP (RAPIDIA-D dimer, Fuji Rebio/MAbCO) is based on a monoclonal antibody (9) which recognizes a conformational epitope on D-dimer fragment of crosslinked fibrin. The specific monoclonal antibody to D-dimer is coupled to latex beads to provide a probe. These antibody-coated latex beads produce visible agglutination with XDP in the plasma or serum specimens, depending on the immunological reaction.

The sensitivity of the reagent was adjusted to give a positive agglutination with samples containing 200 ng/ml XDP or greater. Semi-quantitification of XDP is carried out from the greatest dilution of the sample which shows agglutination.

The whole procedure requires only 5 minutes, after plasma sample preparation.

REAGENTS AND MATERIALS

1 Latex Beads
   0.4% suspension of polystyrene latex beads, coated with the monoclonal antibody to D-dimer in a phosphate buffered saline solution containing 0.01% sodium azide, 10 mg/ml ovalbumin and 5% glycerol. Stored at 2-8 C, it is stable for a minimum of one year from manufacture.
2 Positive Control
   Lyophilized serum containing purified D-dimer and mertholate, which gives a D-dimer concentration of -10 ug/ml, when reconstituted with 0.1 ml distilled water. Once reconstituted, it should be kept frozen and is stable for 3 months. Failure of agglutination with positive control may indicate microbial contamination.
3 Phosphate Buffered Saline
   Lyophilized powder of NaCl (0.800 g), KCl (0.02 g), Disodium-hudrogen phosphate (0.115 g), Potassium dihydrogen phosphate (0.02 g) and Merthiolate (0.01 g). Reconstituting with

100 ml distilled water, a buffer solution of pH 7.4 is given. For semiquantitification, dilute samples with this buffer. Store at 2-8 C.

4 Pipettes or pipette tips of 10, 25, 100 ul and so on.
Glass slides or ceramic tiles. Plastic stirrer. Rotator, if possible.

PROCEDURE

SPECIMEN COLLECTION

PLASMA Freshly drawn citrated, EDTA, heparinized plasma are all suitable for RAPIDIA-D dimer Test. After preparation of plasma with routine centrifugation of the samples the test will be possible immediately. Defibrination of the samples is not required.

SERUM Special procedures or sample tubes are not requested for preparation of serum for the test. Serum separation after 30-60 min, at 20-37 C may be hastened by centrifugal. Caution of false results should be paid in serum, as XDP may be entrapped in clot or, in some cases, elevated from incomplete coagulation.

PROCEDURE

Preparation

1 Add 100 ml of distilled water to buffer salts vial.
2 Reconstitute positive control with 0.1 ml distilled water. Make sure of the complete dissolution of contents before use.

ASSAY PROCEDURE

QUALITATIVE ASSAY

1 Leave the latex beads and samples for a while in room temperature.
2 Invert latex beads several times, rapidly.
3 Holding pipette dropper vertically, place one drop of latex beads on a clean and clear glass slide or ceramic tile.
4 Add 10 ul of undiluted test sample to the drop of latex beads. Positive control (positive) and buffer (negative) may be applied at the same time.
5 Mix the suspension with the plastic stirrer, until an area of 1.5 cm is covered.
6 Rock the slide or tile for 3 minutes, gently. If possible automatic rotator may be applied.
7 After exactly 3 minutes, check the agglutination of latex beads. Read by holding slide 5 cm above a black background, under suitable lighting conditions. Positive agglutination may be confirmed in positive control, and negative result (no agglutination) with buffer solution.

The normal range of plasma and serum XDP in healthy adults is less than 200 ug/ml, and so normal specimens give negative results when tested as described above.

SEMI-QUANTITATIVE ASSAY

Positive agglutination in undiluted sample can normally be obtained with specimens containing more than 200 ng/ml of XDP. By serial doubling dilution of samples in phosphate buffer solutins, followed by testing in the same way as mentioned above, semi-quantitative assay will be done with (200 x maximum dilution) ng/ml.

INTERPRETATION OF RESULTS

I DIC AND PRE-DIC

XDP were assayed together with RAPIDIA-D dimer test and its original EIA. At the same time, FDP were also examined with latex slide test (FDPL test, Teikoku-Zohki Co.) and laser nephelometry (Wako-Junyaku CO.), in 8 cases of clinically defined DIC and 9 cases of so-called pre-DIC, which were anticipated to be overt in 2 days by physicians but withoug hemorrhagic tendency.

It is well confirmed that FDP is elevated in clinically defined DIC. In Fig. 2, results of FDP and XDP, assayed by EIA and latex agglutination in the case of DIC and pre-DIC, which was anticipated by the physician, are shown. In DIC, all specimens showed positive agglutination both in FDP and XDP assay.

II FOLLOW UP IN A CASE OF PRE-DIC

A patient with gastric cancer with strong suspicions of DIC, without bleeding tendency, was under survey of XDP assessment. With positive slide test for XDP, 15,000 u/day heparin was given to him. At almost the same time a slight oozing from the puncture site was recognized. Heparin administration for 2 days resulted in marked reduction of XDP almost to normal range (negative results in slide test) and with discontinuation of heparin, XDP increased again to

500-1000 ug/ml. After all, the patient came to an exaggerated thrombotic and hemorrhagic state several days later and death.

III THROMBOLYTIC THERAPY IN ACUTE CEREBRAL THROMBOSIS

With the collaboration of the neurosurgeon, XDP (slide test and EIA) and fbg assay (Turbidimetry, Iatron Co.) were carryed out in 5 cases of acute cerebral thrombosis under thrombolytic therapy by large doses of Urokinase (Midori-Juji Pharmaceutical Co.).

A large amount of Urokinase (600,000-900,000/day) was given by continuous drip infusion. With a certain interval, fbg and XDP was assayed. Four cases out of 5 showed improvement in clinical and/or roentgenical assessment after 2-3 courses of treatment, while one did not. In Fig. 4, results of XDP and fbg. in cases with and without improvement was shown.

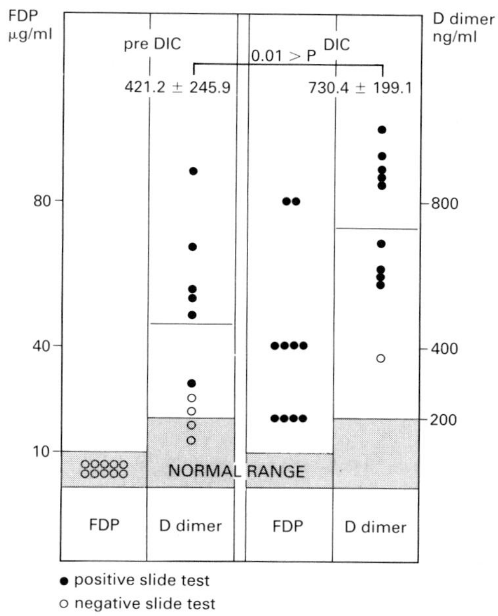

Figure 2 FDP and D dimer in pre-DIC and DIC

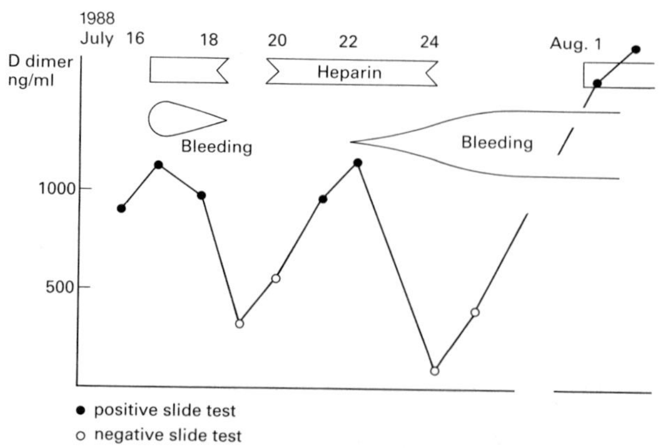

Figure 3 A Case of Gastric cancer with DIC 64Y Males

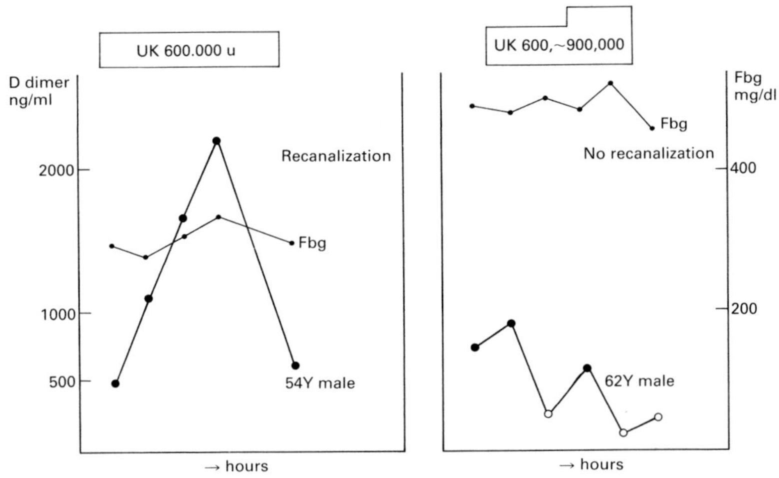

Figure 4 Monitoring in Thrombolytic Therapy in Acute Cerebral Thrombosis

DISCUSSION

With a careful and appropriate timing, XDP assessment may be very useful in the early detection and preventing aggravation of DIC. Monitoring the thrombolytic therapy in cases of cerebral or cardial thrombosis, the specific and sensitive assessment of XDP would be essential to avoid unnecessary medication of fibrinolytic agents.

Limitation in quantitative assessment of the latex slide test, will not lower its availability.

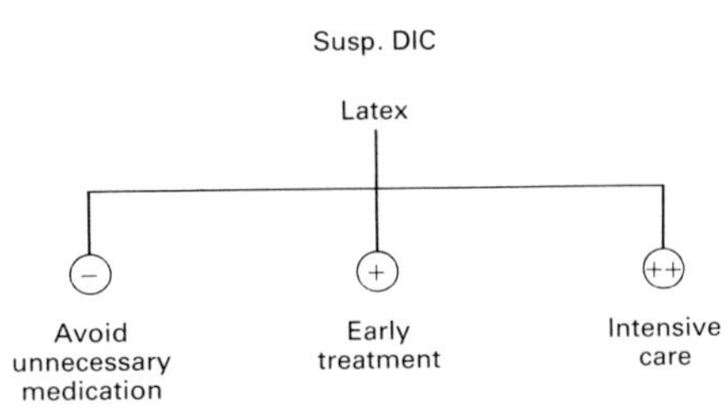

Figure 5 Application of D dimer Slide Test in DIC

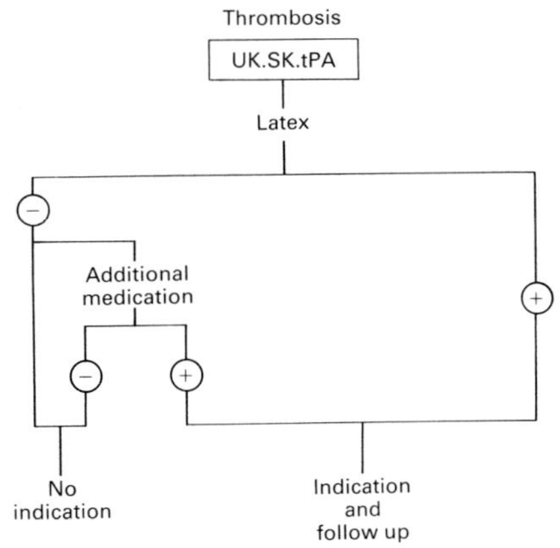

Figure 6 Application of D dimer SLide Test in Thromolytic Therapy

The latex agglutination test depends on the monoclonal antibody specific to D dimer has many advantages; it is applicable both to plasma and serum, as the antibody is specific only to XDP from crosslinked fibrin; heparinized, citrated, EDTA plasma are suitable for the test; it is cost-effective, as it does not request special sample tubes to collect plasma and sophisticated laboratory instruments; it is simple to perform and completed in 5 minutes, and provides an exact, specific and rapid assessment at the clinical decision making of the physician in diagnosing and monitoring thrombotic diseases and thrombolytic therapy.

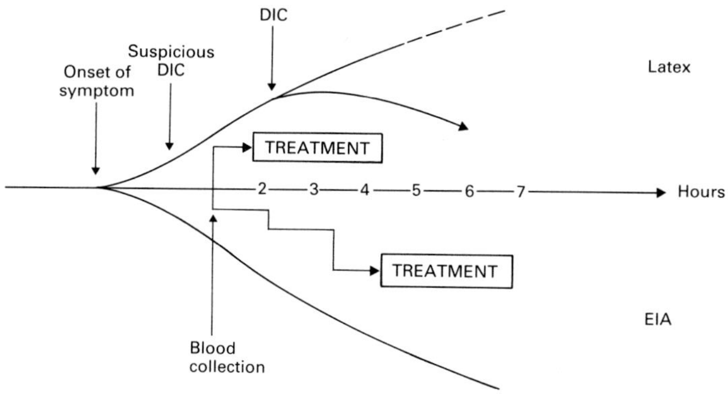

Figure 7 Advantage of Latex Method

REFERENCES

1. Merskey C., Johnson A. J., Lalezari P. Increase in fibrinogen and fibrin-related antigen in Human serum due to lysis of fibrin by thrombin. J. Clin. Invest. 51, 903-911 (1972).

2. Gaffney P.J., and Perry M.J. Unreliability of current serum fibrin degradation project (FDP) assays. Thromb. Haemostas. 53, 301-302 (1985).

3. Donati M.B. Assays for fibrinogen/fibrin degradation products in biological fluids; some methodological aspects. Thrombos. Diathes Haemorrh 34, 652-660 (1975).

4. Kita E. Detection of degradation products from fibrin and fibrinogen. Medical Tech. 13, 341- 346 (1985).

5. Hantgan R.R., Francis C.W., Scheraga H.A., and Mander V.J. Fibrinogen structure and physiology. Haemostatis and Thrombosis 2nd ed., 269-288, J.B. Lippincoll. Philidelphia, Toronto, 198 .

6. Graeff H., and Hafter R. Selection and relevance of crosslinked fibrin derivatives in blood. Semin. Thromb. Haemostas. 8, 57-58 (1982).

7. Hunt F.A., Rylatt D.B., Hart B., and Bundensen P.G. Serum crosslinked fibrin (XDP) and fibrinogen/fibrin degradation products (FDP) in disorders associated with activation of the coagulation fibrinolytic systems. Br. J. Haematol. 60, 715-722 (1985).

8. Mirashahi M., Soria J., Soria C., Perrot J.Y., and Boucheix C. A latex immunoassay of fibrin/fibrinogen degradation products in plasma using a monclonal antibody. Thrombosis Res. 44, 715-728 (1986).

9. Rylatt D.B., Blake A.S., Gottis L.E., Massingham D.A., Fletcher W.A., Masci P.P., Whitaker A.N., Elms M., Bunce I., Webber A.J., Wyatt D., and Bundesen P.G. An immunoassay for human D dimer using monoclonal antibodies. Thrombos. Res. 31, 767-778 (1983).

Ex vivo assessment of the protein C anticoagulant system by monoclonal antibody technology

Armando D'Angelo, Philip C. Comp *, Fletcher B. Taylor Jr.*, Charles T. Esmon *, Pierangelo Bonini, and Silvana Vigano' D'Angelo.

Coagulation Service and Laboratory of Clinical Chemistry, Scientific Institute IRCCS H. S. Raffaele, Milano, Italy
&
Thrombosis/Hematology Research Program, Oklahoma Medical Research Foundation, Oklahoma City, OK, U.S.A.*

Abstract- The protein C system represents a major mechanism of defense against thrombosis. The central protein of this system is protein C, a vitamin K-dependent plasma zymogen, which, once activated, acts as a natural anticoagulant hydrolyzing the activated forms of clotting factors V and VIII and neutralizing the inhibitor(s) of plasminogen activator. The physiological protein C activator is the thrombin-thrombomodulin complex on the endothelial cell surface. For full expression of its biological properties, activated protein C requires a cofactor, protein S, also a vitamin K-dependent protein, which increases the affinity of activated protein C for phospholipid membranes, endothelial cell and platelet receptors. Production and selection of monoclonal antibodies with unique properties has allowed to confirm the pathophysiological relevance of the protein C system in animal models and to develop a new assay for the identification of quantitative and qualitative protein C deficiencies.

INTRODUCTION

Current evidence suggests that the protein C anticoagulant pathway is a major regulatory mechanism responsible for control of coagulation (ref. 1,2,) Paradoxycally, the first component of the protein C anticoagulant system is thrombin. Following disruption of the endothelium on the vessel wall, exposition of subendothelial structures leads to platelet deposition and fibrin formation. Fibrin accretion would proceed uncontrolled if excess thrombin formed at the site of the lesion could not be neutralized by specific mechanisms. A major one is represented by endothelial cell thrombomodulin, which binds thrombin with very high affinity (Kd=0.5 nM) (ref. 3). Once bound to thrombomodulin, thrombin changes its substrate specificity: its ability to cleave fibrinogen is greatly reduced (ref.4, 5) while it becomes a very efficient activator (km=0.5 uM) of protein C (ref. 6), a vitamin K-dependent protein circulating in plasma as a zymogen, hence in a non active form. Activated protein C,through its cofactor protein S (ref. 7, 8), another vitamin K-dependent protein, binds to specific receptors either on the endothelial cell surface (ref. 9) or on platelet membranes (ref. 10) and exerts a number of antithrombotic properties, by inactivating the activated forms of factor V and VIII (ref. 11, 12), by inhibiting platelet prothrombin converting activity (ref. 13, 14)and by stimulating fibrinolytic activity through inactivation of a tpA-inhibitor (ref. 15 - 19). The system is further complicated by the presence in plasma of C4b-binding protein (ref. 20), a regulatory protein of the complement system, reversibly interacting with protein S with high affinity (Kd= 70 nM) (ref. 21). Under normal conditions, about 50% of protein S and C4b-binding protein circulate in the complexed form in plasma. This interaction plays a physiological role as only free protein S can serve as a cofactor for activated protein C (ref. 22 - 24).

The importance of the protein C system has been pointed out in the last few years by a number of reports dealing with clinical aspects of protein C and protein S deficiency (ref. 25). Quantitative congenital deficiencies of protein C and protein S - type I congenital deficiencies - account for 60% to 70% of the congenital abnormalities of blood coagulation observed in patients with venous thromboembolism below the age of 40. Acquired abnormalities can occur in many disease states where thrombosis is a common complication (ref. 26 - 28). The recent advent of monoclonal antibody technology has permitted to confirm the relevance of this system in experimental animal studies and to develop a new assay for a more accurate diagnosis of quantitative and qualitative protein C deficiencies.

MATERIALS AND METHODS

Monoclonal antibody preparation.
Human protein C was purified as previously described (ref. 22). Balb-c mice were immunized i.p. 3 times with 100 ug of protein per injection at two-week intervals. After a two-month rest, they were then injected with 50 ug of antigen and fusion performed 3 days later. A myeloma cell line (p3-X-63-Ag8-653, 15 millions viable cells) was mixed with 170 millions viable spleen cells from one animal and fused by standard procedures using PEG 1500. After selection in HAT medium, culture supernates were tested twice for binding activity by limit dilution. For production of ascites fluid, approximately 5 millions hybridoma cells were injected per Balb-c mouse two weeks after Pristane treatment.

Monoclonal antibody isolation.
The immunoglobulin fractions of the monoclonal antibodies were purified by 50% saturated ammonium sulphate fractionation, QAE anion-exchange chromatography and G-200 gel filtration. For experiments requiring insolubilized monoclonal antibodies, the isolated immunoglobulin fraction was coupled to Affigel 10 (Biorad) to give a final concentration of bound antibody of 5 mg/ml.

Monoclonal antibody characterization.
The monoclonal antibodies directed against protein C were tested for their ion dependency by means of an ELISA technique performed either in the presence or in the absence of Calcium ions. The ELISA technique was carried out as following: 96 microwells plates (Costar) were coated with purified human protein C (50 ul of 5 ug/ml protein) overnight at 4 C. After blocking the plates with 10 mg/ml BSA in 20 mM Tris-HCl, 0.1M NaCl, pH 7.5, the purified immunoglobulin fraction (50 ul of 20 ug/ml, indiluted and diluted 1:2, 1:4, 1:8) was incubated in the presence of either 2 mM Calcium or 2 mM EDTA for 1 hour, at room temperature. The plates were then washed with 0.15 M NaCl, 20 mM Tris-HCl, 0.1% Tween 20 and a peroxidase labelled affinity purified antibody to mouse IgG (Kirkegaard & Perry Laboratories) was added. Finally, the plates were washed again, the peroxidase substrate (ABTS, Kirkegaard & Perry Laboratories))was added and the absorbance was measured at 405 nm. Calcium or EDTA were always present throughout the whole procedure.

The ability of the anti protein C monoclonal antibodies to block activated protein C anticoagulant or amidolytic activity was tested respectively in a coagulometric and in a chromogenic assay (ref. 27).
In the coagulometric assay, to 100 ul of normal pooled plasma at 37 C, 100 ul of cephalin (Sigma) , 100 ul of purified bovine factor Xa and 100 ul of 25 mM CaCl2 were added. The bovine Xa was diluted into 0.1 M NaCl, 0.02 M Tris-HCl, 1 mg/ml BSA, pH 7.5, to give a 30-s clotting time (6ng/ml). The protein C isolated from human plasma and activated with insolubilized thrombin-thrombomodulin complex (20 ul of 4 ug/ml)) was added to the incubation mixture prior to factor Xa. This level of activated protein C gives a 30-35 sec prologation of the clotting time. A standard curve was prepared using serial dilutions of the activated protein C down to 1:8 dilution. A linear relationship was obtained between the concentration of activated protein C and the prolongation of the clotting time.
In the amidolytic assay, 50 ul of the activated protein C were diluted with 400 ul of 0.1 M NaCl, 20 mM Tris-HCl, 1 mg/ml BSA, pH 7.5. Substrate (50 ul of 2 mM S 2238) was then added and the release of paranitroaniline was determined at 25 C by recording the change in absorbance at 405 nm over 3 min in a spectrophotometer.

The ability of the anti-protein C monoclonal antibodies to block protein C activation was tested by activating human purified protein C with the thrombin-thrombomodulin complex (final concentration 90 nM), insolubilized onto Affigel 10 (Biorad) via an anti-rabbit thrombomodulin monoclonal antibody (ref. 27), in the presence of increasing concentrations of the monoclonal antibodies to be characterized or at fixed monoclonal antibody concentrations as a function of activation time. The activation was carried out in the presence of 2 mM Calcium for 60 min at 37 C. The reaction was stopped by centrifuging the Affigel 10 beads and the generated activated protein C was quantitated both according to amidolytic and anticoagulant activity as described above.

RESULTS AND DISCUSSION

One monoclonal antibody showed characteristic of metal ion dependency. This antibody, named HPC4, did recognize protein C only in the presence of Calcium ions. Due to this peculiarity, HPC4 allowed purification of human protein C in large quantities. This, together with the observation of another unique property of HPC4, led us to undertake experiments in animal models to underline the in vivo importance of the protein C system. Activated protein C is a proteolytic enzyme which can be tested by either amidolytic or coagulometric methods, the latter being based on the ability of activated protein C to properly interact with the cofactor protein S on phospholipid surfaces and with the substrates factor Va and VIIIa. In experiments carried out incubating the monoclonal antibodies with activated protein C, none of three different anti-protein C monoclonal antibodies did prove effective in blocking the amidolytic activity of protein C (Fig. 1, left panel). Two monoclonal antibodies (HPC2 and HPC8) blocked the anticoagulant activity of protein C (Fig. 1, right panel).

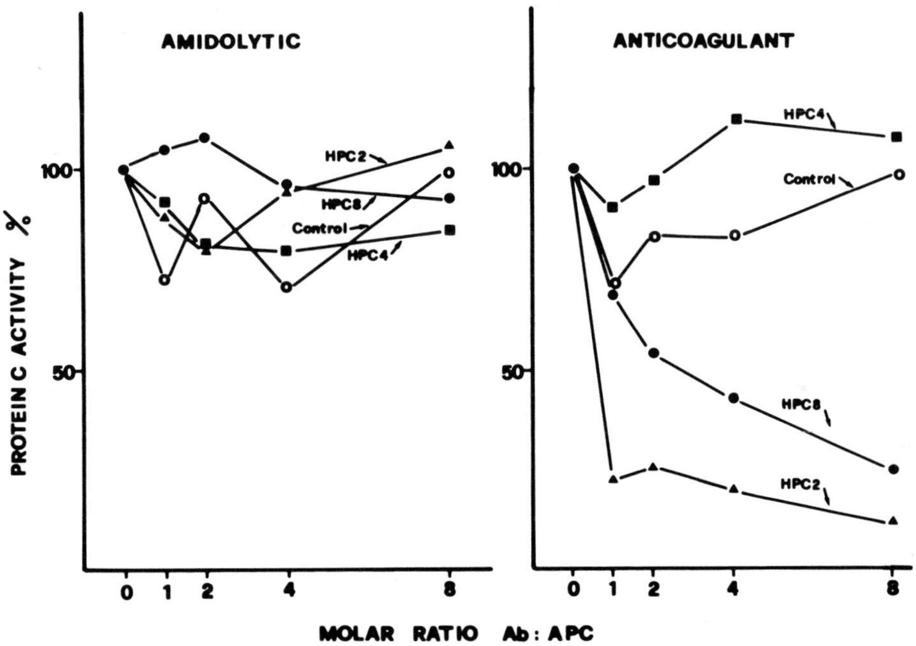

Fig. 1. Inhibition of activated protein C (129 uM) amidolytic and anticoagulant activities by increasing concentrations of monoclonal antibodies. Closed circles: HPC8; squares: HPC4; triangles: HPC2; open circles: control.

The monoclonal antibody HPC4, which did not block any of the activities of activated protein C, could prevent protein C activation. When mixtures of protein C, soluble thrombin thrombomodulin complex in the presence of increasing HPC4 concentrations were incubated for 1 hour at 37 C, activation of protein C - as tested by both amidolytic and anticoagulant activity of activated protein C generated - was inhibited proportionally to the HPC4 concentration with 50% inhibition at approximately 80 ug/ml (Fig 2, left panel).The effect on the initial rate of protein C activation was much more pronounced. When protein C was preincubated with the antibody for 30 min at 37 C, almost 90% inhibition of protein C activation was observed at 15 min at HPC4 concentrations of 40 ug/ml (Fig. 2, right panel).

The observation that virtually identical results could be obtained with human and baboon protein C provided us with a unique tool to evaluate the in vivo physiopathological relevance of the protein C system in an animal

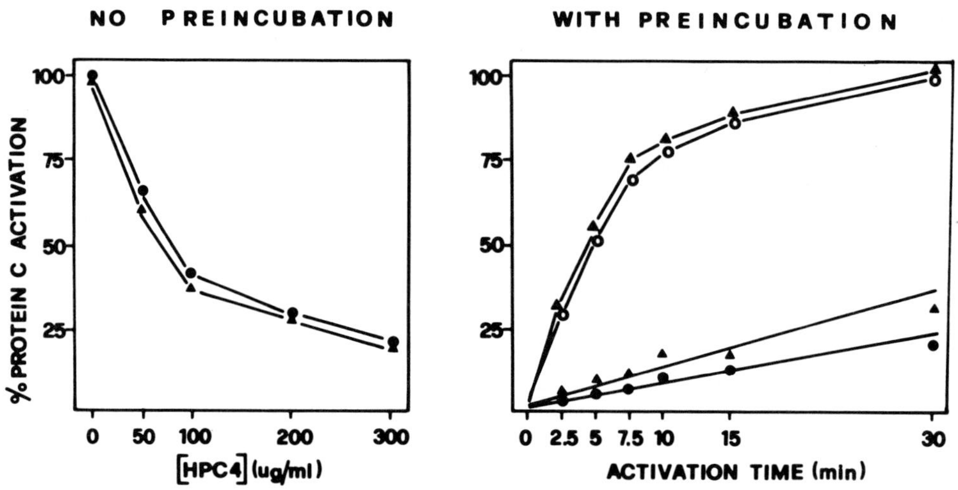

Fig. 2. Inhibition of protein C (81 uM) activation by immobilized thrombin-thrombomodulin complex (90 uM) as a function of HPC4 concentration (left panel). Inhibition of protein C (81 uM) activation by 0 (open symbols) and 40 (closed symbols) ug/ml HPC4 as a function of activation time (right panel). Circles: anticoagulant activity; triangles: amidolytic activity.

model. The injection of sublethal dose of E. Coli in baboons produces an acute phase response in the animal: fibrinogen levels increase while there is no change in protein C. On the other hand, infusion of lethal doses of E. Coli produces a clinical and laboratory evidence of disseminated intravascular coagulation (DIC). Fibrinogen drops to unmeasurable levels within few hours and there is a parallel reduction of protein C (Fig. 3).

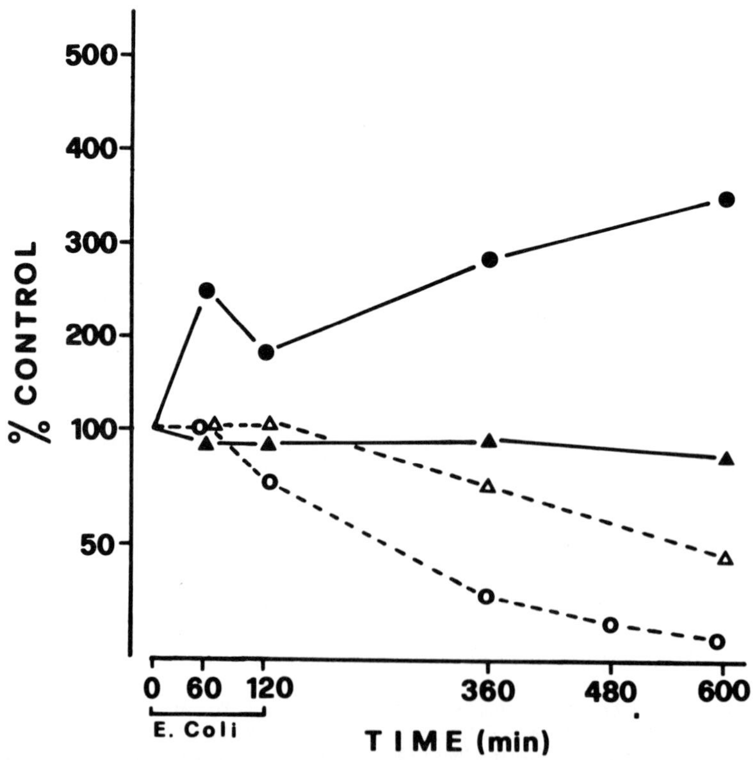

Fig. 3. Response of baboons to infusion of sublethal (closed symbols, continuos line) or lethal (open symbols, dotted line) doses of E. Coli. Circles: fibrinogen; Triangles: protein C/activated protein C.

Due to the short half life of protein C (7-8 hours) and to the severe liver disease induced by E. Coli, it might be wondered if the decrease of protein C is to be attributed to impaired synthesis of the zymogen or to increased protein C activation and consumption (activated protein C has a half life of 10 min in the circulation). To approach the question we infused HPC4 prior to a sublethal E. Coli dose. Inhibition of protein C activation in vivo changed the sublethal dose of E. Coli into a lethal dose, with a drop of fibrinogen within few hours and maintainance of protein C at baseline levels. In additional experiments it was shown that such a picture could be prevented by infusing the animal with previously activated protein C (Fig. 4).

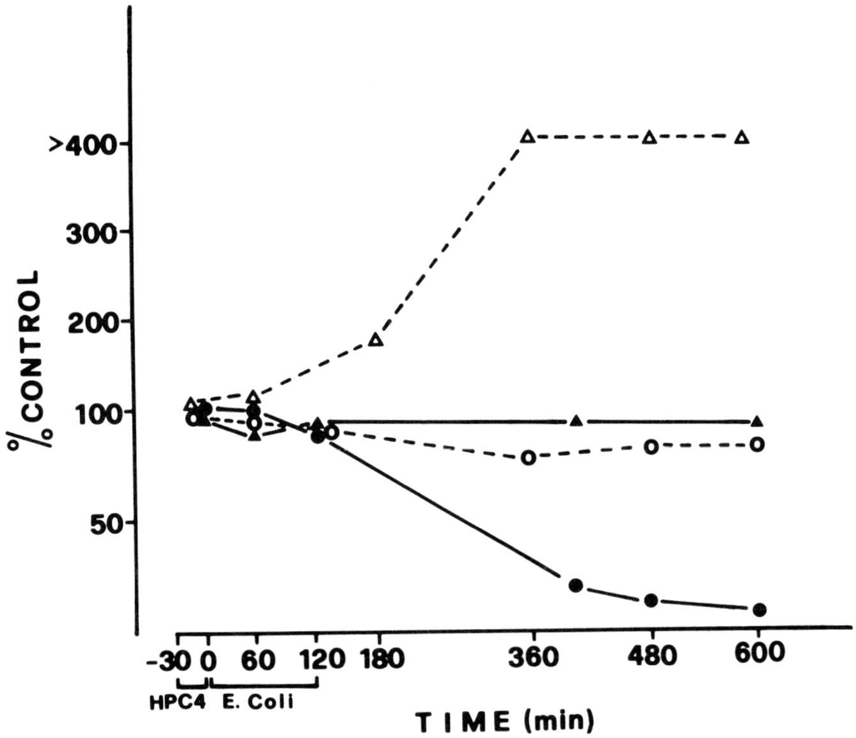

Fig. 4. Response of baboons to the infusion of a sublethal dose of E. Coli preceded by HPC4 (closed symbols, continuos line) and of a sublethal dose of E. Coli and activated protein C preceded by HPC4 (open symbols, dotted line). Circles: fibrinogen; triangles: protein C/activated protein C.

The observation that a sublethal dose of E. Coli is transformed into a lethal dose when protein C activation is blocked, demonstrates that activated protein C prevents the coagulopathic response which follows infusion of E.Coli in sublethal doses . In addition to this ,infusion of activated protein C prevents the lethal effects, thus acting as an effective in vivo anticoagulant.

The Calcium dependency of HPC4 was exploited in setting up a new functional assay for protein C. Similar to all vitamin K-dependent proteins, protein C has a domain, termed the gla-domain, rich in gammacarboxyglutamic acid residues which bind Calcium ions. This domain is critical for the expression of the biological activities of vitamin K-dependent coagulation factors, being implicated in the Calcium dependent binding to phospholipid membranes. Acquired protein C deficiency has been described in association with a- or hypo-carboxylation of the gla-domain (oral anticoagulation). Thus, in order to develop a functional assay for protein C, it was important to know whether the binding of the monoclonal antibody HPC4 involved the gla-domain of protein C. If so, only the fully carboxylated forms of protein C could be isolated. It could be shown that the calcium dependency of HPC4 was not related to the gla-domain of protein C. When protein C was applied to a column of Affigel 10 coupled with HPC4 at 5 mg/ml concentration, in the presence of calcium ions, all the protein bound to the column. Quantitative

Changing trends in hemostatic testing

Jawed Fareed, Ph.D. and Jeanine M. Walenga, Ph.D.

Hemostasis Research Laboratories, Department of Pathology, Loyola University Medical Center, Maywood, Illinois 60153, USA

Abstract - The clinical hemostasis laboratory is undergoing a dramatic phase of development. Routine global assays such as the PT and APTT remain useful for screening of the coagulation factors but current knowledge of hemostatic mechanisms has revealed the added importance of the fibrinolytic system, endothelium, blood cellular elements and numerous regulators. Assays to measure these parameters utilize coagulant, synthetic substrate and immunologic techniques. The measurement of "molecular markers" for sensitive (sub-nanogram/ml levels) and specific evaluation of hemostatic activation are becoming more common. Better knowledge combined with developments in the areas of biotechnology, chemical synthesis, extraction of natural products and pharmacologic concepts have led to the development of more targeted antithrombotic drugs which, unlike warfarin and heparin, can be difficult to monitor. Quantitation of protein C, protein S, factor VII, fibrinopeptide A, prothrombin fragment F 1+2 and thrombin-antithrombin complexes can be used for evaluating venous thrombosis. Platelets and endothelium can be evaluated through platelet release products (platelet factor 4, ß-thromboglobulin), eicosanoids (thromboxane B_2, 6-keto-$PGF_{1\alpha}$) and endothelial release products (t-PA, ACE, growth factors). Fibrinolysis and thrombolytic agents can be monitored utilizing immunologic methods for D-dimer, tPA inhibitor and Bß related peptides. Functional-immunologic ratios of specific coagulant and fibrinolytic proteins and measurement of enzyme-inhibitor complexes can be used to indicate the level of activation. Combining current assay techniques and instrumentation, concepts such as panel profiling of various assays specific for a particular disorder (eg. DIC, bleeding risk, hypercoagulable state) are emerging. In view of the complex mechanisms of thrombogenesis and recognition of specific markers, multiparametric laboratory profiles are being developed which will warrant consideration from both clinicians and laboratorians.

INTRODUCTION

Current advancements in biomedical disciplines have significantly contributed to a clearer understanding of hemostatic mechanisms at a molecular level. The period between 1970 and the early 1980's was explosive in the area of biochemical and molecular techniques which provided a basis for fundamental discoveries. Hemostasis is now known to be a process which encompasses not only coagulation but also fibrinolysis, platelets, endothelium and interacting substances. In fact, hemostasis is no longer regarded merely as an independent system of clotting but rather as a general physiologic response that, when uncontrolled, may contribute to the pathophysiology of inflammatory reactions, heart disease, cancer and other disorders.

Coagulant enzymes, proteins, and activation products (early peptide residues following enzymatic cleavage); circulating enzymes, activation products, and enzyme-inhibitor complexes associated with fibrinolysis; substances and activation products related to platelets; and other substances related to these pathways of which these interacting roles are yet to be clarified are all incorporated in the hemostatic system. Many enzymes have more than one function and can activate several pro-enzymes and/or neutralize various active enzymes (ref. 1-4).

From the standpoint of the current knowledge of the hemostatic system, clinical coagulation laboratories generally only perform basic assays. Global clotting assays (the PT and APTT) are used as screening tests for the coagulation system. More specific assays, using a clotting endpoint, are the thrombin time, fibrinogen assay, fibrin split product quantitation and specific coagulation factor quantitation. Platelet counts are commonly done also. Each of these assays is important for the evaluation of the coagulation system. However, in the past there has been an obvious lack of evaluation of the fibrinolytic system, endothelium and platelet function.

Today with the aid of newer laboratory techniques, the individual components of each phase of the hemostatic system can be identified and evaluated. Beside the clotting techniques which require an intact coagulant system to avoid false results, chromogenic (amidolytic) assays using synthetic substrates, ELISA and RIA assays are now available. Thus, these newer techniques provide more specific and more sensitive diagnostic measures than the routinely used clotting assays (ref. 5).

Using the routine and the newer laboratory methods, on-going clinical events can be more easily defined and treated (ref. 6-8). A hypercoagulable state or a sub-clinical pathologic state in patients at risk of thrombosis can be identified. Equally well, patients at risk of bleeding can be identified and effectively treated. The newly recognized hemostatic parameters, their molecular properties and their significant clinical functions will be described in this manuscript. The well-known common factors will not be discussed. Automation will undoubtedly play a key role in the development, implementation and cost effective use of newer techniques.

HEMOSTATIC PARAMETERS

Coagulation system activators

The enzymes of the coagulation system circulate in blood as pro-enzymes which need to be activated to be functional. All coagulation laboratories measure this, the main system of clotting factors; however, it is now clear that it can be initially activated through many different mechanisms. Thus, any quantitatable change in these factors may represent a chronic and/or severe disorder elsewhere. Furthermore, specific applications of the known clotting factors are under study for the high-risk cardiac and vascular disorders.

Factor VII-VIIa. Although known for many years, the use of FVII-FVIIa in determining a hypercoagulable state has recently come of interest. Ratios of FVII:antigenic to FVII:coagulant may prove to be a relevant marker of hypercoagulable state or atherosclerosis. Similarly, quantitation of circulating levels of tissue thromboplastin (the endogenous activator of FVII) are under investigation as a marker for thrombotic tendency. Factor VII is also activatable by numerous therapeutic agents such as prothrombin complexes, interleukin-II, recombinant erythropoietin and intralipid.

Factor FVIII. Since FVIII is produced in the endothelium, the focus on this factor as a relevant marker for endothelial disorders including atherosclerosis, has emerged. FVIII:antigen also know as Von Willebrand's factor is also being evaluated as a marker of enhanced platelet-endothelium interaction. Increased levels of factor VIII functionality and antigen have been identified as major risk factors in thrombosis.

Complement. Circulating complement system zymogens are activated by antibodies, endotoxin, plasmin, or trypsin (classic pathway) or by bacterial lipopolysaccharides and parasitic antigens (alternative pathway). Complement activation leads to cellular lysis, chemotaxis and phagocytosis, effecting removal of foreign particles from the host. These same factors cause tissue damage when overactivated. The hemostatic system has been linked with the complement system through factor XII and activated leukocytes. In DIC, for example, thrombin cleaves C3 and C5, and several platelet-complement and coagulation-complement interactions have been observed. Considerations for immunotherapy and transplantation are of growing importance.

Fibrinolytic system activators

A large effort to study the fibrinolytic system has taken place in the last several years. As in the coagulation system, both proenzymes, activators and inhibitors comprise this system of clot lysis. Clearly, fibrinolysis is equally important to hemostasis and overall health as is the coagulation system. This has been demonstrated by the extreme interest in the development of thrombolytic agents.

Plasminogen. Plasminogen is the precursor of plasmin, the most significant activator of fibrinolysis. Abnormal plasminogens have been described in persons with thromboembolic disease. Plasminogen deficiencies have been associated with hyaline membrane disease in premature infants, with DIC and with promyelocytic leukemia. Plasminogen measurement is useful for detecting an activated fibrinolytic system. It is essential to have adequate plasminogen levels during thrombolytic therapy for effective treatment.

Plasminogen activator. Plasminogen activators are a heterogeneous group of serine proteases that convert plasminogen to plasmin. They have been commonly isolated from vascular tissue and plasma. Plasminogen activators exist in both zymogenic and active forms. All cleave the Arg_{560}-Val peptide bond of Glu-plasminogen to create plasmin. Urokinase (from urine and kidney tissue culture) has been isolated in two molecular forms: 55,000 daltons (high molecular weight) and 32,000 daltons (low molecular weight). Streptokinase, isolated from ß-hemolytic streptococci, in contrast to urokinase, is not a serine protease. Rather, streptokinase activates plasminogen by forming a 1:1 molar complex. Tissue plasminogen activator (tPA) is of great interest as a measure of endogenous fibrinolytic activity, particularly in association with cardiovascular diseases. It appears to be a serine protease. Increased levels have been shown in certain pathologic bleeding states, particularly in the presence of malignant tumors, and decreased levels of tPA have been correlated with thromboembolic disease.

Coagulation and fibrinolytic inhibitors

Both the coagulation and the fibrinolytic systems, which balance each other in opposing activities, have natural inhibitors to counteract the active state within each system. These inhibitors are indispensable for proper hemostasis.

Antithrombin III. AT III plays a central role in the regulation of the coagulation system, strongly inhibiting thrombin and factor Xa. It also inhibits factors XIIa, XIa and Va, kallikrein, Cl-esterase inhibitor, and plasmin. It is naturally a slow, progressive inhibitor; however, in the presence of heparin, AT III is potentiated 1000-fold to become a fast-acting inhibitor. The therapeutic efficacy of heparin depends on the presence of AT III, such that persons lacking this inhibitor fail to respond to heparin therapy. Qualitative abnormalities and quantitative deficiencies of AT III are associated with an increased risk of thromboembolism, as observed in resistance to heparin therapy, use of oral contraceptives, liver disease, DIC, nephrotic syndrome, and L-asparaginase therapy. Recently, several commercial therapeutic AT III preparations have become available.

Heparin cofactor II. Heparin also interacts with heparin cofactor II (HC II), a plasma inhibitor distinguishable from AT III. This reaction proceeds in a 1:1 molar ratio to inhibit thrombin. Dermatan sulfate a glycosaminoglycan similar to but different than heparin, specifically activates HC II but not AT III.

α_2-Antiplasmin. Several plasma components inhibit plasmin; however, α2-AP (α_2-plasmin inhibitor) is the most rapid and specific of the inhibitors. α_2-AP binds to the light (ß) chain of plasmin to form an inactive complex in a reaction that exceeds the speed of the AT III-heparin-thrombin reaction by 100 fold. The inhibitory activity of α_2-AP is directed against both fluid-phase and fibrin-bound plasmin. α_2-AP has also been shown to directly bind to fibrin, causing interference in the plasmin-fibrin reaction. α_2-AP inhibits serine proteases other than plasmin such as Hageman factor fragment, kallikrein, factor XIa, thrombin, factor Xa and urokinase. In certain disorders of fibrinolysis the level of α_2-AP may be significantly decreased, leading to enhanced fibrinolysis and excessive bleeding. α_2-AP concentration is decreased in hepatic cirrhosis, DIC and during the course of thrombolytic therapy.

α_2-Macroglobulin. α_2-M is a dimeric protein with pairs of subunit chains held together by disulfide bridges. Plasma levels of α_2-M drop from 625 mg/dl in infancy to 250 mg/dl in adults. Increases are observed during pregnancy and oral contraceptive use, whereas decreases are observed during thrombolytic therapy. α_2-M has the widest spectrum of protease inhibiting activity, forming complexes with thrombin, plasmin and kallikrein. Complexes can also be formed with neutral proteases, elastase, collagenase and cathepsin D. Thus α_2-M may play a regulatory role at cell surfaces or on endothelium. The mechanism of action of α_2-M remains unsolved. In comparison to α_2-AP, α_2-M is a slow-acting inhibitor of plasmin.

Cl-Esterase inhibitor. Cl-INH is a plasma protease inhibitor of Cl-esterase (Cl-E, the activated first component of complement), kallikrein, plasmin and factors XIa, XIIa and XIIf. No hemostatic abnormalities have been reported in persons with Cl-INH deficiency, perhaps because of the overlapping inhibitory activity of AT III and plasminogen activator inhibitor. However, observation of decreased levels has been valuable in the diagnosis of angioneurotic edema, a major life-threatening disease.

Protein C. Protein C (PrC) inhibits factors Va and VIIIa and stimulates fibrinolysis. PrC is activated by thrombin, the cofactor protein S (PrS) and thrombomodulin an endothelial cell surface cofactor. It is inhibited by vitamin K antagonists but not by heparin or AT III. Numerous congenital deficiencies of PrC that are directly related to thrombotic complications have been reported. Additionally, PrC contained in prothrombin complex concentrates may be responsible for the undesired anticoagulant activity associated with these treatments.

Protein S. PrS is a vitamin K dependent serine protease that acts as a cofactor (with endothelial surface bound thrombomodulin) in the activation of PrC. It can be quantitated by immunoelectrophoresis.

Plasminogen activator inhibitor. Plasminogen activator inhibitor (PAI), a plasma protein of approximately 75,000 daltons, inhibits factor XIIa and urokinase- or streptokinase-induced activation of plasminogen. However, PAI fails to inhibit plasmin, kallikrein or factors XI, X and IX. Decreased levels of PAI have been associated with bleeding problems. Increased levels of this inhibitor are found in numerous prothrombotic and thrombotic states.

α_1-Antitrypsin. The role of α_1-AT as a protease inhibitor is minor even though its plasma concentration is highest of all protease inhibitors. α_1-AT slowly inhibits thrombin; the rate depends on the molar ratio of α_1-AT to thrombin. α_1-AT also inhibits plasmin, factor XIa, and possibly factor Xa. There is evidence that α_1-AT regulates the actions of white blood cell enzymes. Congenital deficiencies of α_1-AT are not associated with major thrombotic or bleeding tendencies; however, α_1-AT is an acute-phase reactant showing increased levels in inflammatory and necrotic diseases (especially hepatocellular diseases), oral contraceptive use and pregnancy. Proteolytic destruction of pulmonary tissue in congenital α_1-AT deficiency is a direct cause of lung disease.

Serine protease-inhibitor complexes

Activated serine proteases form complexes with their respective inhibitors, for example, FXa-AT III, thrombin-AT III, plasmin-α_2-AP, plasmin-α_2-M, kallikrein-C1-INH, complement-C1-INH, and PrC_a-C_a inhibitor. The presence of formed complexes in circulation indicates hemostatic activation and activated systems can be identified by the specific complexes. Monoclonal antibodies to these complexes are being developed. TAT the thrombin-antithrombin complex has shown under current investigation to be associated with a prothrombotic state in DIC, leukemia and post-surgically.

Platelets

Platelets, the first line of defense against bleeding, are key elements in the balance of hemostatic mechanisms. They react to a wide range of stimuli responding by shape change, adhesion, aggregation and degranulation. Each of these functional responses are quantitatable by laboratory techniques. Several of the new technical applications are given below.

Platelet-associated immunoglobulins. Platelet immunoglobulins may consist of true antiplatelet antibodies binding to platelet Fc receptors or endogenous IgG bound to normal platelets. The increased amount of bound immunoglobulin is responsible for rapid clearance of platelets by the mononuclear phagocytic system, resulting in the clinical manifestation of thrombocytopenia. Platelet associated IgG is elevated in isoimmune neonatal thrombocytopenia, alloimmune thrombocytopenia, idopathic or autoimmune thrombocytopenic purpura and drug-induced thrombocytopenia.

Platelet surface markers. Proteins, phospholipids and glycoprotein receptors provide the make up for the platelet surface. With activation or non-activation the composition of these surface markers will change. Monoclonal antibodies have been developed against these components making it possible to evaluate platelet structure. The presence or absence of receptors for fibrinogen binding (GPIIb, GPIIIa), epinephrine binding (α receptors), or subendothelial binding (GPIb) can be quantitated.

Endothelium

The endothelium is a primary factor in the balance of hemostasis. Although it is of such critical importance, there are few methods of studying its functionality. Several of the herein described parameters are synthesized by the endothelium or found on its surface and are thus being used for its evaluation. These parameters include factor VII:ag and c, factor VIII:ag, t-PA, thromboxane B_2, leukotriene C_4 and certain growth factors.

Molecular markers

The initial activation stages of coagulation, fibrinolysis, platelets or endothelium produce very low molecular weight substances as enzymatic cleavage products or cellular release products. These substances are derived from defined sources by specific processes. For these reasons and since they are only found in ng or pg/ml quantities, they have been collectively termed molecular markers. These markers can be used as sensitive and specific markers of hemostatic activation.

Fibrinopeptide A. Thrombin hydrolysis of fibrinogen yields two small peptides: fibrinopeptide A and fibrinopeptide B (FPA and FPB). As FPA and FPB are released, polymerization sites on the central "D" and "E" domains of the remaining fibrinogen molecule are exposed allowing for the formation of fibrin. Immunoassay of FPA provides an early, specific indication of thrombin activation. The normal plasma FPA range is 0.5 to 3.0 ng/ml. Increased plasma FPA levels are found in DIC, neoplasia, burns, various leukemias and following hip surgery. Decreased levels are seen in antithrombotic therapy.

<u>Bß-related peptides.</u> Plasmin progressively degrades fibrin or fibrinogen to first release a series of peptides from the B chain. These are Bß-related peptides that include Bß1 - 118, Bß1-42 and Bß15-42. Numbers indicate the amino acid region cleaved from the fibrin molecule. Subsequent cleavage yeilds larger fragments X, Y, D and E from the D and E domains. Bß-related peptides are elevated in DIC, primary fibrinolysis and burns. Bß-related peptides are normally present in plasma at a concentration range of 0.5 to 30.0 ng/ml.

Both FPA and Bß peptides are associated with hypercoagulable conditions. However, the specific origins of both substances allow differentiation between primary and secondary fibrinolysis. Primary fibrinolysis associated with plasmin activity will show an increased level of Bß peptides but a normal level of FPA, PF4 and ßTG. Conversely, in secondary fibrinolysis or DIC, the coagulant, fibrinolytic and platelet pathways are activated, producing increased levels of FPA, Bß peptides and platelet release products.

<u>D-Dimer.</u> When fibrin is degraded by plasmin, a fragment is released which is characterized by two D fragments connected by a covalent bond. This D-dimer can be obtained only from fibrin, not fibrinogen, due to the presence of the cross-linking bond from the action of FXIII. Thus D-dimer is a specific marker for the action of plasmin on fibrin. This is in contrast to the fibrin split products (FSPs) which may be derived from fibrinogen or fibrin by the action of thrombin or plasmin. Normal plasma levels are <300 ng/ml.

<u>Platelet factor 4.</u> PF4 is a specific platelet release protein secreted in complex with a proteoglycan carrier. It is stored in the alpha granules and released upon platelet activation. Physiologically, PF4 functions as an antiheparin substance binding to heparin at a site different from the binding site of AT III. PF4 has also been shown to inhibit collagenase and to potentiate granulocyte elastase thus regulating cell growth. Normal plasma PF4 levels are 4.0 to 8.0 ng/ml. Elevated levels have been observed during myocardial infarction, venous thrombosis, myeloproliferative syndrome, diabetes and inflammatory states.

<u>ß-Thromboglobulin.</u> ßTG is a specific platelet release protein stored in the alpha granules. Its physiologic function is considered to be antiheparin. Normal plasma levels are 20.0 to 40.0 ng/ml. Elevated levels have been associated with similar conditions associated with increased PF4 levels.

<u>Prothrombin fragment 1+2.</u> From the action of the prothrombinase complex (FXa-FVa-Ca^+-PL) on prothrombin a peptide fragment, F 1+2, is initially released. Increased levels of F 1+2 can be detected before measurable amounts of thrombin have been generated or before prothrombin is measurably decreased. This is one of the most sensitive markers of coagulation activation.

<u>Eicosanoids.</u> Eicosanoids are unsaturated hydroxylated fatty acids derived from phosphatidylinositol and phosphatidylcholine by the enzymatic action of phospholipases C and A_2, respectively. These substances produce profound effects on all physiological systems at very low concentrations. Prostaglandins are derived from arachidonic acid through the prostaglandin pathways. Leukotrienes are subtances of a similar nature derived from arachidonic acid but through another pathway. Leukotriene C_4 (LtC_4) has been implicated in endothelial function. Preliminary studies have shown possible involvement of eicosanoids in uremia, hypertension, endotoxic shock, ischemic heart disease, diabetes, cerebrovascular disease and atherosclerosis.

Because of the extremely short half-lives (about 8 minutes) of eicosanoids, they are measured by their biologically inactive stable metabolites. Thromboxane B_2 is a stable metabolite of thromboxane A_2 (TxA_2) derived from arachidonic acid through the cycloxygenase pathway. TxA_2 is a very potent vasodilator and a potent platelet aggregating agent. Conversely, prostacyclin (PGI_2 or $PGF_{1\alpha}$), also derived from the arachidonic acid pathway, is a potent vasoconstrictor and inhibitor of platelet aggregation. A homeostatic balance exists between thromboxane production in the platelet and prostacyclin production in the endothelium. Other prostaglandins produced by platelets, such as PGE_2, PGF_2 and PGD_2, are also measurable, although their physiologic roles are less clear. Normal plasma levels of all eicosanoids are 0 to 30.0 pg/ml.

<u>Growth factors.</u> Several growth factors have been identified in relation to platelets and endothelium. Platelet derived growth factor (PDGF) is a smooth muscle cell mitogen which promotes smooth muscle cell growth demonstrated both in vitro and in vivo. Fibroblast growth factor (FGF) has been implicated as a link between the pituitary and the formation of atherosclerotic lesions. Chemotactic and permeability factors have also been isolated from platelets.

ANTITHROMBOTIC THERAPY

Anticoagulants

Anticoagulant therapy to reduce the clotability of blood is possible with warfarin derivatives used orally. This agent modifies the production of factors II, VII, IX and X. Recently, studies have shown that a fixed low dose may provide adequate effect and that the previously used higher dose adjusted by PT values may have been in effect an overdose.

Heparin

Heparin is a naturally occurring anticoagulant widely used as a therapeutic agent. It is a heterogeneous mixture of straight-chain anionic glycosaminoglycans of variable molecular weight (3,000-30,000 daltons), sulfation and saccharidic sequencing. As described previously, heparin potentiates the activity of AT III and HC II, thereby inhibiting numerous proteases, in particular thrombin and factor Xa. Heparin is also suspected in modulating platelet and endothelial cellular activities. The antithrombin action of heparin appears to be highly important for clot inhibition, and it seems to be closely associated with a bleeding tendency. Clinical studies indicate that conventional heparin therapy regulation is best monitored with a clot-based global assay such as the APTT.

Alternate routes of administration of heparin (subcutaneous vs. intravenous), low dose of conventional heparin and newer antithrombotic agents (low molecular weight heparins, dermatans, heparans, synthetic glycosaminoglycans) produce blood levels of heparin and antithrombotic effects that differ from those of conventional heparin therapy (ref. 9). Thus, a more sensitive assay than the APTT is required to monitor these therapeutic regimens. Prophylactic vs. therapeutic treatments are now being tested. Several chromogenic and clotting assays which measure either absolute or functional heparin levels are available based on either thrombin or factor Xa inhibition.

Antiplatelet Agents

Antiplatelet drugs are commonly used in the treatment of arterial thrombotic disorders such as stroke, peripheral vascular disorders and in the prevention of reinfarction. Aspirin and other antiplatelet drugs in combination with thrombolytic agents and oral anticoagulants have also been used to maximize the therapeutic effect. Several newer antiplatelet drugs such as the propionic acid derivative Ibuprofen^R, have also become available. These agents act by inhibiting cycloxygenase thus impairing platelet function. Their therapeutic effects can be monitored by measuring the products of the cycloxygenase pathway, most importantly the generation of thromboxane. Other antiplatelet drugs such as dipyridamole and ticlopidine act by different mechanisms.

Although conventional platelet function tests can be used to monitor the effects of these agents, platelet release proteins have been effectively used as markers of platelet activation (ref. 10-12). These markers can be used for all antiplatelet drugs regardless of their mechanism of action. Both monoclonal and polyclonal antibodies have been used in these assays.

Platelet function is strongly inhibited by stable metabolites of prostacyclin and other analogues. Additionally, W-3 fatty acid rich fish oils have also been used to treat thrombotic complications. Although monitoring is not an important consideration in this type of therapy, various analytical methods such as HPLC can be used to quantitate their levels if desired. The relevance of circulating levels of these agents to the observed therapeutic/toxic effects is not clearly established at this time.

Thrombolytic therapy

An accepted therapeutic measure in the acute treatment of myocardial infarction is lysis of the clot itself. T-PA, streptokinase and urokinase have all proven to be effective thrombolytic agents. Controversy still exists as to which is the better agent for fibrin specificity and whether adjunct heparin therapy to prevent rethrombosis is actually effective.

Developmental agents

Several new prophylactic and therapeutic agents and delivery systems are on the horizon. Hirudin, a specific thrombin inhibitor may replace heparin in certain therapeutic circumstances such as that required during surgery. Endothelial modulators such as ateroid a mixture of various glycosaminoglycans, defibrotide or sequential compression devices are showing beneficial effects. Blood viscosity modulators such as pentoxifylline are under development. Perhaps the most appropriate attitude in the future will be that of polytherapy where specifically targeted agents and dosages tailored to individual needs will be used. Other developments are improved routes of delivery including oral, transdermal and intranasal which are being investigated to replace intravenous and subcutaneous modes.

DISCUSSION

It is often difficult to identify and differentiate hemostatic disorders on the basis of global screening tests such as the PT and APTT and tests of fibrinogen and fibrin(ogen) split products, which were designed only for hemorrhagic disorders and not thrombotic disorders. As a result, relatively high rates of morbidity and mortality associated with thrombotic complications have occurred. Due to an increased understanding of the biochemistry and molecular biology of hemostasis, recent developments in clinical methodology and thus clinical diagnosis have been made.

Although current laboratory monitoring methods employ global tests, with the advent of new drugs which do not produce measurable effects on these global assays, it is necessary to devise newer laboratory methods to monitor the safety/efficacy of these drugs. One of the major targets of newer therapeutic approaches is the endothelium. Both pharmacologic and physical approaches have been used. Endothelial cells are known to produce several biochemically active substances, including tissue plasminogen activator, factor VIII related antigen and prostacyclin. In addition, several other proteins are released from the endothelium which can be used as markers of endothelial activation processes. The difficulty in the assessment of these agents is the relatively small amounts (<ng/ml) of the marker in plasma and their short half-life. The development of highly sensitive immunologic methods has produced a means to perform multiparametric profiling of endothelial cell function. The modulatory effects of endothelium on platelets and blood cells can also be readily observed.

Aside from the obvious bleeding or thrombotic disorders, we are finding activation of the hemostatic system in what were thought to be unrelated circumstances. It is now well recognized that physical and drug treatment of such disorders as cancer, cardiovascular diseases and orthopedic problems can result in significant alterations of the hemostatic system which may also lead to either thrombotic or hemorrhagic states. For example, treatment of cancer with interleukin-II has been found to be associated with stroke, vasculitis and other abnormalities of the hemostatic system. The use of recombinant erythopoietin has been known to produce platelet activation and arterial thrombosis. Numerous other anticancer drugs have been known to produce activation of fibrinolysis resulting in excessive bleeding. Radiation therapy, hyperthermia and mechanical manipulation of the vascular system produce profound alterations of the hemostatic system. These are only some of the examples in which a significant pathologic change in the patient's hemostatic system can be induced by a presumably inert treatment. Recognition of these situations and their prevention by either modifying the therapy or providing adjunct prophylactic measures requires early detection. The laboratory methods described here can be effectively used in these patients for initial diagnosis and then follow-up treatment.

Advanced therapeutic approaches recently introduced are plasma fractions for procoagulant therapy, antiplatelet agents, depolymerized heparins, subcutaneous heparin, and fibrinolytic agents. Furthermore, prophylactic therapies are being developed for those considered at risk to develop thrombosis. Molecular markers or synthetic substrate assays can be used to monitor the effects of these newer treatments.

The concept of polytherapy where more than one drug is used to treat a thrombotic disorder has necessitated the development of newer tests which can correctly predict the clinical effectiveness of combined drugs. In such cases, global and whole blood based assays may be more useful than the single assay for a factor or a platelet related product. It is, however, important to identify the major components of the hemostatic system which are effected by combined drug therapy and relate these to patient care (ref. 13-16). It is also important to develop cost-effective and practical multiparametric assays for both prognostic and diagnostic purposes.

At present, the clinical relevance of the newly identified parameters described must be established in many clinical instances. However, a future can be visualized in which the evaluation of these parameters will be incorporated into clinical laboratory evaluations of the hemostatic system.

REFERENCES

1. R.W. Colman, J. Hirsh, V.J. Marder, E.W. Salzman (eds), Hemostasis and Thrombosis: Basic Principles and Clinical Practice, Lippincott, Philadelphia (1987).
2. J.M. Walenga, Hemostasis and Thrombosis in the Clinical Laboratory, p. 367-416, Lippincott, Philadelphia (1988).
3. A.R. Thompson, L.A. Harker, Manual of Hemostasis and Thrombosis, Davis, Philadelphia (1983).
4. D. Ogston, The Physiology of Hemostasis, Harvard University Press, Cambridge (1983).
5. J. Fareed (ed), Semin. Thromb. Hemost. 9(3 and 4), 139-385 (1983).
6. R. Bick, Disorders of Hemostasis and Thrombosis, Thieme Stratton, New York (1985).
7. O.D. Ratnoff, C.D. Forbes, Disorders of Hemostasis, Grune & Stratton, Orlando (1984).

8. M. Verstraete, J. Vermylen, Thrombosis, Pergamon Press, New York (1984).
9. J. Fareed (ed), Semin. Thromb. Hemost. 11(1 and 2), 1-248 (1985).
10. J. Fareed, H.L. Messmore, E.W. Bermes Jr., Clin. Chem. 26(10), 1380-1391 (1980).
11. J. Fareed, W.H. Baker, A. Hayes, J.M. Walenga, Semin. Thromb. Hemost. 12(2), 102-109 (1986).
12. H.L. Messmore, J.W. Walenga, J. Fareed, Semin. Thromb. Hemost. 10(4), 264-269 (1984).
13. J.M. Walenga, J. Fareed, D. Hoppensteadt, R.M. Emanuele, CRC Critical Review in Lab. Sci. 22(4), 361;-389 (1986).
14. R. Hull, J. Hirsh, Arch. Int. Med. 143, 2061-2063 (1983).
15. J. Fareed, W.H. Baker, J.M. Walenga, H.L. Messmore, Thrombosis and Hemorrhagic Diseases, p. 83-88, Gozlem, Istanbul (1986).
16. P. Theroux, H. Ouminet, J. McCans, Latour, J.G., et al. New Eng. J. Med. 319(17), 1105-1111 (1989).

New diagnostic techniques using saliva: Introduction to the symposium

Rainer Haeckel

Institute for Laboratory Medicine, Zentralkrankenhaus St.-Jürgen-Str. Bremen, W.-Germany

Saliva plays two roles in medicine. On one side it is required for a healthy functioning of the human organism. A complete stop of the salivary flow leads to severe illness and even to death. On the other side it gains increasing importance for diagnostic purposes for several reasons (table 1).

Tab.1: Advantages of saliva as an alternate specimen material for diagnostic purposes

1. Proband
1.1 Less stress
1.2 No anemia risk
1.3 No infection risk
1.4 No thrombosis risk

2. Staff
2.1 No staff training

3. Diagnostic reasons
3.1 Reflexion of unbound plasma fraction
3.2 Reflexion of intracellular concentration
3.3 Better correlation with central compartment
3.4 No volume displacement effect

4. Costs
4.1 Lower costs for sampling

Saliva is easy to obtain. The sampling, which will be discussed at the end of this symposium, usually avoids almost any stress to the patient. Therefore, saliva is especially interesting for those studies which involve the hypothalamic - hypophyseal - adrenocortical - axis. It is well known that repeated venipunctures mask the response of several dynamic function tests.

Furthermore saliva is attractive for all studies which require often sampling as for instance to study biorhythms, ovulation and therapeutic drug monitoring. Furthermore the sampling bears less danger of arteficial anemias, infections or thrombosis.

Because less trained personnel is required the overall costs are lower than for blood sampling. Advantages for diagnostic interpretations will be discussed in the following reports.

These advantages, however, are confronted with two major disadvantages: the limited number of analytes available for diagnostic purposes and the difficulties with the interpretation of saliva/plasma ratios. In the following we will demonstrate which analytes are suited to be determined in saliva for diagnostic purposes and how existing difficulties can be overcome.

Clinical and research applications of salivary steroid analyses

R.F. Walker, G.F. Read, D. Riad-Fahmy, K. Griffiths

Tenovus Institute for Cancer Research, UWCM, Cardiff, CF4 4XX, U.K.

Abstract - Refinements in immunoassay technology have facilitated the determination of neutral steroid hormone concentrations in saliva to the extent that salivary determinations are now a practical alternative to either plasma- or urinary-based investigations. The ease and patient-acceptability of salivary sampling ensures that this technique has a role to play, not only in clinical studies of endocrine dysfunction, but also where intensive multiple-sampling regimens are required for epidemiological investigations.

INTRODUCTION

To those who have practised steroid endocrinology throughout the past three decades, progress during this period of time in the determination of the physiologically important steroid hormones in biological fluids must be considered phenomenal. In the early fifties, only relatively insensitive colorimetric assays were available to assess steroid levels in biological fluids. There was intense excitement in the field of clinical endocrinology when, in 1955, from the laboratories of Professor G.F. Marrian in Edinburgh University, came the announcement [1] of a procedure for the separation and measurement of the urinary oestrogens at levels of only a few micrograms. This work was carried out by J.B. Brown using the Kober reaction. Other group analysis of urinary steroids such as the 17-hydroxycorticosteroids and 17-oxosteroids developed from the work of Norymberski [2]; the specific determination of individual steroid hormones in plasma, however, had to await the arrival of radioactive steroids in the early 1960's, when it became possible to measure plasma levels of aldosterone and testosterone by the tedious double isotope derivative techniques.

Progress in steroid endocrinology was made in the mid-sixties with the development of electron capture gas liquid chromatography and the use of the steroid derivatives, the heptafluorobutyrates, which allowed specific plasma steroids to be measured in the low nanogram - high picogram range. Again, the procedures were complicated and time-consuming but the competitive protein-binding assays, introduced by Beverley Murphy [3], offered a much simpler procedure. The use of antibodies as the protein-binding moiety saw the birth of the radioimmunoassays for steroids in 1969 [4]. Subsequently, as better antisera were produced, sensitive and specific radioimmunoassays for plasma steroids were developed to determine concentrations in the low picogram range. Thus assays were now some 10^6 times more sensitive than in the 1950's. These techniques were comparatively simple and, during the past decade, have been seen to revolutionise the field of steroid endocrinology.

The availability of such sensitive radioimmunoassays for steroids has now allowed the development of yet another exciting era in endocrinology. Pioneering work of Shannon and his colleagues in the mid 1960's [5,6] directed attention to the possible role of salivary steroid analysis to assess adrenal function. Unfortunately, the use of the non-specific Porter-Silber reaction for the determination of 17-hydroxycorticosteroids - present in such low concentrations in saliva, failed to realise the potential value of this form of analysis.

During the last decade, however, using sensitive, specific radioimmunoassays for salivary steroid analysis, research at the Tenovus Institute for Cancer Research in Cardiff has been directed towards establishing the important role such assays will have in future investigations of endocrine function [7,8]. Recent work in other laboratories [9] has now done much to complement these early studies of salivary steroids, directing attention to the value of multiple-sampling regimens [10,11] to investigate endocrine function. Most steroids of diagnostic significance in the routine assessment of endocrine activity can now be measured in saliva, as can various other synthetic steroids used in oral contraception.

IMMUNOASSAYS FOR STEROIDS IN SALIVA

Research at the Tenovus Institute has been concerned with the assessment of the potential value of salivary steroid assays in both clinical endocrinology and in many aspects of endocrine cancer, particularly of breast and prostate. The ease with which saliva can be collected is clearly a major advantage in such studies, the non-invasive procedure providing the opportunity for the development of multi-sampling regimens for intensive investigation of rhythmic hormone production. The inherent fear of tuberculosis is rapidly being overcome, as clinicians realise that it is saliva, not sputum, that is being collected directly into small disposable tubes. Also saliva can, in general, be said to reduce the potential risk of hepatitis infection.

Much of the earlier work has now been reviewed [7,8,9], and the accumulated data indicate that the levels of neutral steroid hormones in whole saliva are identical to those in parotid fluid, and are essentially independent of flow rate. Moreover, salivary levels of neutral steroids relate well to the concentration of plasma free hormone, not bound to circulating proteins and considered the biologically active moiety. However, it has to be recognised that there are steroid metabolising enzyme systems in salivary glands, such as the 11β-hydroxysteroid dehydrogenase (11β-OHSD) [5,12] converting cortisol to cortisone but, providing the assays have sufficient analytical specificity, such determinations are still of clinical value. The unequivocal identification of steroids in saliva demands searching validation techniques and high resolution GLC-mass spectrometry - with selected ion monitoring - is widely accepted as a reference method for the measurement of steroids in plasma [13]. The refinements of high resolution mass spectrometry [14,15] and metastable peak monitoring [16,17], which enhances analytical specificity, have been used by the Institute's Mass Spectrometry Unit to validate immunoassays in saliva.

It has long been appreciated that simple assays to determine the 'free' steroid hormone concentrations in plasma would be of real value. It is well recognised that the difficulties associated with procedures involving equilibrium dialysis or ultrafiltration make them unsuitable for routine use, whereas the salivary steroid assays are technically simple. The data from the Institute, and now from other Centres in the world, thus clearly indicate that the new approach will have a major role to play in clinical endocrinology in the future.

Examples of the use of salivary steroid hormone assays in the routine assessment of endocrine dysfunction are now briefly described and illustrate well the establishment of this new parameter in clinical endocrinology.

HYPOTHALAMIC-PITUITARY-ADRENAL (HPA) AXIS

Cortisol, secreted by the adrenal gland under the control of ACTH, is mainly present in plasma, bound either specifically to corticosteroid-binding globulin (CBG) or, less avidly, to albumin. Only 5-10% of the cortisol circulates as the 'free', physiologically active form which maintains normal homeostasis by a negative feed-back system. Despite the reported activity of the salivary gland 11β-OHSD, an excellent correlation has been found between plasma 'total' cortisol levels and those in saliva, determined by the GC-MS validated assay [18]. Furthermore, infusion of cortisol hemisuccinate into a normal subject whose adrenal gland was suppressed by dexamethasone, with appropriate plasma and saliva collections, indicated an excellent correlation between cortisol concentrations in saliva, plasma free, and total levels in plasma. The administration of a single, i.v. bolus dose of cortisol (5 mg) to another dexamethasone-suppressed volunteer demonstrated a significant increase, within one minute, in the concentration of this steroid in both plasma and saliva.

In the assessment of disorders in the HPA-axis, the capacity of the adrenal glands to secrete cortisol may be determined by a Synacthen stimulation test. The value of using salivary cortisol determinations for this test was clear when elevated levels of cortisol were observed after 60 mins. in both plasma (3-fold increase) and saliva (8-fold increase) in normal volunteers, compared with the lack of cortisol rise in both of these fluids observed in a patient with adrenal atrophy. Determination of cortisol in saliva samples collected at 2-hr intervals during waking hours from normal volunteers showed the characteristic diurnal variation in adrenal activity. Such a circadian rhythm of cortisol secretion is lost in a patient with Cushing's syndrome in whom the basal concentration of cortisol is elevated and is not suppressed by dexamethasone. The potential of salivary steroid analysis to investigate adrenal function is further described elsewhere [7,9] in which it becomes evident that clinical management of such patients can be conducted just as effectively with salivary cortisol measurements as with plasma determinations. For example, dexamethasone suppression tests are frequently used for the differential diagnosis of Cushing's Syndrome; in a patient showing histological evidence of a pituitary tumour, dexamethasone reduced cortisol levels in saliva and plasma but only limited suppression was observed in a patient with ectopic production of ACTH.

Of particular interest, however, have been the studies that clearly highlight the value of salivary assays to investigate adrenal activity in small children and infants. The normal adult range in cortisol concentrations, together with a marked diurnal rhythm, is evident in children aged 3 years or more. Rhythmic activity was less evident in infants of less than 72 hrs age, and the controversy [19,20] as to whether a 12-hr rhythm exists or adrenal activity depends on psychophysiological arousal has been resolved using cortisol determinations in saliva [21].

CONGENITAL ADRENAL HYPERPLASIA

Clinical studies in Cardiff, in which assays for 17α-hydroxyprogesterone (17OH-progesterone) have been used to monitor the treatment of patients with congenital adrenal hyperplasia, are described in detail in a recent report [22]. In a major proportion of cases, the condition results from a disorder in adrenal steroid biosynthesis [23] due to a 21-hydroxylase enzyme deficiency. This leads not only to an accumulation and secretion of 17OH-progesterone, but to the formation of androstenedione and testosterone with the consequent clinical feature of the condition, virilisation. Female infants are born with ambiguous genitalia while males will virilise during infancy if not treated. Urinary pregnanetriol estimations or, more recently, plasma levels of 17OH-progesterone have been used to diagnose the condition, while treatment has been to provide glucocorticoid replacement therapy to suppress ACTH secretion, thereby inhibiting excess androgen synthesis and promoting normal growth through childhood to adolescence.

The treatment has been monitored previously by single plasma sample analysis of 17OH-progesterone, with the inherent problems of interpretation caused by the diurnal rhythmic production of the steroid, the stress of venepuncture and the effect of the regular glucocorticoid therapy on the steroid level. Salivary steroid analysis provides a more patient-acceptable approach to monitoring children with this condition, while serial sampling allows construction of salivary 17OH-progesterone profiles which aid both the monitoring of patient compliance and the assessment of effectiveness of glucocorticoid therapy in achieving clinical control.

In Cardiff, therefore, patients collect saliva samples, at home, during the weekend prior to a visit to the Paediatric Endocrine Clinic. The two consecutive-day 17OH-progesterone profiles are determined to assess adequacy of treatment. A considerable overlap of 17OH-progesterone levels is seen between 1600 and 2200 hrs in patients adequately treated and in those requiring a higher dose of glucocorticoid replacement therapy [9], whereas the early morning concentrations have considerable clinical value. The procedure allows early distinction of children who are over-treated from those who are receiving adequate therapy, such patients previously only being detected when clinical manifestations of glucocorticoid excess appear.

MONITORING OVARIAN FUNCTION IN INFERTILE WOMEN

Early studies at the Tenovus Institute [24] quickly directed attention to the value of serial salivary progesterone analysis to monitor ovarian function in subfertile women. Previously, routine studies of female infertility had to rely on two plasma progesterone analyses, collected at 14-day intervals, assessed in relation to basal body temperature charts.

Preliminary investigations quickly established the close relationship between plasma and saliva progesterone concentrations [7] and a regimen of daily sampling of 15 normal women established a normal pattern of salivary progesterone concentrations through the menstrual cycle. Such daily sampling regimens indicated their value in serial studies to monitor ovulation and luteal function. Women attending the Infertility Clinic, Cardiff, now collect samples at home and these are stored deep frozen in a specially designed container, which eventually is returned to the laboratory. Since there is no evidence of a circadian rhythm of progesterone secretion, saliva sampling need not be restricted to a specific time of day, although in most of the Institute studies, sample collection was around 0900 hrs.

To illustrate the work, profiles of daily salivary progesterone concentrations in a subfertile woman attending the Clinic can show that progesterone levels are only marginally increased in the second half of the cycle, but daily treatment during days 5-9 of the second cycle with 50mg clomiphene citrate produced the required response, such that the subsequent progesterone profile was comparable to that of fertile women. Other patients, however, fail to respond to high (150 mg daily) doses of clomiphene. Certain patients with luteal phase abnormality present with salivary progesterone concentrations similar to those of normal healthy women except the luteal phase is of a short duration (9.2 ± 1.3 days) compared to normal (13.4 ± 1.7 days).

AUTOMATION OF SALIVARY STEROID ASSAYS

It is clear that salivary steroid analyses are just as effective, if not more so, than equivalent plasma determinations in the assessment and treatment of endocrine abnormality. Advantages of salivary analysis are seen where frequent, multiple specimen collection is required, although equally evident from such intensive patient monitoring is the increased laboratory workload. Automation is necessary, and the Institute's work in this field is illustrated by the development [9] of an automated assay for unconjugated salivary oestriol, based upon the continuous-flow, automated system of Ismail and his colleagues [25]. The procedure utilises a radio-iodinated tracer and an antibody coupled to Sepharose solid-phase, while separation of antibody-bound and free radioligand fractions is achieved by on-line filtration across a highly porous nylon membrane, the bound fraction being collected for counting. Output is in the form of a teletype printout and a punched tape which feeds to a data-processing system. A pen recorder allows continual visual monitoring of the output from the radioactivity counter.

There is an excellent agreement between the concentration of unconjugated oestriol in matched samples of plasma and saliva, together with a good correlation between the values of unconjugated oestriol determined by the automated procedure and by a well-validated manual radioimmunoassay [26].

Salivary unconjugated oestriol concentrations increase markedly through the third trimester of an uncomplicated pregnancy. However, although the procedure suggests that the established relationship between abnormal oestriol levels and foetal risk may well be identified using salivary oestriol measurements, it remains to be established whether such assays will be of clinical use in determining the timing of delivery of a patient with a foetus at risk. Certainly, the approach of using daily saliva monitoring is probably the best available to investigate intensively and resolve the controversy surrounding the real clinical value of oestriol analysis. The automated salivary oestriol radioimmunoassay, with an hourly analysis rate of approximately 30, using equipment costing in the order of £7000, offers the means to analyse the large number of specimens that are generated by such a study.

C_{19}-STEROIDS IN SALIVA

As with other steroids in saliva, the concentration of testosterone closely reflects the free, non-protein bound fraction of plasma [27,28] and therefore the index of androgenicity [29]. The circadian rhythm of testosterone production also necessitates multiple sampling schedules to provide a more informative assessment of endocrine status. Now underway are various investigations to assess the potential of salivary androgen analysis [9], but the following exemplify current interest in this field of research. Measurement of testosterone and other androgens in saliva may well be of diagnostic significance in investigations of women with hyperandrogenism. Data reported by James and his colleagues [30] show that androstenedione is a good discriminant in polycystic ovarian disease, with the majority of the patients having elevated levels in both saliva and plasma. Androstenedione production by the ovary has been implicated in the aetiology of the disease, and levels of both androstenedione and testosterone in saliva were decreased following therapy with cyproterone acetate and ethinyl oestradiol.

As part of the Institute's research into the endocrinology of prostatic cancer [31] studies have been directed to the hormonal status of the elderly male. Vermeulen and his colleagues [32] have reported a fall with age, not only in plasma testosterone, but also the plasma 'free' fraction, although the limitations of this latter determination have been well recognised. The steady fall of testosterone levels in saliva with increasing age [33] again illustrates the potential of such assays to investigate this aspect of endocrine cancer. Monitoring of salivary testosterone levels of patients with prostatic cancer whilst undergoing diethylstilboestrol therapy, or currently, after the administration of LH-RH analogues [34], may also provide a valuable clinical use for this analysis.

SALIVARY STEROID ANALYSIS IN RELATION TO CARCINOMA OF THE BREAST

In the past two or three decades, intensive research has been directed to the means by which treatment for cancer of the breast could be improved. It would now seem, however, that although the disease can be palliated by various therapy regimes, and recurrence delayed, there is little evidence to indicate that any of the modifications to well established procedures have subsequently affected survival. It is very reasonable, therefore, that attention should be directed to screening programmes that may identify the women at risk before clinical symptoms of the disease are manifest.

The classic work of Bulbrook and his colleagues [35,36] centred on the analysis of the urinary metabolites of the adrenal steroids, cortisol and DHA sulphate, and directed attention to the possible relationship of androgens to the aetiology of breast cancer; low androgen production appearing to constitute a high-risk factor. When analysed [37] with other well-established risk factors - age at menarche, family history, age at first-term birth - these, together with the low urinary C_{19}-steroid excretion, were found to have cumulative effects on a logistic scale for the probability of developing breast cancer. However, the weight of evidence was not considered adequate enough to instigate a national screening programme to identify those women at risk and hence requiring more careful clinical screening.

In relation to this, a study was undertaken to determine whether this reported abnormality of androgen secretion, identified by analyses of plasma and urine, was reflected in steroid levels in saliva [38]. Samples of saliva were collected over two days from normal women and from postmenopausal women with breast cancer, since it was believed that, if differences existed, discrimination may be improved by considering the rhythmic variability. Cortisol and DHA sulphate levels showed considerable between-subject variability both in cancer patients and in control subjects. Cortisol concentrations in both groups exhibited circadian rhythmicity, but values were higher in the saliva of patients. Although a less pronounced circadian rhythmicity was seen with DHA sulphate levels, with lower concentrations observed in breast cancer patients, and with the ratio of cortisol/DHA sulphate separating the groups, the value of the analysis in a screening programme must be considered low.

Although the role of the various hormones in the aetiology of breast cancer remains to be elucidated, it appears reasonably clear that the ovarian steroid hormones oestradiol-17 and progesterone are implicated. Early menarche and late menopause, which effectively increases the reproductive period of the female, have been reported to increase the risk of breast cancer [39], presumably related to the number of menstrual cycles and the changes in concentrations of ovarian hormones to which the maturing breast is subjected. With the well-accepted protective effect of early first-term birth [40], it would seem that these steroids are involved in the aetiology of the disease between menarche and first full-term pregnancy, a period that has been referred to as 'the first window' [41]. The 'second window' relates to the 5-10 year period prior to the menopause when abnormal cycles are frequently observed.

In these various arguments, oestradiol has generally been considered to promote the growth of breast cancer, whereas accumulated data from investigators with uterine tissue suggests that progesterone has a protective effect. It was of interest therefore that Mauvais-Jarvis and his colleagues [42] determined the luteal phase oestradiol and progesterone levels in plasma of 109 premenopausal women with various breast mastopathies and in 50 normal women. It was reported that in women with benign breast disease, the progesterone concentrations were subnormal, thus inferring inadequate luteal function. This initiated a similar study at Tenovus involving the measurements of salivary progesterone levels in premenopausal women with a history of benign breast disease, in women with primary breast cancer, and comparison with a group of age-matched controls [43]. Samples were collected, twice daily for one complete menstrual cycle, from 18 subjects in each group. Luteal dysfunction, as assessed by comparison with progesterone profiles of parous, mature premenopausal women, was not observed in women with a previous history of benign breast disease or in those with primary breast cancer.

Studies are currently underway [44] to obtain more detailed data on hormonal patterns in the postmenarchal girl during the period referred to as the first window. Salivary steroid analysis allows accurate assessment of ovarian function, together with timing of the establishment of ovulatory cycles in schoolgirls in the U.K. compared with those in Bangkok, Thailand, where the incidence of breast cancer is lower. Clearly, analysis of steroids in saliva is the only ethical and practical approach for such an investigation and, once again, illustrates the versatility of this new approach to steroid endocrinology.

REFERENCES

1. J.B. Brown, Biochem. J. 60, 185-193 (1955).
2. J.K. Norymberski and R.D. Stubbs, Biochem. J. 64, 176-178 (1956).
3. B. E.P. Murphy, W. Engelberg and C.J. Patee, J. Clin. Endocr. Metab. 23, 293-300 (1963).
4. G.E. Abraham, J. Clin. Endocr. Metab. 29, 866-870 (1969).
5. F.H. Katz and I.L. Shannon, Acta Endocr. (Copenh.) 46, 393-403 (1964).
6. I.L. Shannon, S.C. Beering and R.L. Jenson, J. Clin. Endocr. Metab. 26, 967-970 (1966).

7. D.R. Fahmy, G.F. Read, R.F. Walker and K. Griffiths, Endocrine Revs. 3, 367-395 (1982).
8. G.F. Read, D.R. Fahmy, D.W. Wilson and K. Griffiths, Commentaries on Research in Breast Disease 3, 61-92 (1983).
9. G.F. Read, D.R. Fahmy, R.F. Walker and K. Griffiths, (Eds.) Immunoassays of Steroids in Saliva. Proceedings of the 9th Tenovus Workshop, Alpha Omega Publishing Ltd., Cardiff (1984).
10. J.W. Goldzieher, T.S. Dozier, K.D. Smith and E. Steinberger, J. Clin. Endocr. Metab. 43, 824-830 (1976).
11. J.E. Buster, P.J. Meis, C.J. Hobel and J.R. Marshall, J. Clin. Endocr. Metab. 46, 907-910 (1978).
12. F.X. Galen, P. Pesquies, J. Menard and P. Corvol, Ann. Biol. Clin. (Paris) 31, 459-465 (1973).
13. H. Breuer and L. Siekmann, J. Steroid Biochem. 6, 685-688 (1975).
14. D.S. Millington, J. Steroid Biochem. 6, 239-245 (1975).
15. S.J. Gaskell and A.W. Pike, In 'Quantitative Mass Spectrometry in Life Sciences', A.P. De Leenheer, R.R. Roncucci and C. Van Peteghem (Eds.) Elsevier, Amsterdam, p.181-189 (1979).
16. S.J. Gaskell and D.S. Millington, Biomed. Mass Spectrom. 5, 557-558 (1978).
17. S.J. Gaskell, A.W. Pike and K. Griffiths, Steroids 36, 219-228 (1980).
18. R.F. Walker, In "Frontiers of Oral Physiology Vol. 5, Steroid Hormones in Saliva", D.B. Ferguson (Ed.) Karger, Basel, p33-50 (1984).
19. R.P. Zurbrugg, In 'Monographs in Paediatrics' Vol. 7. F. Faulkner, N. Kretchmer and E. Rossi (Eds.) Karger, Basel, p.1-83 (1976).
20. T.F. Anders, E.J. Sachar, J. Kream, H.P. Roffwarg and L. Hellman, Pediatrics 46, 532-537 (1970).
21. S.J. Francis, R.F. Walker, D.R. Fahmy, D. Hughes, J.F. Murphy, O.P. Gray, J. Pediatr. 111, 129-135 (1987).
22. I.A. Hughes, J. Dyas, J. Robinson, R.F. Walker and D.R. Fahmy, In 'Congenital Adrenal Hyperplasia', M.I. New (Ed.) Annals of The New York Academy of Sciences, Vol. 458, p193-202 (1985).
23. K. Griffiths and E.H.D. Cameron, Advances in Steroid Biochemistry and Pharmacology Vol. 2, Academic Press p223-265 (1970).
24. D.R. Fahmy, G.F. Read, R.F. Walker, S.M. Walker and K. Griffiths, J. Rep. Med. 32, 254-272 (1987)
25. A.A.A. Ismail, P.M. West, D.J. Goldie and A.C. Poole, Ann. Clin. Biochem. 18, 287-294 (1981).
26. P.L. Truran, G.F. Read and S. Walker, Clin. Chem. 28, 2393-2397 (1982).
27. R.G. Smith, P.K. Besch, B. Dill and V.C. Buttram, Fertil. Steril. 31, 513-517 (1979).
28. P.M. Baxendale, H.S. Jacobs and V.H.T. James, Clin. Endocrinol. (Oxf.) 16, 595-603 (1982).
29. A. Vermeulen, T. Stoica and L. Verdonck, J. Clin. Endocr. Metab. 33, 759-767 (1971).
30. V.H.T. James and P.M. Baxendale, In 'Immunoassays of Steroids in Saliva' G.F. Read, D.R. Fahmy, R.F. Walker and K. Griffiths, (Eds.) Alpha Omega Publishing Ltd., Cardiff, p.193-201 (1984).
31. K. Griffiths, P. Davies, M.E. Harper, W.B. Peeling and C.G. Pierrepoint, C.G. In 'Endocrinology of Cancer' Vol. 2, D.P. Rose, (Ed). CRC Press, p1-55 (1979).
32. A. Vermeulen, R. Rubens and L. Verdonck, J. Clin. Endocr. Metab. 34, 730-735 (1972).
33. G.F. Read, M.E. Harper, W.B. Peeling and K. Griffiths, Int. J. Androl. 4, 623-627 (1981).
34. K.J. Walker, A.O. Turkes, R.I. Nicholson, A. Turkes, K. Griffiths, M. Robinson, E. Dris and Z. Crispin, Lancet 2, 413-415 (1983).
35. R.D. Bulbrook, Adv. Steroid Biochem. Pharmacol. 1, 387-413 (1970).
36. R.D. Bulbrook, J.L. Hayward and C.C. Spicer, Lancet 2, 395-398 (1971).
37. V.T. Farewell, Cancer 40, 931-936 (1977).
38. G.F. Read, D.W. Wilson, F.C. Campbell, H.W. Holliday, R.W. Blamey and K. Griffiths, Eur. J. Cancer Clin. Oncol. 19, 477-483 (1983).
39. A. Kalache, Br. J. Surg. 68, 797-799 (1981).
40. B. MacMahon, P. Cole, T.M. Lin, et al. Bull. WHO 43, 209-221 (1970).
41. B.M. Sherman and S.G. Korenman, Cancer 33, 1306-1312 (1974).
42. P. Mauvais-Jarvis, R. Sitruk-Ware, F. Kuttenn et al, In 'Commentaries on Research in Breast Disease' R.D. Bulbrook and D.J. Taylor, (Eds.) Alan R. Liss Inc., New York, Vol. 1, p.25-29 (1979).
43. G.F. Read, J.A. Bradley, D.W. Wilson, W.D. George and K. Griffiths, Europ. J. Cancer Clin. Oncol 21, 9-17 (1985).
44. G.F. Read, D.W. Wilson, I.A. Hughes and K. Griffiths, (1984) J. Endocr. 102, 265-268 (1984).

Interpretation of salivary drug concentrations

Rainer Haeckel

Institute for Laboratory Medicine, Zentralkrankenhaus St.Jürgen-Str., Bremen, W.-Germany

Abstract - Although the use of saliva has great advantages in comparison with venous blood, it is not generally accepted yet, mainly because of problems with the interpretation of the results.

Usually blood and saliva conentrations are compared with each other by calculating the saliva/plasma ratio. At least eight factors have been identified which can influence the saliva/plasma ratio: transfer mechanism, pH-partition theory, salivary flow rate, phenomenon of fluctuating arterial-venous differences, linear elimination kinetic molecular weight, solubility and protein binding.

Several drugs are already known of which the therapeutic monitoring in saliva is caffeine, carbamazepine, citrofloxacin, diazepam, digoxin, ethanol, lithium, metoprolol, ofloxacin, oxprenolol, paracetamol, phenobarbital,phenytoin, procainamide, quinine, theophylline, tolbutamide.

INTRODUCTION

The determination of salivary drug concentrations is one of the major domaines for the application of saliva in laboratory medicine.

Phenytoin is one of the most accepted examples. This drug is more than 90 % bound to plasma albumin, and binding is commonly reduced in renal failure, hepatic disease, infancy, pregnancy, overdose and by drug interactions. In many epileptics, therefore, monitoring of total plasma phenytoin is invalid and should be replaced by measuring free plasma or total saliva concentration, which both correlate very well which each other (1).

Although the use of saliva has several advantages in comparison with venous blood, it is not generally accepted yet for many other drugs, mainly because of problems with the interpretation of the results.

The results from saliva are usually interpreted in comparison with results obtained from venous blood simply by considering the saliva/plasma ratio (S/P ratio). This ratio varies from analyte to analyte inter- and intra-individually. Various factors can influence the S/P ratio:

1. Transfer mechanism 2. Degree of ionisation 3. Flow rate
4. Protein binding 5. Molecular weight 6. Solubility
7. Linear elimination kinetics 8. Phenomenon of fluctuating arterial venous differences 9. Metabolism by salivary glands

The most important determinant for the S/P ratio is the transfer mechanism by which blood constituents are transfered from the intravasal compartment through the salivary cells into saliva. The mechanism can be divided into an intracellular and an extracellular route. Diffusion is the most commonly encountered intracellular mode and ultrafiltration, which occurs between the cells, the most common extracellular mode. A few substances are probably excreted into saliva, as for instance lithium and penicilline.

Most drugs pass into saliva by simple diffusion, which mainly depends on 3 factors: (1) The molecular weight appears to play a minor role. (2) The major determinant for free diffusibility is the solubility in water and/or lipids. Lipophilic substances more easily diffuse than lipophobic molecules. (3) The degree of ionisation plays an important role because of the partition theory.

According to the partition theory only the unionized fraction is able to pass the lipoid barrier between the 3 compartments: plasma, intracellular space and salivary fluid. Because the pH-value differs between the extra- and intracellular space (2), the total concentration as the sum of the ionized and unionized fraction varies on both sides. Acidic drugs tend to be lower and basic drugs to be higher in the cellular and salivary side than in the intravasal space.

The reverse situation occurs if the salivary pH-value is higher than the blood pH-value as for instance after a strong stimulation of the saliva flow rate or as usually observed in goats and cows which both have a salivary pH-value of about 8.0 (3). Under these conditions a saliva/plasma ratio of 3.3 was found for phenobarbital (in man it is about 0.32).

The saliva/plasma ratio of stronger acids and bases depends on variations of the salivary pH-value while the saliva/plasma ratio for weak acids with pK_a-values above 8.5 or weak bases with pK_a-values below 5.5 are almost unaffected by alteration of the salivary pH value in the range between 6 and 8. Consequently neutral drugs such as digoxin, ethanol, antipyrine and acetaminophen are pH-independent.

The protein binding of drugs is a further factor determining the S/P ratio. The protein bound fraction of drugs cannot pass the cell membrane. Therefore, the salivary drug concentration directly reflects the free plasma fraction.

Another factor which can influence the S/P ratio is the salivary flow rate, eventually because it affects the salivary pH value. Therefore, it is important to study the influence of the salivary flow rate on any constituent which is determined in saliva.

The next problem with the interpretation of the S/P ratio is its inconstancy during the 3 pharmacokinetic phases (absorption, distribution and elimination). At least three reasons can be identified: the phenomenon of fluctuating arterial-venous differences, the elimination kinetics and the concentration-dependent protein binding.

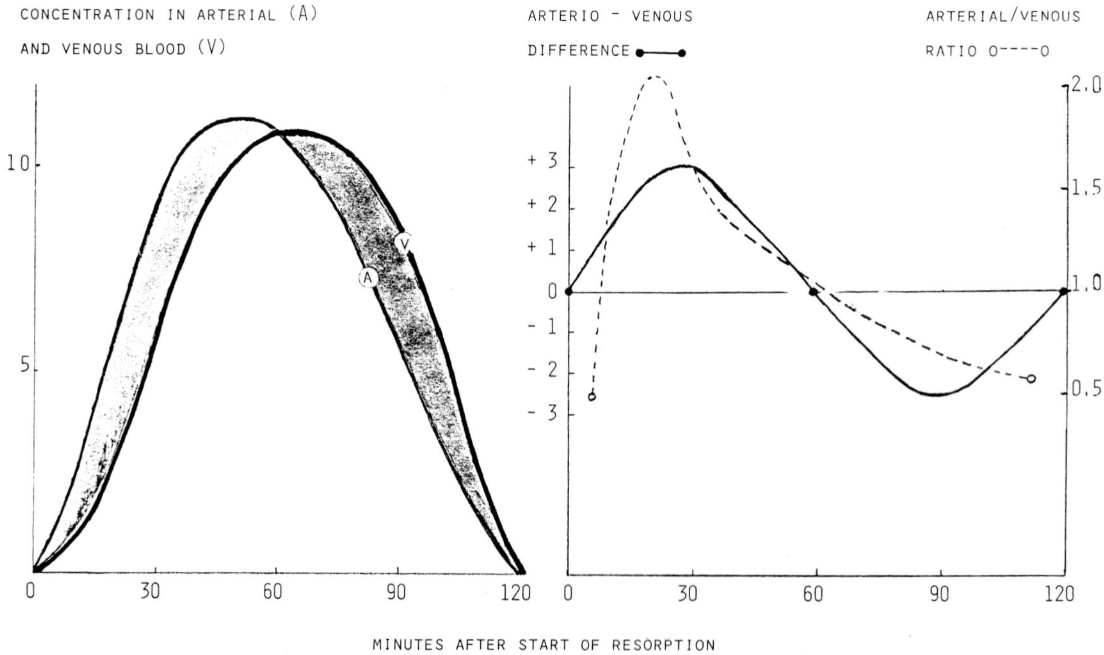

Fig. 1. Theoretical example of the arterial and venous blood concentration of freely diffusible drugs in the peripheral compartment with relatively low blood flow volume. The concentration is given in arbitrary units. The corresponding arterial-venous difference and ratio are shown on the right side.

The first reason has been termed by us the phenomenon of fluctuating arterial-venous concentration differences (4). The various organs differ with respect to the volume of the blood flow, one group has a high (e.g. liver, kidney, brain, salivary glands) and one has a relatively low flow volume (e.g. skin, resting skeletal muscle, fat).

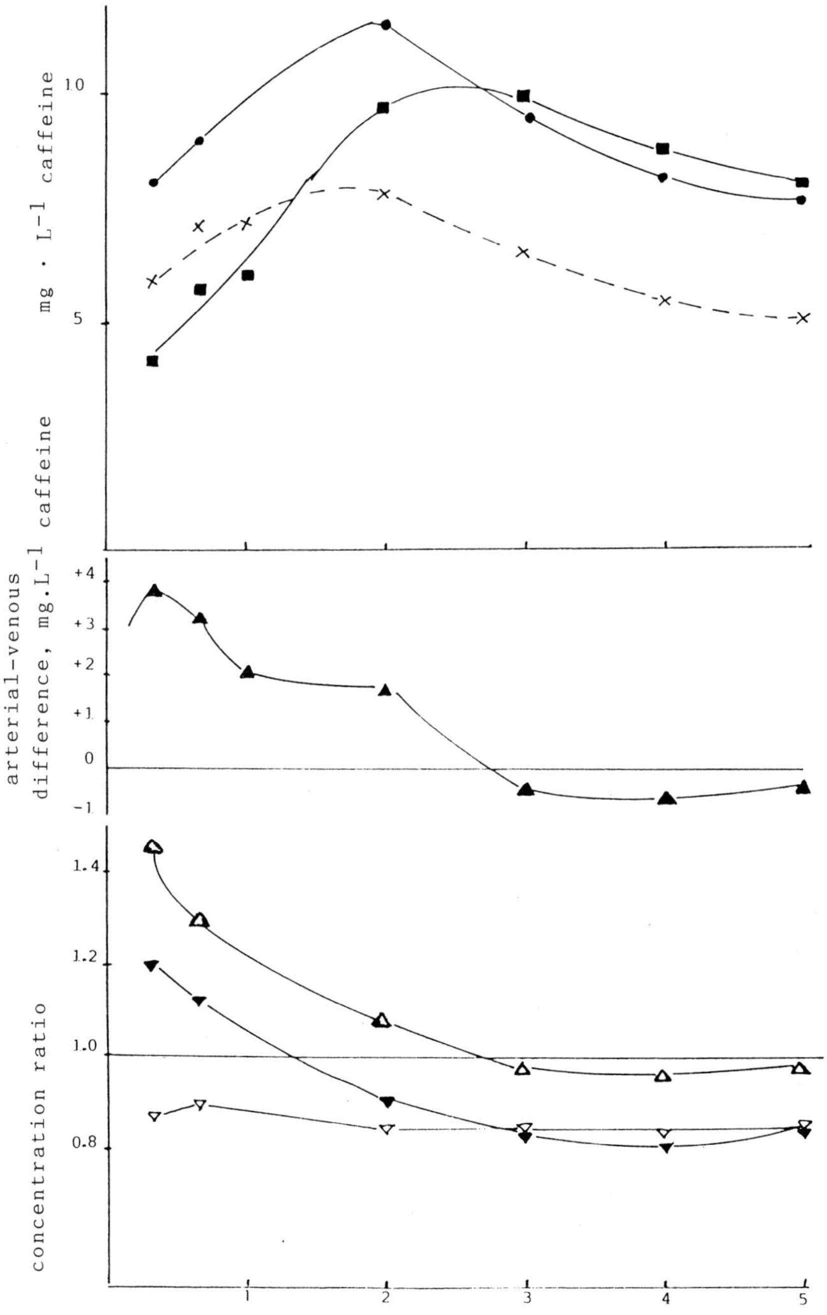

Fig. 2. Total caffeine concentration in venous blood ■---■, capillary blood ●---● and saliva x---x after the oral uptake of one capsule with 350 mg caffeine. The concentration ratios were calculated from capillary/venous blood ▲---▲, salivary/capillary blood ▽---▽ and saliva/venous blood ▼---▼. The three male subjects (20-30 years) had fasted 12 hours. The "arterial" blood was taken from hyperaemised ear lobes, the venous blood from the cubital region.

In pharmacokinetics the first group is often considered as a central compartment and the second as a peripheral compartment. The pharmacokinetics of freely diffusible substances have been described as a coupled convention-diffusion transport phenomenon. This model (4,5) represents theoretical concentration differences in the various parts of the blood circulation system for free diffusible substances.

A theoretical example is demonstrated in figure 1 for the peripheral compartment with relatively low blood flow. After the uptake of an orally applied substance from the intestine the arterial blood (left hand side) first has a higher concentration than the venous blood (positive arteriovenous difference). If the resorption is finished and the substance is not metabolised (or only metabolised to a minor extent) in the particular organ, the situation is reversed because the substance rediffuses from the cell into the blood (negative arteriovenous difference in the elimination phase). From the two curves the behaviour of the arteriovenous difference can be derived (right hand side). This behaviour indicates a fluctuation.

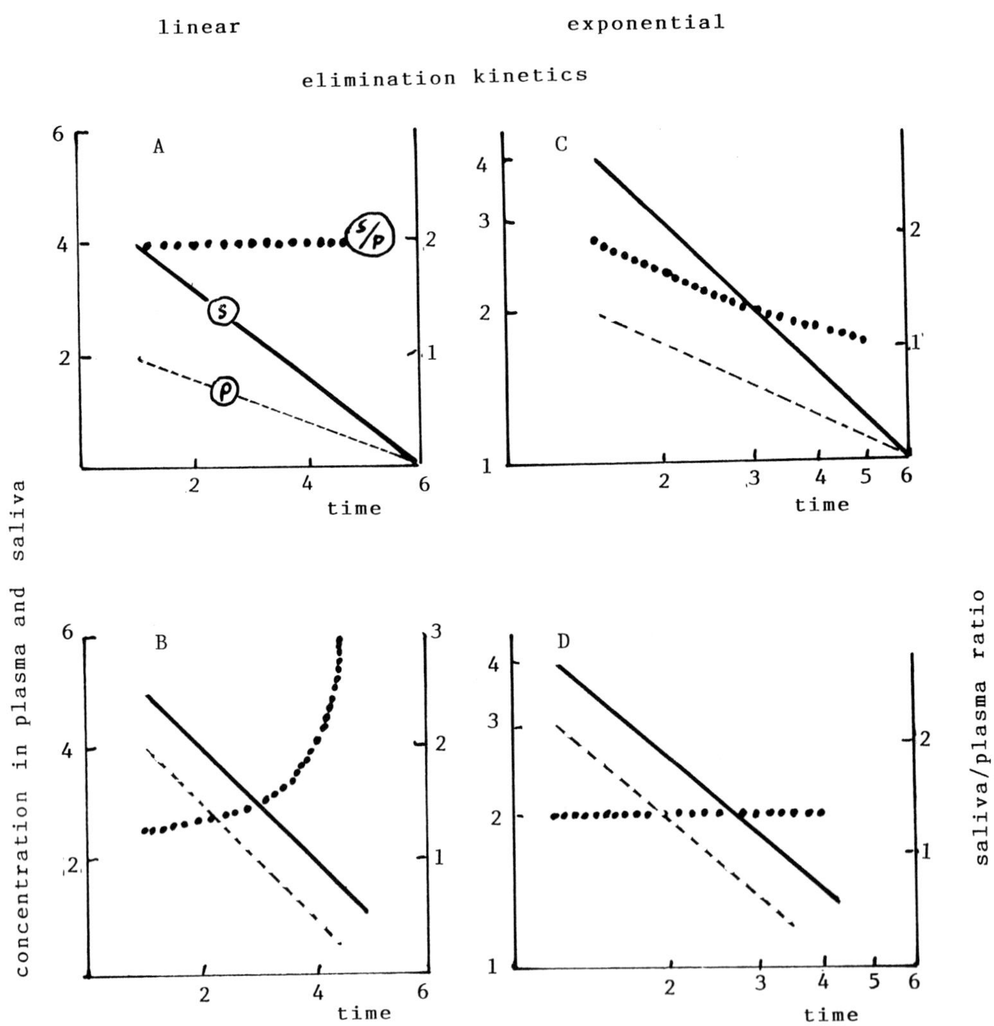

Fig. 3. The relation between the saliva/plasma ratio (S/P...) and the type of drug elimination kinetics. A, C analyte concentration differs between plasma (---) and saliva (——); B, D parallel decline of the analyte concentration.

Salivary glands have a high blood flow volume. Therefore, the arteriovenous difference of freely diffusible substances is relatively small. This must be considered if saliva concentrations are compared with blood concentrations derived from cubital venes belonging to the peripheral compartment.

Poor correlations between both compartments which have been reported in the literature may be at least partly explained by the neglection of the phenomenon described.

In those cases where the phenomenon mentioned exists the salivary concentration may reflect the cellular situation in organs with a high flow volume better than the concentrations determined in blood from cubital venes. So far we have shown the existance of this phenomenon in 3 examples: ethanol, caffeine (fig.2) and theophylline. All 3 substances easily diffuse into saliva and are neutral or at least largely unionized.

The phenomenon described can explain why the saliva/plasma ratios derived from venous and arterial blood can differ in many cases.

Independent from the phenomenon of fluctuating arterial-venous differences the saliva/plasma ratio cannot be expected to be constant in all pharmacokinetic phases. In all cases where the saliva/plasma ratio deviates from 1.0 it depends on the pharmacokinetic behaviour. If the elimination occurs linearly and with the same velocity in plasma and saliva (parallel decline), the ratio must be inconstant (left hand side in fig.3). In the case of exponential elimination kinetics (right hand side in fig.3) the ratio remains constant with a parallel decline of the drug concentration in both plasma and saliva.

A third reason for an intraindividual inconstancy of the S/P total concentration ratio has been mentioned by Derendorf et al. (6). With some cases the degree of protein binding depends on the plasma concentration of the particular drug. If the free drug fraction varies with the plasma concentration, the S/P ratio cannot remain constant during all pharmacokinetic phases.

If the factors mentioned above are considered for the interpretation of the saliva/plasma ratio, then salivary drug concentrations can be clinically more meaningful than the presently used total plasma concentrations.

REFERENCES

1. Reynolds F, Ziroyanis PN, Jones NF, Smith SE. Salivary phenytoin concentrations in epilepsy and in chronic renal failure. The Lancet 2, 1976, 384-386.

2. Baron DN. Intracellular clinical chemistry. Clin.Chem.18, 1972, 320-329.

3. Rasmussen F. Salivary excretion of sulfonamides and barbiturates by cows and goats. Acta Pharm.Tox.21, 1964, 11-19.

4. Haeckel R, Bucklitsch I. The comparability of ethanol concentration in peripheral blood and saliva. The phenomenon of variation in saliva to blood concentration ratio. J.Clin.Chem.Biochem.25, 1987, 199-204.

5. Wehner HD, Rittner Ch, Delius R, Heifer U. The resorption of ethanol in the coupled convection-diffusion system of the circulation. Blutalkohol 20, 1983, 131-143.

6. Derendorf H, Rohdewald P, Möllmann H, Rehder J, Barth J, Neveling D. Pharmacokinetics of prednisolone after high doses of prednisolone hemisuccinate. Biopharm.Drug Disp.6, 1985, 423-432.

Correlation of metabolites in the saliva and blood

Kiyoshi Okuda

Department of Laboratory Medicine, Osaka City University Medical School, Osaka 545, Japan

Abstract – There is increasing emphasis on saliva as a biological specimen for laboratory testing because of advantages of saliva over blood samples. The salivary levels of some metabolites are suggested to be indicators of blood levels. The relationship between the levels of some metabolites in the saliva and the blood was assessed.
Saliva is convenient specimen for bed-side testing and a dry chemistry technique to assay is also suitable for this purpose. We have developed and used a dry chemistry system to measure both salivary and blood urea nitrogen. A gargle reduced the salivary urea nitrogen levels but they returned to the original levels within 10 min. A high correlation was seen between blood and salivary urea nitrogen in healthy subjects and patients with kidney diseases. The salivary concentration of alcohol is also known to be a good indicator of the blood alcohol concentration. The saliva/blood alcohol ration is constant for several hours after ingestion of alcohol and profiles of blood and saliva levels are similar. The correlation coefficient between blood and saliva concentrations of ketone bodies was not so high as compared with urea nitrogen or alcohol. The animal experiment showed that the changes in the salivary ketone body were about 10 min later than those in the serum when β-hydroxybutyric acid was infused. Recently immunoreactive insulin was shown in the saliva and it peaked about 30 min later than serum levels during a glucose loading test in healthy subjects. However, it seems that salivary insulin is not a reliable index of serum insulin in diabetic patients because of the large discrepancies in each case.

INTRODUCTION

Saliva has been used as a convenient specimen in assessing some materials in body fluids. It was already known in the nineteen-fifties that the saliva contained various materials, including ions, relatively small chemical compounds, carbolydrate, proteins, lipids, and so on. In this paper, the correlation of the levels of some metabolites in the saliva and the blood is referred from our experiences.

UREA NITROGEN

We have been interested in analytical systems to evaluate various metabolites in blood, which systems are non-invasive, easy to operate, and quick in giving results. In 1969, we developed a dry chemistry system including reflectometry to estimate urea nitrogen. The relationship of the salivary urea nitrogen measured by the strip method to the blood levels was studied and a high correlation coefficient was seen between them. However, the salivary levels were about 15% lower than the blood levels and we found a problem in this dry strip system. So we improved this system and developed a new dry regent strip for urea nitrogen measurement (ref. 1). The reaction principles of the reagent layer and indicator layer are: salivary urea is hydrolyzed by urease to produce ammonium hydroxide and carbon dioxide, then the ammonia hydroxide produces ammonia gas under alkaline conditions, which changes the color of the bromcresol green in the indicator layer from yellow to blue. The results of the evaluation of precision in the assay of specimens of saliva showed that within-run CVs were 5.9 to 8.0%, day-to-day CVs were 2.6 to 9.0%.
In this assay system, ammonia which is produced by bacteria in the mouth might affect the results and a gargle is recommended to remove ammonia. The effect of a gargle on the urea nitrogen concentration in the saliva in shown in Fig. 1. A gargle reduced the salivary urea nitrogen concentration to 60% of the original levels. However, the concentrations was restored within 10 min. The levels of the salivary urea nitrogen measured by our strip method and these by the urease-indophenol method were compared in healthy control subjects, patient with kidney diseases, and patients under hemodialysis. The correlation coefficient was 0.98 between the levels measured by the dry and the wet chemistry techniques. The relationship between blood and salivary

concentrations of urea nitrogen in these sabjects is shown in Fig. 2. A high correlation was seen between blood and salivary urea nitrogen in both the healthy subjects and the patients with kidney diseases.

We compared urea nitrogen concentrations in serum, saliva, and pancreatic juice in four dogs. The dogs were infused with 20ml of 50% urea from the abdominal aorta, and urea nitrogen levels were measured. In two dogs, serum urea nitrogen peaked first, pancreatic juice second, and saliva last, but in other dogs these levels peaked at the same time. However, after 2 hours, the serum and salivary levels were not very different in the different dogs (ref. 2).

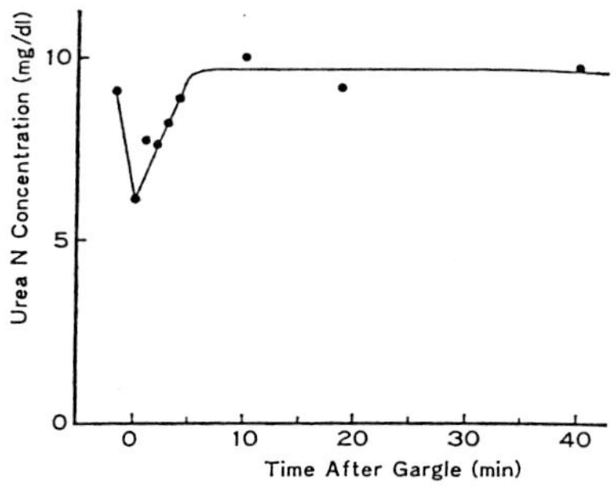

Fig. 1. Effect of gargle on urea nitrogen concentration in saliva.

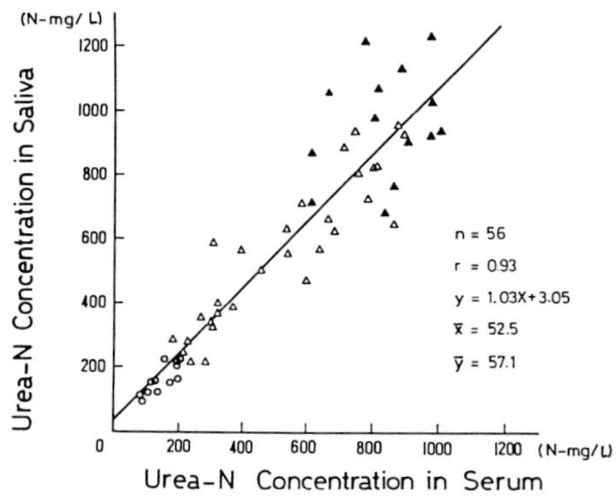

Fig. 2. Relationship between serum and salivary concentrations of urea nitrogen. ○ healthy subjects, △ patients with kidney diseases, ▲ patients under hemodialysis.

ALCOHOL

The salivary concentration of alcohol has been reported to be a good indicator of the blood alcohol concentration (ref. 3). In experiments concerned with the fate of alcohol in the body, many studies have focused on calculation of the blood/body fluid alcohol ratio. Jones (ref. 4) reported that the saliva/blood alcohol ratio was remarkably constant. He investigated the components of variation in saliva/blood alcohol ratio in 48 men after they drank 0.72g of ethanol per kilogram of body weight. Saliva and blood ethanol profiles were monitored for 7 hours after intake. He showed that the analytical component of variation in an estimate of the saliva/blood alcohol which was expressed as coefficient of variation was 1.75%. Also the constant saliva/blood alcohol ratio and almost overlaping pattern in the blood and salivary alcohol concentrations were seen.

KETONE BODIES

Measurement of ketone bodies in the urine and blood is used in the diagnosis and management of diabetes. At times, however, it is difficult to collect blood or urine specimens for this measurement because of dehydration or anuria. We measured ketone bodies in the saliva and tried to estimate ketone bodies in the blood using these measurements. Fig. 3 shows the relationship between serum and saliva concentrations of acetoacetate. The coefficient of correlation was 0.70. The relationship between the sum of acetoacetate and β-hydroxybutyric acid in serum and saliva is shown in Fig. 4. The correlation coefficient between the serum and saliva levels was 0.53.

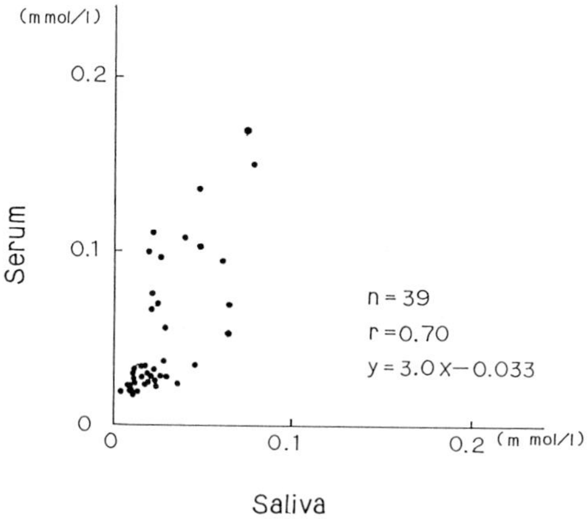

Fig. 3. Correlation between serum and salivary concentrations of acetoacetate.

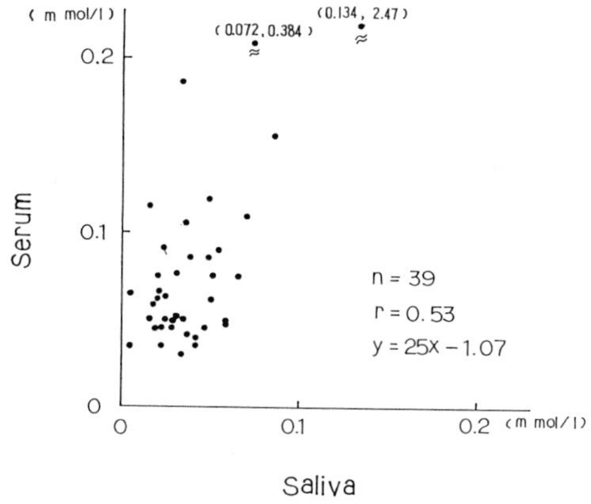

Fig. 4. Correlation between serum and salivary concentrations of sum of acetoacetate and β-hydroxybutyric acid.

We compared the serum and salivary concentrations of β-hydroxybutyric acid in an animal experiment. An anesthetized dog was continuously infused with β-hydroxybutyric acid intravenously and the dose was increased step by step. The changes in the salivary β-hydroxybutyric acid concentrations were about 10 min later than those in the serum (Fig. 5). The increase in the salivary concentration began when the serum concentration reached about 0.5 mmol/L. The correlation between serum β-hydroxybutyric acid levels and salivary levels 10 min later was high with the correlation coefficient of 0.88.

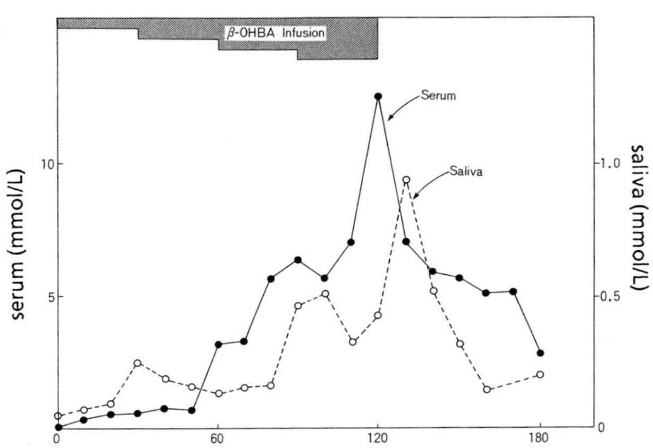

Fig. 5. Serum and salivary β-hydroxybutyric acid (β-OHBA) in dog during intravenous infusion. ● — ● Serum β-OHBA, ○---○ salivary β-OHBA

INSULIN

A recent report has shown that immunoreactive insulin is present in the saliva of normal subjects (ref. 5). Pasic and Pickup (ref. 6) studied the relationship between serum and salivary immunoreactive insulin in normal subjects and insulin-dependent diabetic patients to see whether salivary insulin might be an indicator of serum insulin. When normal subjects were glucose-loaded orally, salivary insulin levels increased with a delay in peak concentration of ~45 min in comparison with serum levels. There was a significant correlation (r=0.81) between mean serum insulin and the salivary insulin 30 min later. However, in diabetic patients, the individual profiles showed marked discrepancies between serum and salivary levels.

REFERENCES

1. T. Akai, K. Naka, C. Yoshikawa, K. Okuda, T. Okamoto, S. Yamagami, T. Inoue, Y. Yamao and S. Yamada, Clin. Chem. 29, 1825–1827 (1983).
2. K. Okuda, T. Akai and A. Tani, Jpn. J. Clin. Chem. 9, 411–419 (1980).
3. B. B. Goldwell and H. W. Smith, Can. J. Biochem. Physiol. 37, 43–52 (1959).
4. A. W. Jones, Clin. Chem. 25, 1394–1398 (1979)
5. G. Vallejo, P. M. Mead, D. H. Gaynor, J. T. Devlin and D. C. Robbins, Diabetologia 27, 437–440 (1984).
6. J. Pasic and J. C. Pickup, Diabetes Care 11, 489–494 (1988).

Sampling techniques and advantages of saliva over blood

Terence D. Geary,

Institute of Medical and Veterinary Science, Adelaide, South Australia, 5000

Abstract - With the introduction of commercial collection vessels the process of obtaining a specimen of saliva has been simplified and made more acceptable to the patient. Where there is a need for repetitive or serial sampling and with the growing interest in patient self monitoring collection of saliva provides a means of obtaining a specimen suitable for analysis. The suitability of saliva as a specimen depends upon the concentration of the analyte and the relationship between the salivary and blood levels. This relationship and the concentration is determined by flow rates, pH, mixed saliva concentrations, and the transfer across the cell membrane. The use of stimulants to increase the flow rate are known and if possible the collection of the specimen should proceed without the use of stimulants.

INTRODUCTION

In this section of the symposium it is intended to discuss the collection of saliva and the advantages it provides as a non-invasive technique.

Interest in the composition of saliva stemmed from the work of dental researchers who, in their investigations determined the concentration of inorganic ions and protein components. As in other areas of clinical investigation progress followed developments in technology. Initially, progress was made with the introduction of flamephotometry, leading to other more sensitive techniques like atomic absorption. With the widespread use of immunoassay, the ability to quantify the low levels of drugs and hormones which may be present has opened up new avenues.

Although a number of recent publications have emphasised the interest in the use of saliva for the measurement of steroids and drugs (ref. 1,2,3), the techniques have not been utilised to the extent that they warrant. This may be because the reporting of investigations is often not selective and the results obtained by useful tests are buried among those where difficulties have been and will continue to be encountered. In addition there was certain stigma associated with the collection of saliva. However, as a non-invasive technique it allows for the collection of serial samples by the patient and provides means of extending the tests which can be performed by the patient. The evolution of thought on the role of patient self monitoring has been quickened by the development of analytical instrumentation and techniques that enable an enlarged menu of compounds to be tested. The measurement of glucose is widely accepted in this environment and it is to be expected that, because of this acceptance, efforts will be made to extend the range of tests which can be performed by the patient.

The following methods have been described for the collection of saliva from various sources (ref. 4):

Parotid	Polyethylene catheter
	Suction cup
	Combined catheter and suction cup
Submandibular	Polyethylene catheter
	Segregator appliance
	Suction cup
Sublingual	Segregator appliance
Mixed	Spitting
	Drainage
	Suction
	Cotton wool rolls
Minor	Capillary tubes

For the use of saliva to be of practical use it is imperative that the simplest technique of collection should be used. This is the collection of mixed saliva.

With the introduction of specimen collection vessels by some commercial companies the process of obtaining an appropriate specimen has been simplified and the procedure made more acceptable to the patient. The Salivette produced by Sarstedt which incorporates the cotton wool plug into a sealed centrifuge tube has advantages of simplicity of use. This has overcome much of the social stigma against the collection of this form of sample. The problems associated with the use of stimulants to increase the flow rate are known and if possible the collection of the specimen should proceed without their use. Stimulation to the flow rate causes an increase in metabolism to provide the energy necessary. The resulting increase in bicarbonate elevates the pH of the saliva from a resting value of 6.5 up to 8.0.

If one should list the disadvantages and advantages of the collection of saliva these would include:-

Emotional - As mentioned previously there is a stigma associated with the collection of saliva which has been reduced by the collection vessels which now are available commercially.

Effect of Flow Rate - The flow rate does affect the concentration of some analytes.

Metabolism in the Saliva - There may be enzyme degradation in the saliva. This needs to be determined in the case of each analyte.

Low Concentration of Analyte - The saliva is an ultrafiltrate and the level of an analyte may reflect the free concentration in the blood. Methods with low limits of detection may be required in those cases.

However, there are advantages

Collection Costs - There is a reduction in costs associated with the collection of saliva. Non-skilled labour or the patients themselves instead of trained nurses may be only required. The separation techniques are simplified and this means that the patient can take repeat specimens without the expense of travelling to a clinic.

Monitoring of Certain Drugs of Abuse - the technique allows for the simplification of the task of positively identifying the specimen collected from clients in a screening programme.

Patient collection - repeated sampling can be made by individuals at home which provides many advantages. The collection of blood from children has always presented a problem which may be largely overcome by the use of saliva specimens.

Selected Group of Patients - the technique, by avoiding the stress associated with venepuncture, is useful when collecting specimens for corticosteriods. It assists as well in any group of patients who may be stressed already for one cause or another, e.g. in a psychiatric ward, to prevent the false elevation of cortisol which may cloud the underlying pathological response.

Ultrafiltrate - in many cases, the level in the saliva reflects the free levels in the blood. The saliva is largely protein free and presents an ideal matrix for many tests.

The expanded use of Breathalyser Units has increased the number of motorists apprehended for driving under the influence of alcohol but has not addressed the problem of intoxication due to other drugs. Peel et al (ref. 5) studied the instance of drugs other than alcohol in a group of impaired drivers stopped for breathalyser testing. The use of saliva in this situation proved to be of considerable value.

There are a number of important drugs and hormones which meet the criteria of being unaffected by flow rate and alteration in the pH of saliva and having adequate saliva to plasma ratios. With the increasing interest in patient self monitoring, the use of non-invasive sampling and improvement in analytical techniques, the use of body fluids other than blood and urine presents an attractive proposition. The collection techniques for saliva have improved to the stage where the specimen is suitable for the measurement of a number of analytes.

REFERENCES

1. R.F. Vining, and R.A. McGimley, CRC Critical Reviews in Clinical Laboratory Sciences, 23,2, 95-146 (1986).

2. Front. Oral Physiol., 5, 1-162 (1984).

3. O.R. Idowu and B. Caddy, J. of Forensic Sci., 22, 123-135 (1982).

4. D.K. Mason and D.M. Chisholm, Salivary Glands in Health and Disease, W.B. Saunders Co. Ltd., 249-260 (1975).

5. H.W. Peel, J. of Forensic Sci., 29, 185 (1984).

Biosensors: principles and applications

MASUO AIZAWA

Department of Bioengineering, Tokyo Institute of Technology
Ookayama,Meguro-ku, Tokyo 152, Japan

Abstract - Biosensors are exemplified by enzyme sensors and immunosensors of which principles and performances are described. Great emhasis was placed on clinical applications of enzyme immunosensors using oxigen electrode, bioaffinity sensors with preformed metastable ligand-receptor complex, and electrochemical luminescence-based optical immunosensors.

1. INTRODUCTION

Advances in sensor technology have opened the way for new and sophisticated measurement techniques and instrumentation for biotechnological process control, environment control, and medical diagnosis. Among various sensors, a biosensor can offer high selectivity for a specific substance, which has not been attained by synthetic sensor materials. The new breed of biosensors will present a unique combination of matrix-bound biochemical, transducer, and microelectronic components to allow almost instantaneous determination of substrate, analyte, or ligand concentrations[1-5].

Molecular recognition of substrates by enzymes, organelles, microorganisms or tissue slices is followed by conversion into the corresponding products which are detected and recorded by the electronic device. The physico-chemical changes associated with molecular recognition caused by binding of the substance to be determined or by the enzymatic substance conversion are transduced by potentiometric or amperometric electrodes, thermistor, field effect transistors (FET), optoelectronic detectors, optical fibers, or other devices into an electric signal. Biosensors are classified into enzyme sensors, microbial sensors, immunosensors, and others.

2.ENZYME SENSORS

Ever since Clark and Lyons presented the first enzyme electrode in 1962, many workers have been occupied with the development of enzyme electrodes in general. The enzyme electrode, which consists of matrix-bound enzyme and an electrochemical measuring device, has found wide application in various fields. In a similar manner to the enzyme electrode, matrix-bound enzyme has recently been coupled with electronic devices such as a thermistor, field effect transistor(FET), and photodiode to construct biosensors. The term "enzyme sensor" is used to describe these sensors.

Enzymes are commonly used in a matrix-bound form. Several methods have been established to immobilize enzymes onto the matrix; (1)Covalent,(2)Entrapment,(3)Adsorption, and(4)Encapsulation methods. Polymer membrane matrices are widely used to couple the immobilized enzyme with an electrochemical measuring device. Enzymes should retain sufficient activity in the matrix-bound form. It is required that the polymer membrane matrix should provide permeability to the corresponding substrate and products. The performance of an enzyme sensor may reflect these properties of matrix-bound enzymes.

Enzyme sensors may be classified as:

(1)Electrochemical enzyme sensor
(2)Enzyme thermistor
(3)Enzyme transistor
(4)Enzyme field effect transistor(ENFET)

(5)Enzyme photodiode
(6)Optical enzyme sensor
The selectivity of all of these enzyme sensors depends on the molecular recognition of the matrix-bound enzyme.

Electrochemical enzyme Sensors for Glucose. An enzyme electrode sensor for glucose installed in a glucose analyzer became commercially available in the mid-1970s. In the early 1980s, extensive development of glucose analyzers, which have been developed for clinical use, require 5-20 l of serum sample for blood glucose analysis.

The sensor consists of a glucose oxidase(GOD) membrane and a Clark-type oxygen electrode. GOD selectively catalyzes the following reaction:

$$\beta\text{-D-Glucose} + O_2 + H_2O \rightarrow \text{D-Gluconate} + H_2O_2$$

Glucose in a sample solution is oxidized with the resulting consumption of oxygen when contacted with the membrane-bound GOD. The decrease of dissolved oxygen is sensitively detected with the oxygen electrode. The output change of the sensor reflects the concentration of glucose in solution.

Hydrogen peroxide is formed in the GOD-catalyzed reaction. A GOD membrane may be coupled with a hydrogen peroxide electrode to form another type of glucose sensor. Both oxygen electrode and hydrogen peroxide electrode-based glucose sensors are now commercially available.

Glucose oxidase has been immobilized onto various matrices. Gel entrapment and cross-linking with bifunctional agents, e.g.,glutaraldehyde, in mixtures with an inert protein are frequently used immobilization methods for enzymes. Polyacrylamide, gelatin, and collagen are representative for entrapping enzymes. The method of covalent coupling, e.g., to nylon netting or collagen membrane, has also proven effective. The operation of the electrode requires the diffusion of the analyte from the immobilization medium of the enzyme, and subsequent detection of the reaction product by the electrode before the product diffuses back into the solution.

Shinohara et al. modified the platinum electrode surface with a GOD-entrapped polyaniline thin layer[6]. The modification was accomplished by the electropolymerization of aniline in the presence of GOD in a neutral aqueous solution. The GOD-entrapped polyaniline membrane rejects the permeation of chemicals except gas molecular such as dissolved oxygen. A micro-enzyme sensor is fabricated by the electrochemical polymerization.

Despite the emphasis on amperometric determination of either oxygen or hydrogen peroxide, there are some disadvantages in using an oxygen-coupled glucose assay. Variations in oxygen tension of the sample may introduce fluctuations into the electrode response at low oxygen tension. The upper limit of linearity for the current response may be reduced. In commercial analyzers, this is usually circumvented by predilution of the sample into oxygenated buffer. Higgins et al. developed an alternative amperometric detection method, based on glucose oxidase, that is not dependent on oxygen as a mediator of electron transfer[7]. The electrode uses a substituted ferricinium ion as a mediator of electron transfer between immobilized glucose oxidase and a graphite electrode.

In the condition of diabetes mellitus, the determination of blood glucose levels rapidly, conveniently, precisely, and economically is important for its diagnosis and effective management. The bedside-type artificial endocrine pancreas, the closed-loop control system used in the treatment of diabetic patients, has revealed that insulin delivery in response to measured blood glucose concentrations on a minute-by-minute basis can normalize glycemia in diabetic patients following various stimuli. However, the problems associated with long-term venous access and the size of the artificial endocrine practice. The miniaturization of a glucose monitoring system is an essential requirement for its clinical application. Shichiri et al. have developed a needle-type glucose oxidase[8]. The current output was not significantly altered by changes in the oxygen tension of the solution in the range from 25-150mmHg. The glucose sensor was connected with a microcomputer system to calculate the insulin infusion rate and a syringe-driving system to deliver insulin. The sensor was inserted into the subcutaneous tissue of pancreatectomized dogs, and renewed every forth day. The artificial endocrine pancreas has kept effective in diabetic dogs with a glucose range of 5-9.5mmol^{-1} for 7 days.

Electrochemical Enzyme Electrodes for Enzyme Activity. Enzyme electrodes are sometimes mistaken for electrodes which measure enzyme activities. There are electrode systems which are specifically designed to assay for enzyme activity such as the use of the NH_3 gas electrode for kinetic determination of trypsin activity based on the hydrolysis of a synthetic substrate. However, most enzyme electrodes couple an amperometric device with a specific enzyme that acts upon selected substrates. An enzyme electrode for pyruvate, which consists of membrane-bound pyruvate oxidase and an oxygen electrode, was coupled with immobilized oxaloacetate decarboxylase to determine glutamate pyruvate transaminase(GPT) and glutamate oxaloacetate transaminase(GOT) activities[9].

Enzyme FET Sensors. A family of new biosensors has been studied in the last decade using the MOSFET structure[10]. The new biosensors consist of immobilized enzyme attached to ion-sensitive field effect transistor without a metal gate. The operation of the ISFET is similar to that of the insulated gate FET in that the reference electrode and the electrolyte constitute the modified gate. The interfacial potential at the electrolyte/insulator interface produced by the ions in solution will affect the channel conductance of the ISFET in the same way as the external gate voltage applied to the reference electrode. The advantages of these bioelectronic sensors, including enzyme FETs and enzyme transistors, are the possibilities of miniaturization and direct integration with microelectronics. It should even be possible to develop multichannel devices with several different enzymes combined with different sensitive areas on the chip[11,12,13].

Optical Enzyme Sensors. The term optrode, formed by combining "optical" and "electrode" emphasizes that the use of optical sensors is very similar to that of electrodes. The devices involve a molecular recognition part on the end of a fiber optic. In operation, interactions with the determinant lead to a change in optical properties of the molecular recognition part, which is probed and detected through the fiber optic. Depending on the particular device, the optical property measured can be absorbance, reflectance, luminescence, or something else.

Seitz et al. reported various enzyme optrodes sensitive to enzyme substrates[13]. A fluorescence-based, competitive optrode for glucose has been described[14]. The specific glucose-binding reagent is concanavalin A immobilized on Sepharose. The competing ligand is dextran labeled with fluorescein.

Aizawa et al. utilized enzymatic luminescence to detect hydrogen peroxide and glucose[15]. A photodiode or phototransistor is coupled with immobilized enzyme which catalyzes a luminescent reaction. The device is termed enzyme photodiode (or transistor). The concentration of hydrogen peroxide is determined by counting photons at a constant concentration of luminol. Peroxidase was immobilized onto a Si photodiode to form an enzyme photodiode sensitive to hydrogen peroxide. A glucose sensor was constructed by incorporating glucose oxidase together with peroxidase onto a Si photodiode.

3. IMMUNOSENSORS

The interaction between antigen and antibody molecules may be extremely specific under favorable condition as a consequence of binding geometries. Immunoassay, which relies its high selectivity and sensitivity on the molecular recognition of antibody is classified into two categories: non-labeling and labeling ones. Since the pioneering work of Yalow and Berson radioisotopes have been employed as the label of choice. However, a number of nonisotopic alternatives have been developed including electron spin resonance for detecting radical labels, nepherometry, fluorescence, chemiluminescence and enzyme labels. moreover, immunoassay with an electroactive label has become attractive due to the wide dynamic range and low detection limits of modern electroanalytical methods. On the basis of these immunoassays, there have been proposed variety of immunosensors, which are classified as follows:

(1) Non-labeled Immunosensors
a) Transmembrane potential
b) Electrode potential
c) Piezoelectric
d) Polarographic
e) FET

f) Surface plasmon
g) Capacitance

(2) Labeled Immunosensors
a) Enzyme-linked amperometry
b) Enzyme-linked potentiometry
c) Enzyme-linked luminescence
d) Electrochemical luminescence
e) Fluorescence
f) Other optical labels
g) Electro chemically active labels

Enzyme Immunosensors Using Oxygen Electrode: An enzyme immunosensor is an analytical device which is dependent on the immunochemical affinity for selectivity and on the chemical amplification of a labeling enzyme for sensitivity.

In case that catalase, which catalyzes the evolution of oxygen from hydrogen peroxide is a labeling enzyme for an antigen, the enzyme immunosensor is constructed by assembling an antibody-bound membrane and an oxygen sensing electrode. In heterogeneous enzyme immunoassay, the labeling enzyme is measured by amperometry with the oxygen sensing device. The enzyme immunosensor requires an extremely short time for measuring the labeling enzyme. Consequently, rapid and highly sensitive enzyme immunoassay may be accomplished with the enzyme immunosensor.

The enzyme immunosensor is prepared by attaching the antibody-bound membrane to a Clark-type oxygen electrode which has an oxygen permeable plastic (e.g. Teflon) membrane on the cathode surface and responds sensitively and rapidly to oxygen.

Ochratoxin A (OTA), a secondary metabolite of Aspergillus ochraceus, Penicillium viridicatum and strains of some other species of both genera, causes nephropathy in animals and most probably in man. Recently also carcinogenicity has been demonstrated in feeding experiments. Its occurrence specially in grains seems to be prevailing in not only European and North American countries but Asian countries. OTA has most commonly been determined by chemical analysis which requires a tedious separation from a sample. Bioassay and radioimmunoassay have also been conducted with problems in operation. A simplified and rapid analysis of OTA is urged to be developed. An enzyme immunosensor for OTA has recently been developed.

The toxin sensor consists of an amperometric oxygen electrode and an OTA-bound membrane. Catalase-labeled OTA, which is added at a fixed amount to a sample solution, may competitively react with membrane-bound OTA and free OTA to be determined. The sensor is then assayed for amperometric determination of catalase activity. OTA was selectively and sensitively determined by measuring the sensor output. Competitive immunoassay of OTA was carried out using the immunosensor for OTA. OTA was determined under a constant concentration of catalase-labeled antibody. Sensor response was obtained for each concentration of free OTA, where the experiment was carried out in the PBS buffer at 35°C. The change of sensor output decreased with the addition of free OTA to be determined. The standard curve shifted to the lower concentration range with a decrease in antibody concentration. The minimum detection limited was in the order of 10^{-10} $g \cdot ml^{-1}$, when the concentration of labeled antibody was fixed at 20 $g \cdot ml^{-1}$.

Bioaffinity Sensors with Preformed Metastable Ligand-Receptor Complex: A new biosensor has been designed on the basis of bioaffinity difference between two ligands, i.e., one a determinant and the other an analogue compound in a given binding reaction. In general an analogue compound shows lower affinity to the binding protein than a determinant does. Therefore, one can expect the following displacement reaction when a membrane-bound analogue compound complexed with its binding protein is exposed to a determinant molecule. The binding protein is displaced from the membrane-bound analogue molecule. The displacement is supposed to depend on the bioaffinity difference of an analogue molecule and a determinant as well as the determinant concentration. The determinant concentration may be easily measured by detecting the residual molecular complex which remains on the membrane surface. High sensitivity can be attained by chemical amplification by the usage of an enzyme catalyst as a label. A biosensor based on the above principle may be termed "Bioaffinity sensor".

A bioaffinity sensor for thyroxine (3,5,3',5'-tetraiodothyroxine: T_4), a thyroid hormone, is composed of membrane-bound T_4 and enzyme-labeled antibody, i.e., thyroxine is chemically immobilized on a membrane. The membrane-bound T_4 is undergone immunochemical reaction with enzyme-labeled anti-T_4 antibody to form an immunocomplex. Membrane-bound T_4 has less affinity to the antibody than free T_4 in solution. Attachment of the membrane where antigen-antibody complex is formed on the surface of a galvanic-type oxygen electrode results in a bioaffinity sensor for T_4. When the sensor is immersed in a solution containing free T_4 to be determined, the antigen-antibody complex will be dissociated upon exposure to T_4. The dissociation may be enhanced with an increase in the analyte concentration. The released enzyme-labeled antibody will then form a stable complex with T_4. Consequently, T_4 can be determined by measuring the enzyme activity of enzyme-labeled antibody on the T_4 membrane.

In case of a bioaffinity sensor for bovine insulin, porcine insulin is used as the analogue compound. A porcine insulin-bound plate is undergone immunoreaction with peroxidase-labeled anti bovine insulin antibody to form an immunocomplex. When the plate on which surface the immunocomplex is formed is immersed on a solution containing free bovine insulin to be determined, the complex may be dissociated. The dissociated enzyme-labeled antibody then forms a stable complex with bovine insulin in a solution. Insulin is thus determined by measuring peroxidase retained on an immunoplate. The luminol-H_2O_2 system is employed to detect peroxidase activity. The emitted light is transferred to a photomultiplier through an optofiber.

Electrochemical Luminescence-Based Optical Immunosensor: The authors aimed at employing aromatic hydrocarbon such as pyrene as an electroactive label for immunoassay. It was found, however, that the electrochemical luminescence of the label was extremely sensitive to immunochemical reaction. The new findings have lead us to establish a novel immunosensor for homogeneous immunoassays. The electrochemical luminescence immunoassay is based on the following principle. The antigen (human serum Albumin) labeled with an aromatic hydrocarbon (aminopyrene) was prepared. The pyrene-labeled HSA emits luminescence by electrochemical technique, while the labeled HSA complexed with antibody generates less luminescence depending on the antibody concentration. This may probably be caused by the steric hindrance to the access of the aromatic hydrocarbon to the electrochemical luminescence (ECL) detection. In the further investigation, luminol was found to exhibit electrochemical luminescence in an aqueous solution. Luminol was also employed as an electroactive label for immunoassay. In addition, an optical fiber electrode has been developed to improve the ECL measurement. The optical fiber electrode is an optically transparent electrode which is fabricated on thc top of an optical fiber. Any electrochemically induced optical changes can sensitively be detected with the optical fiber electrode. Such a device should pave the road to optical chemical sensors and biosensors.

Future Aspects of Immunosensors : Immunosensors have been realized by fascinating combination of immobilized antibody (or antigen) with an electronic device. High selectivity may be attained by both non-labeled and labeled immunosensors due to specific affinity of antigen to the corresponding antibody. However, the immunochemical reaction of matrix-bound antibody (or antigen) is influenced by non-specific adsorption of coexisting substances onto the matrix. There have been proposed several methods to present the non-specific adsorption, although they are not satisfied. It is stressed that further research should be concentrated on the development of improved material for immunosensors.

Non-labeled immunosensors are characterized by high selectivity with simple operation. Most of these sensors are based on potentiometric measurement. Further investigation is required to seek for novel non-labeled immunosensors with high selectivity and sensitivity.

In contrast with non-labeled immunosensors, labeled immunosensors have been succeeded in enhancement of sensitivity with retaining high selectivity. Enzyme labels have successfully been incorporated into the immunosensor to work as effective chemical amplifier. The lower limit of detection ranges in the order of 10^{-11} $g \cdot ml^{-1}$. Further improvement of sensitivity appears promising.

FIBER-OPTIC LUMINESCENCE BIOSENSORS

We recently developed in our group a novel fiber-optic biosensor based on solid phase bio- or chemiluminescence reactions (ref. 20). The device consists of a 1-meter long glass fiber bundle of 8 mm internal diameter. One end is equipped with a screw-cap which maintains an enzymatic polyamide disk in close contact with the surface of the fibers (Fig. 1).

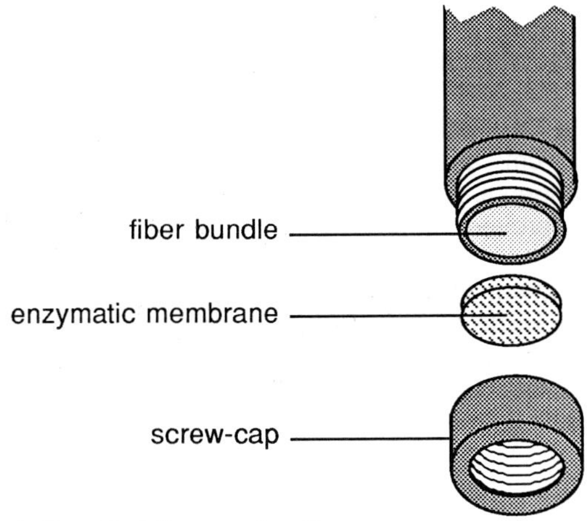

Fig. 1. Detail of the sensing tip.

The sensing tip is immersed in a light-proof thermostated vessel in which samples are injected through a septum. The light emitted at the membrane level is conducted through the glass fibers to the other end of the bundle which is connected to the photomultiplier tube of the luminometer (Fig. 2).

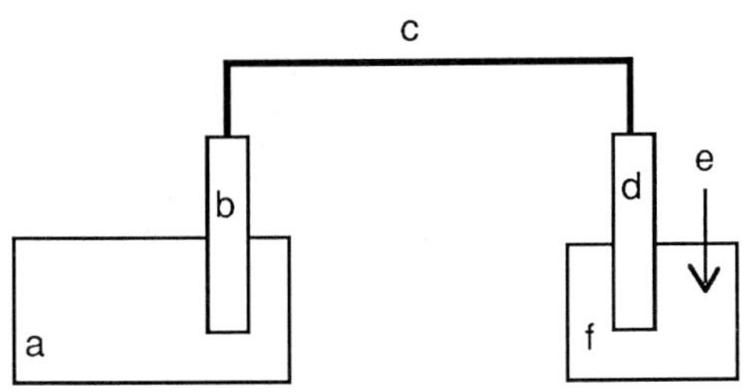

Fig. 2. Block diagram of the fiber-optic luminescence biosensor arrangement. (a) luminometer; (b) connection to the photomultiplier tube; (c) fiber bundle; (d) enzymatic sensor; (e) septum; (f) light-proof thermostated reaction cuvette.

Monitoring of generic species

Hydrogen peroxide, ATP and NADH could be determined using the fiber-optic biosensor covered with an immobilized enzyme membrane involving either the horseradish peroxidase, firefly luciferase or the luminescent bacterial system respectively (ref. 20,21). Performances of these systems are presented in Table 1. It must be stressed that amounts as low as 70 pmol/assay, 1.0 pmol/assay and 1.3 pmol/assay for H_2O_2, ATP and NADH could be detected respectively.

Coupled dehydrogenase reactions with the bacterial luminescent system

A promising analytical application of the bacterial luminescent system is the possibility of coupling various NAD(P)-dependent enzymes in order to determine other analytes. This can be done using our sensor after coimmobilizing on the same membrane the selected dehydrogenase with the bacterial system (Fig. 3). Such a tri-enzyme membrane has been prepared for the assay of ethanol using alcohol dehydrogenase. A linear calibration was obtained in the range 4×10^{-7} - 7×10^{-5} M with a precision of 5.4 % (for ten replicates at 5.7×10^{-6} M). The detection limit was 1.8 nmol/assay.

TABLE 1. Performances of the luminescence fiber-optic sensor.

Metabolite	H_2O_2	ATP	NADH	
Membrane type	Immunodyne	Immunodyne	Immunodyne	NAZ
Detection limit (M)	2×10^{-8}	2.8×10^{-10}	3×10^{-10}	1×10^{-8}
Linearity (M)	2×10^{-8} - 2×10^{-5}	2.8×10^{-10} - 1.4×10^{-6}	1×10^{-9} - 3×10^{-6}	1×10^{-8} - 2×10^{-5}
Coefficient of variation (%)	6.8 (a)	3.7 (a)	4.8 (b)	6.0 (b)
Response time (min) at the steady-state	1	1 at 2.8×10^{-10} M 6 - 7 at 3×10^{-6} M	2	3

Note a : on the entire linear range; Note b : for ten replicates at 4×10^{-8} M.

Concerning the stability of such a system, it could be demonstrated that on storage 100 % of the initial activity was retained after at least 3 months when the membranes were kept at -20 °C in a medium containing 20 % glycerol, 1 % BSA and 0.2 mM dithiothreitol. The system exhibited a quite good operational stability with an acceptable precision when calibration was performed every ten assays.

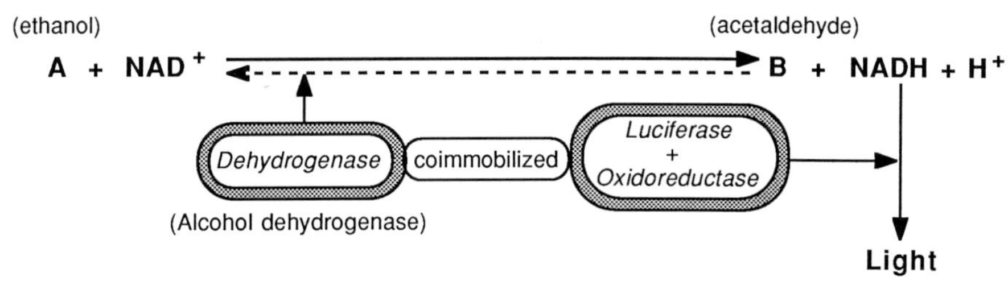

Fig. 3. Principle of assays using a coupled dehydrogenase reaction with the bacterial luminescent system.

The analysis of other compounds is now under investigation and promising results have been recently obtained using sorbitol dehydrogenase and malate dehydrogenase for the measurement of sorbitol and oxaloacetate respectively (ref. 22).

CONCLUSION

The possibility of designing a novel optical biosensor based on luminescent reactions has been demonstrated. Further improvements should involve the use of entrapped co-reactants or the setting of a control delivery system in order to propose a self-contained operational biosensor.

REFERENCES

1. P.R. Coulet, Analytical Uses of Immobilized Biological Compounds for Detection, Medical and Industrial Uses, p. 319, D. Reidel, Dordrecht, Holland (1988).
2. J.M. Engasser and P.R. Coulet, Biochim. Biophys. Acta 485, 29-36 (1977).
3. D.R. Thevenot, R. Sternberg, P.R. Coulet, J. Laurent and D.C. Gautheron, Anal. Chem. 51, 96-100 (1979).
4. M. Arrio-Dupont and P.R. Coulet, Biochem. Biophys. Res. Commun. 89, 345-352 (1979).

5. P.R. Coulet, R. Sternberg and D.R. Thevenot, Biochim. Biophys. Acta 612, 317-327 (1980).
6. P.R. Coulet, J.Carlsson and J. Porath, Biotechnol. Bioeng. 23, 663-668 (1981).
7. G.G. Guilbault and P.R. Coulet, Anal. Chim. Acta 152, 223-228 (1983).
8. G.Bardeletti and P.R. Coulet, Anal. Chem. 56, 591-593 (1984).
9. C.H. Assolant-Vinet and P.R. Coulet, Anal. Letters 19, 875-885 (1986).
10. G.Bardeletti, F. Séchaud and P.R. Coulet, Anal. Chim. Acta 187, 47-54 (1986).
11. L.J. Blum and P.R. Coulet, Biotechnol. Bioeng. 28, 1154-1158 (1986).
12. B. Maïsterrena, L.J. Blum and P.R Coulet, Biochem. J. 242, 835-839 (1987).
13. N.N. Ugarova and O.V. Lebedeva, Appl. Biochem. Biotechnol. 15, 35-51 (1987).
14. P.R. Coulet and L.J. Blum, Analytical Uses of Immobilized Biological Compounds for Detection, Medical and Industrial Uses, p. 237, D. Reidel, Dordrecht, Holland (1988).
15. P.R. Coulet and L.J. Blum, Fluorescence Analysis in Biology and Medicine, Dekker, New York, in press.
16. P.R. Coulet, J.H. Julliard and D.C. Gautheron, Biotechnol. Bioeng. 16, 1055-1068 16. (1974).
17. L.J. Blum, P.R. Coulet and D.C. Gautheron, Biotechnol. Bioeng. 27, 232-237 (1985).
18. L.J. Blum and P.R. Coulet, Anal. Chim. Acta 161, 355-358 (1986).
19. L.J. Blum, J.M. Plaza and P.R. Coulet, Anal. Letters 20, 317-326 (1987).
20. L.J. Blum, S.M. Gautier and P.R. Coulet, Anal. Letters 21, 717-726 (1988).
21. S.M. Gautier, L.J. Blum and P.R. Coulet, Biosensors, in press.
22. S.M. Gautier, L.J. Blum and P.R. Coulet, J. Biolum. Chemilum., submitted.

New directions for decentralization

Marvin A. Genshaw

Miles Inc., Diagnostic Division, P.O. Box 70, Elkhart, IN 46515, U.S.A.

Abstract - The decentralization of testing of clinical samples is being driven by a number of factors. Among these are the availability of new technologies for use in the small laboratory, the desire or need for a rapid turnaround from sample drawn to result, and fiscal considerations. Test sites now include the hospital ward and emergency room, small clinic, doctor's office, and even the patient's home.

Past technologies required centrifugal separation of serum from blood with analysis by an autoanalyzer or a relatively complex manual or semi-automated system. The current and emerging technologies use new and simple to use dry reagent and electrochemical technologies. These technologies have permitted the development of compact instrumental systems providing whole blood assays.

INTRODUCTION

Decentralized testing is not a new phenomenon. A century ago nearly all testing was decentralized. The centralization of testing resulted from the development of analytical systems giving efficiency from economy of scale. Now various factors are completing the cycle of testing sites with a trend away from testing in central laboratories to testing in decentralized sites.

We may divide diagnostic testing sites into laboratories of various sizes. The largest laboratories include government laboratories such as CDC and NIH labs in the USA, research and teaching hospital labs, large hospitals and diagnostic centers as well as larger commercial laboratories such as MetPath. Intermediate sized laboratories are found in small hospitals, clinics and large group practices. Small laboratories are found in decentralized testing sites. Decentralized testing, the concern of this discussion, occurs in small group practices, individual doctors' offices, hospital wards or emergency rooms, screening programs and even in the patients' homes.

A number of factors promote decentralized testing (ref. 1-2). These factors include the need for an immediate result, fiscal factors and the availability of appropriate technology.

NEED FOR IMMEDIATE RESULT

In a number of medical emergencies, a rapid test result is needed to confirm a diagnosis. Appropriate therapeutic measures can then commence. Waiting for a result from a distant laboratory is not consistent with good patient care when immediate therapy is needed. Thus, an immediate diagnostic test at the decentralized site, where the patient is seen, can readily be justified as providing better patient care (ref. 3).

Rapid test results can also aid busy physicians. Frequently a preliminary diagnosis can be made when a patient is first seen. This diagnosis is based on the history and physical exam. However, a diagnostic test is often needed to confirm the diagnosis and eliminate the possibility of alternate syndromes with similar symptoms (ref. 3-4). To perform the test, a blood sample is drawn and sent out to the reference laboratory. Sometime later, the result is received by the physician. The patient must then be contacted and appropriate therapy begun. Contacting the patient consumes time for the physician. A significant amount of time is required to collate laboratory results with the patient file, and contact the patient to discuss the results of laboratory tests.

This evolution from simple testing near the patient to an increasing sophistication in instrumentation and complexity of analytical procedures has led naturally to a change in the manner in which laboratory services have been provided. A point made by Doctor Burtis in his plenary lecture, that is, the role played by the clinical laboratory is influenced by technology, management and medical practice, is an appropriate starting point for any discussion on the impact of instrumentation on the laboratory.

Technology and the demands of medical practice influence the manner in which the clinical laboratory functions and management needs to be constantly changing to provide the organisation necessary to optimise the benefit accruing from advances in clinical laboratory technology. The optimisation of laboratory service is a function of management which will lead to the use of resources to provide improved patient care. The impact of instrumentation on the laboratory will be discussed from this management position.

One of the aims of management is to take advantage of all the tools available to cope with the increasing workload and increasing costs with ever diminishing resources. In order to achieve this aim it is important to define for each laboratory situation the factors which will affect the effective use of available resources. One of these factors is testing outside the traditional laboratory environment and there is a need to determine the cost/effectiveness and benefit of this for patient care. To do this each situation should be considered carefully by a team consisting of the laboratory staff and appropriate staff from the end user location. The team should consider ways in which the existing and new services external to the laboratory can be effectively integrated. This should lead to the most effective use of staff and funds, a plan for maintenance of analytical quality and a programme for education and re-education of end user staff.

To achieve its aim the team should look at

1. Justification for service.
2. How the purchase of the analytical system is to take place.
3. Handling of specimens.
4. Interaction with the laboratory staff.
5. Quality assurance.
6. The cost effectiveness of any move away from the traditional way in which the services are being provided.

I would like to consider each of these points. Under justification there needs to be a review of the clinical needs of each location. Some will need a reduction in the turnaround time of analytical results for diagnostic purposes, but others will be mainly monitoring treatment.

If the location of the service is in the hospital environment then the purchase should be made with the assistance of laboratory staff and the instrument should meet the needs for:

1. The technical skills of the operators.
2. The tests required in the environment.
3. The number of specimens to be tested.
4. The maintenance requirements.
5. The stability of and storage requirement for the reagents.

The acquisition should follow a set protocol. At the second Asian and Pacific Congress of Clinical Biochemistry held in Singapore the IFCC Commission on Analytical Systems presented a symposium on the Selection of Instrumentation for the Clinical Laboratory. A point made by Professor Haeckel was that more than one instrument may satisfy the analytical needs and often non monetary criteria and subjective assessment determine the instrument to be purchased. Assuming that this is the case, a clear definition of requirements for each location is needed. Published reports and full evaluations carried out at the Institute of Medical and Veterinary Science indicate that with very few exceptions the analytical performance of the small instruments commercially available meet the performance criteria necessary for adequate patient care and the reports which have appeared indicating unacceptable performance often relate to technical errors which in turn relate to education of the end user. It is important to note that manufacturers have a need to maintain the quality of their product for regulatory as well as competitive reason and to do this they perform exhaustive quality control checks.

Quality assurance is always important but the need for quality assurance and the help provided by an adequate quality programme must be clearly understood by non-laboratory trained operators. If the manufacturer is selling analytical systems to locations remote to laboratories then they should assume much of the responsibility for the quality program.

As part of quality assurance the team or the responsible organisation must

1. provide adequate information on such matters as

    1.1 patient preparation
    1.2 safety in handling specimens
    1.3 specimen storage
    1.4 training, documentation of results, information on interpretation of results

2. give due thought to the educational background of the staff who may be using the system.

3. decide who will be operating the system.
   Whether the laboratory staff are seconded on a rotational basis or will staff from several locations be allowed to perform their own tests.

4. provide a maintenance programme for the instrument.

5. ensure that interaction with trained laboratory staff is established.

The above discussion concerned the establishment of a service in an environment which is external to the central laboratory but within a hospital complex. The same principles apply to any other location, however remote to the central laboratory. There is need for support to assist with the successful establishment and continued running of such a service. There are many areas where service to the patient can be improved by the appropriate use of small instruments and each such situation presents an organisational problem to the laboratory which needs to be resolved carefully.

The introduction of these extended services may lead eventually to the central laboratory staff concentrating their skills on specialised analytical procedures to assist with the diagnosis and treatment of specific patient populations instead of handling the broad spectrum of patient groups and procedures which we do currently. Further it may lead to an increase in the number of patient beds under the direct supervision of laboratory staff that in effect will mean that the patient and not the specimen is brought to the laboratory for specialist diagnostic testing.

In conclusion small instrumentation has and will continue to change the manner in which laboratories are organised and managed by providing ways to add flexibility to the existing testing procedures. But the contribution will depend upon the establishment of a management structure and skills to effectively take advantage of all facilities available.

The following points should be re-iterated:

1. New management skills need to be learnt in order to take full advantage of the flexibility of the instruments.

2. The small instruments
    2.1 are easy to operate and maintain
    2.2 give acceptable analytical performance
    2.3 have an important role to play

3. Many of the errors which occur are related to training not to the analytical system used and so are due to the handling of the patient, or collection and treatment of the specimen.

Instrumentation in primary care

Peter M.G. Broughton

Wolfson Research Laboratories, Queen Elizabeth Medical Centre,

Birmingham B15 2TH, UK

Abstract - A wide range of commercial systems and instruments is now available for use in primary care. Several surveys have shown that the quality of some results obtained with these is poor, mainly due to the influence of the operator. Proposals are made for improvements in instrumental design which would lessen the effect of operator-dependency. Scientists in clinical laboratories need to become more involved in improving the quality of testing in primary care by helping with training and quality assurance, as well as evaluating and advising on selection of equipment. There are opportunities for research and development of new instruments and systems, and of quality control materials and techniques. Close collaboration between the physician, manufacturer and laboratory staff is needed to ensure that instruments are effectively and efficiently used in primary care.

INTRODUCTION

Although simple laboratory tests have beeen performed by doctors in primary care for many years, the recent development of commercial kits and instrumental systems has made it possible to do a much wider range of tests nearer the patient (refs. 1, 2, 3). The convenience and simplicity of these methods enable a relatively unskilled operator to obtain a result within a few minutes. In many countries these systems are being increasingly used in doctors' offices, and in the USA it has been estimated that 90% of primary care physicians perform some office testing (ref. 4).

This form of testing is claimed to have 3 main benefits (ref. 5): patients can be investigated and treatment prescribed in a single visit; clinical decisions can be made more rapidly; and the test provides a source of income for the physician. In addition, there are commercial pressures for the wider use of this type of testing, and an increasing awareness of the needs and importance of primary care, particularly in developing countries and rural areas which are remote from hospitals and their laboratories.

Many laboratory workers view these developments with concern because they believe that the quality of tests performed nearer the patient is often inferior to that which they can achieve, and because they have no responsibility for or involvement with testing in primary care. However, the problem will not go away, and it is more constructive to consider how both laboratory staff and manufacturers can contribute to improving the use of instruments in primary care.

ANALYTICAL SYSTEMS FOR PRIMARY CARE

The range of commercial systems available is expanding rapidly, and cover chemistry, haematology, microbiology and immunology (ref. 1). When these are used in primary care the traditional boundaries between disciplines disappear: the test becomes just another measurement, often made by a nurse who measures the blood pressure as well. The role of the operator then becomes paramount.

These systems can be divided into 3 main groups:

1. Qualitative and semi-quantitative tests requiring little or no instrumentation. These include dipsticks (e.g. for urine testing), kits (e.g. for pregnancy tests), and a variety of novel devices, such as enzyme immunochromatography for therapeutic drug monitoring.

2. Dedicated instruments for performing common tests, such as measurement of blood haemoglobin, glucose and, recently, cholesterol.

3. Versatile instruments capable of performing several different tests one at a time.

All of these will be further developed by industry. The choice betweeen them will be dictated mainly by clinical demands and by financial considerations, rather than the quality of results obtained with them.

Different problems arise in developing countries, where the clinical needs are both greater and different, but finance is lacking, so that the new technology being used in developed countries is having little impact (ref. 6). This is illustrated by the choice between the immunological kit and the microscope, which is probably the commonest instrument used in developing nations for detecting common bacterial and parasitic infections. The relative merits of these two techniques may be summarised as follows:

Capital cost of the microscope is relatively high, but is small for a kit.

Running costs for reagents and consumables are low for the microscope but much greater for kits.

Labour requirements: use of the microscope requires skill, training and some maintenance, which the kit does not.

Versatility: the microscope can be used to identify different organisms in several types of specimen, but a different kit is usually needed for testing for each antigen, which will increase running costs.

Sensitivity: direct comparison is difficult, but the kit is probably better.

The choice between the two therefore depends on several conflicting factors, the most important being the availability of finance and a skilled operator.

THE INFLUENCE OF SKILL

Most published evaluations of equipment which might be used in primary care have been made by trained staff in clinical laboratories. Only rarely is data given on the influence of the operator on the quality of results. Drucker, Williams and Price (ref. 7) found that the quality of results obtained with a typical blood glucose meter used on hospital wards and in doctors surgeries was inferior to that obtained in the laboratory, and 63% of measurements made in general practice could be considered unsatisfactory. Other reports (refs. 8, 9) of two dry reagent systems found that non-technical operators obtained results with significantly worse precision and accuracy than trained laboratory analysts. Proficiency testing for a variety of analytes measured in a group of physicians' office laboratories showed significant error rates, in some cases as high as 40% (ref. 4).

It is clear that improvements are needed if legislation to control laboratory testing in primary care is to be avoided. Both manufacturers and laboratory staff have important roles in bringing about this improvement.

INSTRUMENT DESIGN

"User-friendly" instruments tend to encourage more operators to use them, thereby increasing the need for the manufacturer to make the instrument as foolproof as possible. Design features which would reduce the number of operator-dependent steps and manipulations which could lead to errors include the following (ref. 10):

(1) Use urine or whole blood specimens which do not require an independent centrifuge and the need for separation of plasma.

(2) Avoid the need for accurate measurement of sample and reagent volumes.

(3) Use pre-prepared and stable reagents which will usually need to be matched to the instrument. The advantage of using a system, rather than an independent instrument and reagents, is that a single manufacturer will then be responsible, which is simpler for the user in primary care.

(4) Use procedures which will prevent the use of outdated or incorrect reagents, which are a comon source of error with simplified systems. Manufacturers could encourage this by offering a rebate for unused reagents which had passed their expiry date.

(5) Make calibration automatic with pre-prepared calibrants.

(6) Avoid the need for accurate timing and, when this is necessary, make all timing steps automatic.

(7) Provide stable liquid quality control materials whenever reagents are purchased or, better, build quality control systems into the instrument, with a lockout device to prevent the display of incorrect results whenever there is a malfunction.

(8) Simplify the operation of the instrument by minimising the number of control switches and knobs.

(9) Replace the conventional operating manual (which is often not read or lost) by suitable software, so that the user can operate the instrument, check that it is performing correctly and locate simple faults merely by pressing a yes/no button.

Many of these features have been incorporated into modern ion selective electrode systems and blood gas analysers, enabling relatively unskilled staff to use them satisfactorily. One consequence of this is that the responsibility for ensuring reliable results is transferred from the user to the manufacturer, and there is little scope for the user to modify the method or reagents. Closer collaboration with clinical laboratories is needed to ensure that the same standards of accuracy apply, wherever the test is performed.

MEASUREMENT OF PLASMA CHOLESTEROL IN PRIMARY CARE

In several countries increasing numbers of plasma cholesterol measurements are being made outside the clinical laboratory as part of community health programmes concerned with the prevention of coronary heart disease, and for opportunistic screening in primary care (refs. 11, 12). In addition to the benefits of near-patient testing mentioned earlier, the drama of seeing the test performed and being given a rapid result seem to have a powerful effect in motivating the patient to comply with dietary or other advice which can be given during the same visit. At least 5 instruments are currently available with which a nurse or other non-technical person can obtain a cholesterol result on a capillary blood specimen within a few minutes (ref. 13). Although several recent reports suggest that most of these instruments are satisfactory when used by trained laboratory staff, it should not be assumed that they are equally reliable when used by non-technical personnel.

In the UK we have recently made some external quality assessment (EQA) surveys of cholesterol measurements made by extra-laboratory users of one instrument (Boehringer Reflotron) (ref. 14), and will be extending these on a regular basis to include any other instruments which may come into widespread use in the community. The Figure shows some typical results obtained when 67 users analysed the same serum specimen. In this example, the dispersion of results (coefficient of variation = 6.4% after exclusion of results >2 S.D. from the mean) was greater than that usually found in surveys of cholesterol assays made in hospital laboratories. More detailed analysis of the data suggested that some users consistently obtained results close to the target values, but others did not. The commonest cause of error appeared to be poor technique and, in some cases, the use of reagent strips which had passed their expiry date.

So far, we have mostly used reconstituted lyophilised serum specimens in these surveys. These can show matrix effects with the reagent strips used with this instrument (ref. 15), so that the accuracy of results obtained on these specimens cannot be compared with that of conventional laboratory methods. However, when a serum specimen from a patient with hyperlipidaemia was analysed the mean result obtained by participants agreed with that found by reference laboratories. This, and other published reports (refs. 15, 16), suggest that the instrument per se is accurate when used with patients' specimens. The variability of results illustrated in the Figure can therefore only be blamed on the instrument in that it allows the unskilled operator sufficient latitude to get wrong results: that is, it is not foolproof.

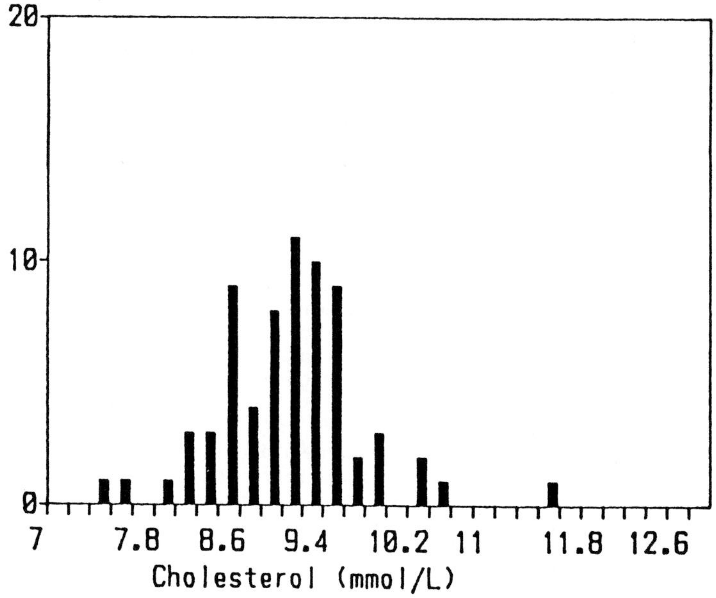

Fig. Distribution of cholesterol results obtained on a reconstituted lyophilised serum by 67 extra-laboratory users of the Reflotron. (Mean = 9.14 mmol/L, range 7.4-11.6 mmol/L)

In these surveys most of those who performed the test were nurses, with little or no laboratory experience or knowledge of quality assurance, and most had no contact with a recognised laboratory. Arising from these experiences we prepared some simple guidelines to help inexperienced users obtain reliable results with the Reflotron. With the full cooperation of the manufacturer these have been circulated to all owners and new purchasers of the instrument. The main recommendations of the guidelines are that users should (1) establish contact with a local clinical chemistry laboratory for help in training, quality control etc, and for advice in following up patients who may have a lipid disorder; (2) join an EQA scheme; and (3) contact the manufacturers if results are unsatisfactory.

HOW LABORATORY STAFF CAN HELP IN PRIMARY CARE

The experiences gained during the operation of this EQA scheme suggested that many users of instruments in primary care need and welcome help and advice. Some of the ways in which laboratory staff can provide this are summarised below (see also ref. 17):

1. Get involved: testing in primary care will inevitably increase, and provides many opportunities and scientific challenges for the laboratory worker.

2. Advise on the selection of suitable instruments and check that these give results which agree with those of the laboratory. Test experimentally whether results depend on the skill and experience of the operator.

3. Advise on test strategies suitable for use in primary care, and provide back-up for confirming doubtful results and any further investigations required.

4. Advise on reference ranges and on the interpretaion of results.

5. Ensure that all who use the instrument are fully trained. Consider the issuing of certificates of competence to operators who pass suitable practical tests (e.g. obtain satisfactory results on a series of quality control specimens).

6. Arrange for internal quality control to be performed regularly, scrutinise the results and ensure that appropriate action is taken when necessary. Test lyophilised specimens to ensure that there are no matrix effects. Arrange for the regular interchange of patients' specimens to ensure that results agree with those obtained in the laboratory.

7. Ensure that all instruments are regularly maintained in collaboration with the manufacturer.

8. Ensure that adequate records are kept, including quality control results.

9. Organise EQA schemes such as those described for glucose (ref. 7), cholesterol (ref. 14) and a variety of other simple tests performed in primary care (ref. 18). Encourage all users in primary care to participate and ensure that appropriate action is taken.

CONCLUSIONS

If instruments are to be used efficiently and effectively in primary care, there needs to be closer collaboration between the physician, the manufacturer and the clinical laboratory, and a better understanding of the roles and responsibilities of each.

For the physician the main consideration is not whether it is possible to do a test in primary care, but whether it is worth doing and, if so, where it can best be performed with the speed and quality required. If the physician decides to do the test, he alone will be responsible for the quality of the results. His initial contact is likely to be the manufacturer's representative, but he lacks the knowledge and experience to distinguish a good instrument from a poor one, or even to realise that there are important differences, and that none is foolproof. The physician therefore needs help, although initially he may not realise this.

Manufacturers should provide more realistic specifications of the performance of their instruments when used in primary care, expressed in terms which a non-technical purchaser can understand and relate to his needs. Better instruments are required, incorporating design features which minimise the influence of the operator's skill on the quality of results. However, accuracy must not be sacrificed by the requirements for speed and simplicity. Usually the manufacturer will provide training for one operator, and perhaps offer quality control materials, but is unlikely to follow up each newly installed instrument to make sure that it is performing satisfactorily. At this stage, collaboration between the physician, manufacturer and clinical laboratory becomes essential.

Often laboratory staff only become aware that tests are being done locally in primary care when they are asked to deal with problems such as equipment failure or an obviously incorrect result. It would be much better to involve the laboratory at the earliest possible stage. For laboratory staff there are opportunities to become involved with different types of clinical problems, for evaluating and advising on the selection of equipment, and for research and development on new types of instrumental systems, quality control materials and techniques.

REFERENCES

1. R. Belsey, D. Baer and D. Sewell, J. Amer. Med. Ass., 255, 775-786 (1986).
2. V. Marks and K.G.M.M. Alberti, Clinical Biochemistry Nearer the Patient, Churchill Livingstone, Edinburgh (1985).
3. V. Marks and K.G.M.M. Alberti, Clinical Biochemistry Nearer the Patient II, Balliere Tindall, London (1986).
4. M.J. Bloch, G.S. Cembrowski and G.J. Lembesis, J. Amer. Med. Ass., 260, 230-235 (1988).
5. B.E. Statland and M.A. Moskowitz, Clin. Lab. Med., 6, 205-209 (1986).
6. M. Cheesbrough, Brit. Med. J., 288, 1978-1982 (1984).
7. R.F. Drucker, D.R.R. Williams and C.P. Price, J. Clin. Pathol., 36, 948-953, (1983).
8. P.M.S. Clark and P.M.G. Broughton, Ann. Clin. Biochem., 20, 208-212 (1983).
9. R. Belsey, M. Vandenbark, R.K. Goitein and D.M. Baer, J. Amer. Med. Ass., 258, 357-361 (1987).
10. P.M.G. Broughton and B.M. Buckley, Scand. J. Clin. Lab. Invest., 47, 99-104 (1987).
11. H.K. Naito, Clin. Chem., 34, 444-449 (1988).
12. J.I. Mann, B. Lewis, J. Shepherd, A.F. Winder, S. Fenster, L. Rose and B. Morgan, Brit. Med. J., 296, 1702-1706 (1988).
13. T.R. Koch, U. Mehta, H. Lee, K. Aziz, S. Temel, J.A. Donlon and R. Sherwin, Clin. Chem., 33, 2262-2267 (1987).
14. D.G. Bullock, P.M.G. Broughton and R. Cramb, in preparation.
15. G.J.M. Boerma, I. van Gorp, T.L. Llem, B. Leijnse, J. Bellm and C.A. Carstensen, Clin. Chem., 34, 1124-1127 (1988).
16. C.P. Price and P.U. Koller, J. Clin. Chem. Clin. Biochem., 26, 233-250 (1988).
17. V. Marks, Ann. Clin. Biochem., 25, 220-225 (1988).
18. S. Landaas and A. Juell, Scand. J. Prim. Health Care, 4, 169-173 (1986).

The use of enhanced chemiluminescence in immunoassay

Thomas P. Whitehead

BUPA Medical Research, Battle Bridge House, 300 Gray's Inn Road, London, WC1X 8DU, England

Abstract - A method of immunoassay has been developed as an alternative to radio-immunoassay in which the peroxidase label in an enzyme-immunoassay is detected and quantified by luminescence. The luminol reaction is considerably enhanced by the addition of p-iodophenol to the reaction which is sensitive, specific and produces a light output which persisits for several minutes. A variety of methods of detection of photons have been studied including photographic film.

INTRODUCTION

The use of chemi- or bioluminescence in clinical analysis has a relatively short history compared with that of colorimetry or fluorescence. Colorimetry is concerned with the absorption of light, fluorimetry with emission of light at a wavelength different from the excitation wavelength. Luminescence results from a chemical reaction in which light is produced without the production of heat.

In the Wolfson Research Laboratories, Department of Clinical Chemistry, University of Birmingham, UK, we began to investigate various immunoassay labels as alternatives to radioactive labels in 1970. Before a label that met all our requirements was found we studied three alternatives. Enzymimmunoassay in our hands in the early 1970's was not sensitive enough to compete with radioactivity as an alternative. Background interference was a major problem in the use of fluorescent labels. Time decay fluorescence, an extremely elegant technique, provided the necessary sensitivity and specificity but the preparation of the rare earth chelates gave us considerable problems which we failed to solve.

LUMINESCENT IMMUNOASSAYS

In studying substances that could be made to luminesce in chemical reactions, three approaches were possible.

Labelling the antigen or antibody with (1)luminescent labels such as luminol analogues; (2)products from enzyme labels such as NADH or ATP; (3)using a catalyst for luminescent reactions eg peroxidase, haem, metal complexes.

We investigated all three methods. The first of these approaches we investigated using luminol and some of its derivatives but found that the quenching of the light output by the proteins, inevitably present, considerably reduced the sensitivity. Additional disadvantages were that the reaction took place at a high pH and fast precise pipetting was required. A sophisticated light measuring device was required to measure the resultant "flash" of light and because of this the final "trigger" solution had to be added in front of this measuring device. It was difficult to obtain high specimen throughput. The first of these disadvantages has been overcome by the Cardiff group using acridinium ester labels but the others still remain.

In attempting to use marine bacteria culture as a source of bioluminescent labels we soon realised that we would have overwhelming problems in quality controlling the biological reagents required.

The third approach was the one that we adopted but only after we had observed the phenomenum of enhanced luminescence.

If hydrogen peroxide is added to luminol in alkaline solution light is produced but the amount is extremely low. If the enzyme peroxidase is added to this reaction it acts as a catalyst and the emission of light is greater.

Peroxidase is a commonly used label in enzymimmunoassays and therefore its potential for taking part in luminescent reactions is considerable.

However it was still not sensitive enough to challenge the very high sensitivity of radioimmunoassay. In attempting to increase this sensitivity we observed that if luciferase as well as luminol was incorporated into the reaction then the light produced was increased by several magnitudes compared with luminol and peroxidase alone. In fact we had a sensitivity equal to or greater than radioactivity.

Specificity of enhanced reactions. Enhanced reactions in addition to being sensitive are also very specific with "low" background.

Light output from enhanced reactions. A considerable advantage ofenhanced luminescent reactions is the character of the light output. In reactions where luminescent substances such as the acridinium esters are used as labels the light output is a "flash" reaching a peak in seconds and then decaying quickly. With the enhanced reaction the light reaches a peak over a period of a few minutes and then remains relatively constant for several minutes; it "glows" rather than flashes.

The reaction conditions. The optimal pH of the reaction is 8.7 thus avoiding the high pH required by other luminescent labels. All reactions can take place at room temperature and the reaction, similar to other luminescent reactions is not temperature sensitive within the usual ambient range.

If maximum sensitivity for a particular reaction is required then optimisation of the reaction is recommended, merely increasing an enhancer molar concentrations beyond the very small concentrations required may reduce light output. High quality chemicals, particularly luminol are required. In the course of the investigation of the use of enhanced luminescence in routine immunoassays no interfering substances were encountered.

Solid phases. During the course of these investigations a wide variety of solid phases were successfully used. These included beads, tubes, microparticles, microtitreplates and micropins.

Luminometers. Additionally several different luminometers were employed of varying sensitivity. These included conventional luminometers both manual and automatic using photomultiplier tubes, photocurrent and photocounting. We also used microtitre plate readers, photographic methods of detection and also a hand held battery operated luminometer using a silicon photodiode.

The enhancer. Although the original observation of enhancement was made with luceferin further investigation showed that other 6- hydroxybenyothiazoles, phenols such p-phenylphenol and also naphthols enhanced the reaction. The most powerful enhancers were the halophenols particularly p-iodophenol. The light emitted from a reaction enhanced by p-iodophenol is almost nine times that produced by phenylphenol which itself enhances the non-enhanced reaction by a factor of 70. In some immonassay we have investigated too high a sensitivity caused problems so that in practice a variety of enhancers were employed.

Use of enhanced immunoassay reactions. Enhanced luminescent immunoassay results have been compared with both radio and enzyme-immunoassay results and for several assays equivalent accuracy and precision were obtained.

Commercial development. Amersham International of the UK are the first to commercialize an immunoassay system dependent on enhanced luminescence under the trade name Amerlite. It comprises a microtitre plate, loading and washing system, an incubater/shaker, a microtitre plate reader and appropriate computer software.

All assays can be completed in less than two hours.

Conclusions. Enhanced luminescence has the following advantages

- prolonged relatively constant light emission
- intense light
- uses inexpensive shelf stable reagents widely available
- speed
- sensitivity
- high signal to background ratio
- performed under mild conditions
- signal is amplified

This work was carried out whilst the author was Professor of Clinical Chemistry at the University of Birmingham UK and Director of the Wolfson Research Laboratories where this work was carried out.

REFERENCES

1. T.P. Whitehead, G.H.G. Thorpe, T.J.N. Carter, C.J. Groucutt and L.J. Kricka, Nature, Lond., 305, 158 (1983).
2. G.H.G. Thorpe, T.P. Whitehead, R. Penn and L.J. Kricka, Clin. Chem., 30, 806 (1984).
3. T.P. Whitehead, G.H.G. Thorpe, L.J.Kricka, J.E.C. Gibbons and R.A. Bunce, Eur.Patent Pub., 110610 (1983).

Bioluminescence and chemiluminescence in clinical microbiology and chemistry

Philip E. Stanley

Consultant Scientist, 48 Glisson Road, Cambridge CB1 2HF, England

Abstract - Assays based upon bioluminescence or chemiluminescence offer sensitivities often between the picomole and femtomole level. With present luminometers the use of firefly luciferase permits the assay of a femtomole of adenosine triphosphate (ATP) whilst bacterial luciferase can be used to assay tens of femtomoles of NAD(P)H.

Rapid microbiology using ATP and firefly luciferase have been applied with success to bacteriuria screening (10 minutes) and antibiotic susceptibility testing (2-3 hours). The basis of the test is to selectively extract and measure ATP from the microorganisms. Susceptibility testing also involves assessment of changes in microbial ATP levels.

A light-based technology involving specific phages permits the assay of particular species of microorganisms. Included within the phage is a bacterial luciferase gene which can be expressed after the phage enters the target cell. The light is then measured.

Kinetic and end-point assays for a wide range of metabolites and enzymes of clinical importance may be made using coupled reactions with firefly luciferase (ATP) or bacterial luciferase (NAD(P)H). Reactions based upon peroxidase may be measured using luminol.

Immunoassays based upon chemiluminescence end-points are finding increasing use and several companies now market kits for a wide range of hormones and proteins of clinical importance.

Luminometers are now commercially available with automation suited to clinical microbiology and clinical chemistry.

INTRODUCTION

Chemiluminescence (CL) may be simply described as light generated by a chemical reaction whereas bioluminescence (BL) is light produced as a result of a protein catalysed reaction. The reaction promotes the production of product molecules in an excited state and their decay to ground state is accompanied by the emission of a photon. The quantum efficiency of the process varies from nearly 100% for the firefly luciferase system to 1% for the luminol system and often many magnitudes smaller for other CL reactions. The photons are generally in the visible portion of the spectrum. An example of a reaction producing CL is that of luminol with peroxide and for BL the action of the enzyme firefly luciferase on adenosine triphosphate (ATP) and D-luciferin. Many reactions generating BL or CL are oxidative processes.

BL and CL based assays offer sensitivities better than those afforded by conventional spectrometric and fluorometric procedures and are often comparable with or exceed those offered in radionuclide-based techniques. In round terms this means that it is often possible to measure down to a femtomole (10^{-15} mole) of analyte.

It is only in recent years that BL and CL have found a place in the clinical laboratory and this to a large extent has been due to a lack of protocols and commercial reagents and instrumentation. The situation is now changing quickly with the introduction of new reagents and suitable instruments. Luminescence based immunoassays for a range of clinically relevant analytes have recently been introduced as replacement technology for radioimmunoassay. The measurement of microbial ATP provides a very rapid (10 minutes) method for bacteriuria screening. Phagocytosis by neutrophils produces luminescence and this is another fruitful area for investigation of chemiluminescence processes.

For the reader wanting general reading in the area of CL (and associated chemistry) the volume by Gundermann and McCapra (ref. 1) is recommended and for both BL and CL the volume edited by Van Dyke (ref. 2) will provide a comprehensive coverage. In the series Methods in Enzymology, two volumes have been devoted to BL and CL (refs. 3-4) and there have been several specialised symposia (refs. 5-9). Two volumes on clinical and biochemical uses of luminescence (refs. 10,11) are particularly relevant.

BIOLUMINESCENCE AND RAPID MICROBIOLOGY

In the clinical microbiology laboratory those techniques capable of providing results within the time range of a few minutes to a couple of hours, have a central role to play in contributing better health care. It is clearly more advantageous to be able to provide an antibiotic susceptibility result within a couple of hours rather than a whole day or to screen for bacteriuria within 10 minutes rather than 24 hours.

Instrument based rapid microbiology tests are finding increasing use and indeed the enumeration of microbes can in certain cases be obtained using bioluminescence (ref. 12). These technique utilise the intrinsic ATP of microorganisms and its reaction with firefly luciferase to produce a number of photons which can be related to the number of microbial cells in the sample. ATP is of course present in all living cells and is not only important as an energy source but also as a regulator of many enzymes. Consequently the amount of cellular ATP remains rather steady and it is this fact which makes it very useful as an indicator for microbial numbers. The "average" bacterium contains around 10^{-15} g ATP per cell and with present reagents and instruments it is possible to assay around one thousand bacteria per test cuvette.

Should the physiological status of the microbe change then there may be a change in ATP content, an example would occur when a bacterium goes from stationary phase into exponential growth. Even so this change may not be sufficiently large to disqualify the use of the technique especially when it is used for a screening test or when it is compared to a conventional microbial growth assay where some microbes may be missed because they fail to grow.

At least two bioluminescence based protocols are worthy of note for the microbiologist; bacteriuria screening (refs. 13,14) and antibiotic susceptibility testing (refs. 15,16) and I shall discuss in general terms the basic protocols which are applied.

The extraction of ATP from cells is normally straightforward but a number of sample formats should be kept in mind (ref. 17) since they may require special treatment. Sample pretreatment is an important step since nearly all samples will contain ATP of non-microbial origin. This is especially true of urine which contains leukocytes, perhaps erythrocytes and certainly free ATP in solution. The treatment of urine involves addition of a non-ionic detergent for example, to lyse the non-microbial cells (sometimes called somatic cells) and to release ATP from these cells into the surrounding liquid. The released ATP as well as free ATP is then hydrolysed by addition of an ATP-ase such as apyrase. This is an important step since the amount of somatic ATP is often greatly in excess (perhaps many thousand-fold) of the microbial ATP. (Any somatic ATP remaining after ATP-ase treatment will carry over and contaminate that ATP derived later from the microbes). The microbial ATP is then extracted using an acid or perhaps a quaternary detergent. This takes just ten seconds or so and is followed immediately with a volume of firefly luciferase which reacts with the microbial ATP to produce photons. This light is measured over a ten second time interval and the reading obtained compared with the threshold value used for the bacteriuria screen. Notice that there is no need to convert the light reading to ATP. All that is required is the light reading threshold or cut-off reading to distinguish between positive or negative specimens and this will have previously been derived by comparing results for a few hundred urine samples assessed using the BL method and also with the conventional technique previously used in the laboratory.

Antibiotic susceptibility testing involves growing the organism in the standard range of antibiotics for a number of hours (2-6 hours) and measuring the ATP in each culture and comparing it with a control without antibiotic (refs. 15,16). In many species of susceptible organism the ATP level will rapidly diminish as compared to the control. A decrease of 50% is often used to signify susceptibility. In this procedure somatic and free ATP are not usually present and the non-ionic detergent treatment followed by apyrase is unnecessary.

Recently a new bioluminescence approach to detecting and enumerating bacteria has been described by Ulitzur and co-workers (ref. 18). Genetic engineering has been the key to this strategy. Bacteriophages which are specific to particular species or groups of species or strains have been derived and lux genes from luminescent bacteria have been inserted into the phages. Lux genes are responsible for the cellular production of luciferase (and oxidoreductase) and which produce light in the presence of NAD(P)H. In broad terms the protocol is as follows. The sample is inoculated with the phage which is specific for the microbe being sought. If it is present the phage enters the microbial cell and begins to synthesise luciferase and in doing so produces light. That light can of course be detected and measured and indicates not only the presence of the species in question but also gives an indication of numbers of microbial cells. The test takes just a few hours.

BIOLUMINESCENCE AND CLINICAL CHEMISTRY

The enzymes which are relevant in this section are (a) firefly luciferase which is specific for ATP and (b) bacterial luciferase (and its associated oxidoreductase) which may be used for measuring NAD(P)H and flavin mononucleotide (FMN). Conventional enzyme coupling procedures may be utilised for measurement of metabolites and enzymes which utilise or produce ATP, NAD(P)H or FMN. In addition a number of studies have demonstrated the use of immobilised luciferases is effective in coupled reactions.

Lack of space precludes a thorough review of the many dozens of analytes for which BL protocols have been described. Instead I will mention just a few as examples and the interested reader should look at references 2-11 for a wider range and references 19-22 for examples and lists of analytes.

As an illustration of an ATP based protocol there is perhaps no better clinical example than that for creatine kinase isoenzymes (ref. 23). Purified ADP and creatine phosphate are the substrates and the product ATP is continuously monitored with firefly luciferase, the light being measured in real time. Specific determination of each of the isoenzymes in serum is achieved using selective immunoinhibition or by chromatographic separation.

Bacterial luciferase may be used for the assay of NAD(P)H and analytes conjugate with it and such a procedure opens a very wide range of possibilities including metabolites such as malate (ref. 24), bile acids (refs. 25,26), D-3-hydroxybutyrate (clinical marker for monitoring ketosis) (ref. 27) and dehydrogenases. Standard enzyme coupling procedures are used and light output is measured with a suitable luminometer. The bacterial luciferase is also unusual in that it requires the presence of a long chain aldehyde cofactor. As the bacterial luciferase technique requires the presence of the oxidoreductase the ratio of these two enzymes is important since this will determine to a large extent the kinetics of the photon output. Whilst the firefly luciferase reaction gives a more a less instantaneous response to the ATP concentration the bacterial luciferase gives a light output which rises gradually to a plateau within 10 to 90 seconds depending on the ratio mentioned earlier. It is possible to determine analyte by reference to this plateau light level or by measuring the slope of the light output line at early in the reaction. Many such assays are capable of measuring femtomole amounts of metabolites and amounts of dehydrogenases far below those attainable by conventional spectrophotometry of fluorometry.

CHEMILUMINESCENCE IN CLINICAL CHEMISTRY

Whilst a number of chemiluminescent assays have been described for compounds of clinical interest such as uric acid (ref. 28) the main interest now firmly centers upon the field of luminescence immunoassay. The need to replace radionuclide labels in clinical immunoassays has been voiced for a number of years.

Chemiluminescence offers the sensitivity achieved in the most sensitive radioimmunoassays and provides the user with a kit which has a long shelf life and obviates the problems generated by the necessity of radionuclide disposal. Several companies (Amersham International, Mallinckrodt, Ciba-Corning) now offer kits covering a wide range of clinically important compounds.

A broad range of papers about various formats of luminescent immunoassays may be found in references 7-9. The topic is also covered more extensively elsewhere in this volume.

CHEMILUMINESCENCE DETECTION IN HPLC

This is a powerful, extremely sensitive and relatively inexpensive way of detecting certain compounds as they elute from the column. By adding a post-column mixing pump it is possible to admix a reagent which produces CL. Many such reagents are somewhat non-specific that is they will react with a class of compounds and this is a particular advantage when one is separating congeneric compounds such as for example dansylated amino acids. The reaction of the latter with TCPO (bis(2,4,6-trichlorophenyl) oxalate) provides a ready means for detecting them. The instrumentation is also somewhat simpler than other HPLC detectors in that a photomultiplier operated in photon counting or current measuring mode is all that is required. Special optics other than good light collection, are not required and the signal is always a positive one against a blank of a darkened reaction flow cell. A fluorometer with the excitation light source switched off makes an excellent detector for use this technique. See reference 29 for more details.

CELLULAR CHEMILUMINESCENCE

It has been known from work in the USSR in the early part of this century that many living cells produce low levels of light. It is only in the last fifteen years or so that the biochemical basis has been investigated. In the clinical field perhaps the subject which has received most attention is that luminescence associated with phagocytosis by neutrophils and macrophages. The oxidative processes which accompany the so-called respiratory burst (hexose monophosphate shunt) during the "killing" process have been shown to be important.

The generation of free radical oxygen and chlorine species is also known to occur at this time in the phagocytic process and be associated with the subsequent production of photons. The pioneering work of Allen and co-workers (ref. 30) is notable, however the literature is extremely wide and the subject still requires fuller elucidation. To date there is no routine clinical laboratory test associated with this phenomenon although several papers appear each week. For a comprehensive text see reference 31.

INSTRUMENTATION - LUMINOMETERS

In the early studies of luminescence and of luminometric assays workers were obliged to build their own luminometers or to modify instruments used by physicists for light measurement. This inevitably led to difficulties in comparative work because of a lack of uniformity of performance and facilities.

In the mid-1970's several companies came to the marketplace with specialised reagents suitable for bioluminescent analyses together with protocols for their use and luminometers for light measurement. For review see references 32-34.

Most of the instruments were based upon a photomultiplier although a few had a solid state detector. The latter whilst being relatively inexpensive and portable and without the need for high voltage power supply, lacked high sensitivity. Clearly, analyses based upon BL and CL are particularly useful where extreme sensitivity is required and lower sensitivity can be obtained by use of a fluorometer for example. Consequently the solid state devices were not a commercial success although certain present day photodiodes are achieving the required performance at room temperature but are restricted in terms of sensitive working surface.

Today there at least twenty models of luminometer available on the commercial market some of which are used for a specific task with the manufacturers protocols and reagents. Manufacturers include:- Dynatech Instruments (Billingshurst, UK), Hamilton Bonaduz AG (Bonaduz, Switzerland), Berthold (Wildbad, Federal Republic of Germany), Lumac BV (Landgraaf, The Netherlands), Turner Designs (Mountain View, California, USA), Foss Electric (Hillerod, Denmark), Microbics Corporation (Carlsbad, California, USA), Amersham International (Little Chalfont, UK), Flow Laboratories (Rickmansworth, UK), Nivarox (St Oulens, Switzerland), Pharmacia-LKB (Turku, Finland) and Aloka (Tokyo, Japan).

Luminometers are available with a wide range of facilities and options. Present prices vary from £5000 to ten times this amount although most lie in the range £10-20,000.

The sensitivity of instruments range from 0.1 pg ATP to about 50 pg ATP and in general terms the more expensive instruments offer better sensitivity as well as more facilities. The higher sensitivity is more than adequate for the currently available commercial immunoassays based upon chemiluminescence. The efficiency of light collection from the sample cuvette and the detection of those photons by the photomultiplier are both important in determining that sensitivity. Most photomultipliers used in todays luminometers have an optimum sensitivity (quantum efficiency) to blue photons around 400 nm but are still quite usable for photons produced in the firefly luciferase-ATP reaction (yellowish, peak at 560 nm).

The sample chamber is a light tight device holding the cuvette close to the photomultiplier. Facilities on most instruments include automatic injection of reagents into the sample cuvette to permit measurement of light which is produced as a flash over a few seconds, e.g. acridinium based immunoassays. In assessing the injection facility attention should be paid to the efficacy of mixing in the cuvette as well as the lack of splashing of reagents into the upper part of the cuvette where reactants may not be seen by the photomultiplier. For an instrument to be used in rapid microbiology it is important that the injector and its associated plumbing be of a type which is easily cleaned and sterilised.

Some instruments have temperature control of the sample chamber and in most cases is just a simple heater which may have shortcomings when operating at temperatures close to ambient. In other instruments a Peltier element may be incorporated and this will also cool the chamber to a limited extent whilst in others temperature control is effected by circulation of water from a thermostatted supply. Cuvettes are usually constructed of plastic (size generally around 12 mm x 50 mm) and the poor thermal conductivity of this material precludes rapid temperature equilibration its contents with the outside chamber. The volume of the cuvette is generally about 3 ml whilst the volume of reactants in the range 0.1 ml to 0.5 ml.

A number of new luminometers has recently been introduced and models are available from Amersham, Dynatech and Flow. These instruments are based on the microtitre plate format so that 96 samples can be accommodated at one time. An X-Y table moves each of the wells sequentially in front of the photomultiplier and the instruments are favorably suited to immunoassays and to studies involving cellular luminescence such as phagocytosis.

Most other luminometers have facilities for handling samples in a semi-automatic fashion or fully automatic way. The semi-automatic units, e.g. Lumac M2500, will automatically process a single sample whilst an instrument such as the Berthold LB950 can incubate and process several hundred samples in an unattended mode.

All instruments have a RS232 computer interface to allow data transfer to an external device and many of the more sophisticated luminometers have software which either (a) fixed (e.g. Hamilton Lumicon, which has excellent graphics associated with the programme), or (b) user programmable (e.g. Pharmacia-LKB 1251, which is IBM-compatible, and uses an emulator program for user written software and which is particularly flexible).

Two other kinds of instrumentation should be mentioned. First the camera luminometer marketed by Dynatech (ref. 35) in which light is recorded on instant film. This unit is useful for microtitre plate measurements and is of course portable and without the need for electrical supply. The other instrument is the imaging luminometer which has been developed and used in astronomical work but which has obvious possibilities for high sensitivity luminometry where imaging is important. Work with samples on microtitre plates has been described (ref. 36).

Subsequent to the presentation of this lecture a new volume was published which comprehensively covers the applications of chemiluminescence in biology and medicine (ref. 37).

REFERENCES

1. K.D. Gundermann and F. McCapra, Chemiluminescence in Organic Chemistry, Springer-Verlag, Berlin (1987).
2. K. Van Dyke, Ed., Bioluminescence and Chemiluminescence: Instruments and Applications, in 2 vols, CRC Press, Boca Raton (1985).
3. M. DeLuca, Ed., Methods in Enzymology, vol 57: Bioluminescence and Chemiluminescence, Academic Press, New York (1978).
4. M.A. DeLuca and W.D. McElroy, Eds., Methods in Enzymology, vol 133: Bioluminescence and Chemiluminescence, Part B, Academic Press, Orlando (1986).
5. E. Schram and P. Stanley, Eds., Proceedings International Symposium on Analytical Applications of Bioluminescence and Chemiluminescence, State Printing & Publishing Westlake Village, CA 91361 (1979).
6. M. DeLuca and W.D. McElroy, Eds., Bioluminescence and Chemiluminescence: Basic Chemistry and Analytical Applications, Academic Press, New York (1981).
7. L.J. Kricka, P.E. Stanley, G.H.G. Thorpe and T.P. Whitehead, Eds., Analytical Applications of Bioluminescence and Chemiluminescence, Academic Press, Orlando (1984).
8. J. Scholmerich, R. Andreesen, A. Kapp, M. Ernst and W.G. Woods, Eds., Bioluminescence and Chemiluminescence: New Perspectives, John Wiley & Sons, Chichester, UK (1987).
9. M. Pazzagli, E. Cadenas, L.J. Kricka, A. Roda and P.E. Stanley, Eds., Proceedings 5th International Symposium on Bioluminescence and Chemiluminescence, Florence, September 1988, John Wiley & Sons, Chichester, UK (in press).
10. M. Serio and M. Pazzagli, Eds., Luminescent Assays. Perspectives in Endocrinology and Clinical Chemistry, Raven Press, New York, (1982).
11. T.J.N. Carter and L.J. Kricka, in: Clinical and Biochemical Luminescence, L.J. Kricka

and T.J.N. Carter, Eds., p.135, Marcel Dekker, New York, (1982).
12. M.J. Harber, in: Clinical and Biochemical Luminescence, L.J. Kricka and T.J.N. Carter, Eds., p. 189, Marcel Dekker, New York, (1982).
13. A. Lundin, H. Hallander, A. Kallner, U. Karnell Lundin and E. Osterberg, in: Rapid Methods and Automation in Microbiology and Immunology, p. 455, K.O. Habermehl, Ed., Springer-Verlag, Berlin (1985).
14. G.D.W. Curtis, H.H. Johnston and A.R. Hack, Eur. J. Clin. Microbiol., 6, 275-280 (1987).
15. L. Nilsson, S.E. Hoffner and S. Ansehn, in: Bioluminescence and Chemiluminescence: New Perspectives, J. Scholmerich, R. Andreesen, A. Kapp, M. Ernst and W.G. Woods, Eds., p. 503, John Wiley & Sons, Chichester, UK (1987).
16. P.F. Wheat, J.G.M. Hastings and R.C. Spencer, J. Med. Microbiol., 25, 95-100 (1988).
17. P.E. Stanley, Meth. Enzymol., 133, 14-22 (1986).
18. S. Ulitzur and J. Kuhn, in: Bioluminescence and Chemiluminescence: New Perspectives, J. Scholmerich, R. Andreesen, A. Kapp, M. Ernst and W.G. Woods, Eds., p. 463, John Wiley & Sons, Chichester, UK (1987).
19. P.E. Stanley, in: Bioluminescence and Chemiluminescence: Basic Chemistry and Analytical Applications, M.A. DeLuca and W.D. McElroy, Eds., p. 275, Academic Press, New York (1981).
20. A. Lundin, in: Clinical and Biochemical Luminescence, L.J. Kricka and T.J.N. Carter, Eds., p. 43, Marcel Dekker, New York (1982).
21. T.P. Whitehead, L.J. Kricka, T.J.N. Carter and G.H.G. Thorpe, Clin Chem, 25, 1531-1546 (1979).
22. F. Gorus and E. Schram, Clin. Chem., 25, 512-519 (1979).
23. A. Lundin, W. Gerhardt, K. Lindberg, T. Lovgren, R. Norlander, O. Nyquist and I. Styrelius, Clin. Biochem., 12, 214-215 (1979).
24. P.E. Stanley, Meth. Enzymol., 57, 181-188 (1978).
25. J. Scholmerich, G.P. Van Berge Henegouwen, A.F. Hofmann and M. DeLuca, Clin. Chim. Acta, 137, 13-20 (1985).
26. A. Roda, S. Girotti, S. Ghini, B. Grigolo, G. Carrea and R. Bovara, Clin. Chem., 30, 206-210 (1984).
27. R.P. Raunio, P.V. Leivo and A.M. Kuusinen, J. Biolum. Chemilum., 1, 11-14 (1986).
28. F. Gorus and E. Schram, Arch. Intern. Physiol. Biochem., 85, 981-982 (1977).
29. K. Imai, K. Miyaguchi and K. Honda, in: Bioluminescence and Chemiluminescence: Instruments and Applications, Vol 2, K. Van Dyke, Ed., p. 65, CRC Press, Boca Raton (1985).
30. R.C. Allen, in: Bioluminescence and Chemiluminescence: New Perspectives, J. Scholmerich, R. Andreesen, A. Kapp, M. Ernst and W.G. Woods, Eds., p. 13, John Wiley & Sons, Chichester, UK (1987).
31. K. Van Dyke and V. Castranova, Eds., Cellular Luminescence (in 3 vols), CRC Press, Boca Raton (1987).
32. P.E. Stanley, in: Clinical and Biochemical Luminescence, L.J. Kricka and T.J.N. Carter, Eds., p. 219, Marcel Dekker, New York (1982).
33. P.E. Stanley, Meth. Enzymol., 133, 587-603 (1986).
34. K. Van Dyke, in: Bioluminescence and Chemiluminescence: Instruments and Applications, Vol 1, K. Van Dyke and V. Castranova, Eds., p. 83, CRC Press, Boca Raton (1985).
35. L.J. Kricka and G.H.G. Thorpe, Meth. Enzymol., 133, 404-420 (1986).
36. D.H. Leaback and C.E. Hooper, in: Bioluminescence and Chemiluminescence: New Perspectives, J. Scholmerich, R. Andreesen, A. Kapp, M. Ernst and W.G. Woods, Eds., p. 439, John Wiley & Sons, Chichester, UK (1987).
37. A.K. Campbell, Chemiluminescence: Principles and Applications in Biology and Medicine, Ellis Horwood, Chichester (UK) (1988).

Recent advances in chemiluminescence immunoassay systems for clinical laboratory

A. TRUCHAUD.[1], Y. GARCERA.[1], G. THORPE[2]. and R. MASSEYEFF[3]

1. Hopital de Meaux, 77104 MEAUX FRANCE
2. Wolfson Research Laboratories Birmingham B 152 TH , UK
3. Immunologie, Faculté de Médecine 06034 NICE FRANCE

Abstract - Recent luminescent immunoassay are presented as complete systems. We classified this systems among the immunoassay systems using fluorescent labels. Recent Technologic improvements in practicability, photon counting measurements and data processing were reviewed and we made proposals concerning further automatisation for quantitative immunoassays. Photographic detection allows qualitative and semi-quantitative screening determinations with a permanent visual record.

INTRODUCTION

During the last 3 decades, biochemists and chemists have unravelled many of the complicated processes underlying fluorescence, bioluminescence and chemiluminescence, but it is only in recent years that light producing labels have been used in immunoassay systems for the clinical laboratory (Table 1).

The main reason is the development of complete systems including reagents, consumables and an adapted instrumentation, presented to the clinical chemist as a ready-to- use package.

TABLE 1 IMMUNOASSAY SYSTEMS USING LABELS PRODUCING LIGHT

SYSTEM	DETECTION	INTRODUCTION
TDX (ABBOTT)	FLUORESCENCE POLARISATION	1983
ARCUS (PHARMACIA)	TIME RESOLVED FLUORIMETRY	1985
STRATUS (BAXTER)	FRONT SURFACE FLUORIMETRY	1985
AMERLITE (AMERSHAM)	CHEMILUMINESCENCE	1987
MAGIC LITE (CORNING)	CHEMILUMINESCENCE	1987
IMX (ABBOTT)	FRONT SURFACE FLUORIMETRY	1988
CYBER FLUOR	TIME RESOLVED FLUORIMETRY	1988

About the analytical process, many confusing abbreviations have been proposed by manufacturers to characterize their products.

CLASSIFICATION

In France Pr MASSEYEFF, proposed recently a classification that allows to present visually immunoassay systems and to predict analytical capabilities and performances.
This classification is based on three items :

1. The principle of the reaction :

* competitive methods by introduction in the mixture of a little amount of labeled reagent, the signal being modified by the analyte in a direct or reverse way.
* In the other hand, with extraction-saturation methods, a large excess of immunologic reagent is used to react with most of the molecules of the analyte in a first immunologic reaction step (EXTRACTION).

The second step is the specific recognition by a large excess of labeled immunochemical reagent ("SATURATION"). Competitive methods will be more used for little molecules like some hormones, drugs and now antibodies.

2. The second item is the nature of the variation of the signal which is measured : in so-called "homogeneous methods", the signal is modulated by immunological reaction. In "heterogeneous methods", a physical separation is necessary before the measurement of the total remaining signal.

3. The third item is the kind of label, but there is often an intermediary step, by example an enzyme revealed by fluorescence or luminescence.

These three items help to classify immunoassay systems and to predict analytical flexibility and performances, through a possible three-dimensional representation (Fig 1).

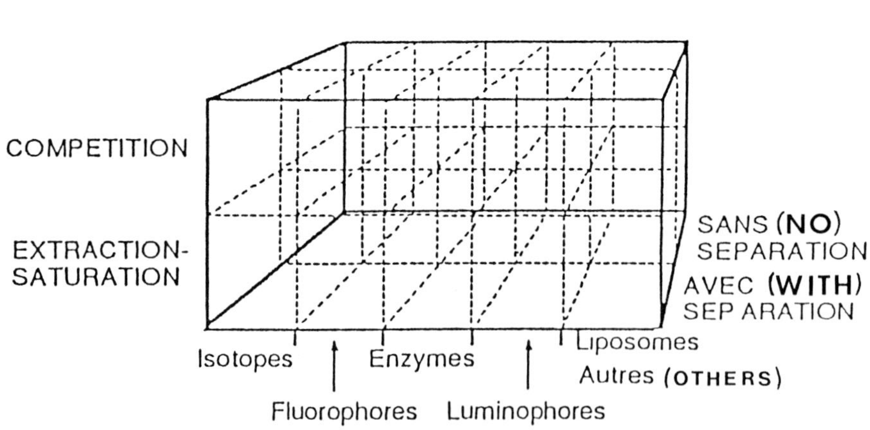

Fig 1 : Three dimensional representation of immunoasay systems.

QUANTITATIVE IMMUNOASSAYS USING LUMINESCENT LABELS

Two immunoassay systems using luminescent labels are actually available : the Amerlite developed by Amersham (Little Chalfont, Buckinghamshire, HP 79 NA, UK.) and the Magic Lite developed by Ciba-Corning (East Walpole, Massachussets 02032,USA).
We will discuss here only the differences between the two systems and make some proposals for improvements from the user's point of view.
If we follow the proposed classification, the AMERLITE system allows reactions by competition or by extraction-saturation : this allows determinations of molecules of a large range of size and concentration.

TABLE 2. Amerlite : available parameters.

CEA, AFP

TOTAL T_4, FREE T_4, TBG

TOTAL T_3, T_3 UPTAKE, FREE T_3

ULTRASENSITIVE TSH

DIGOXINE, FERRITINE

CORTISOL, OESTRADIOL, HCG

LH, FSH, PROLACTINE, PROGESTERONE

A separation step is required and a mixed label with an enzyme and then a fluorophore is used to produce the light.
Preparation of the batches in individual strips of coated wells is helped by an ergonomic work station with pipetters and dispensers ; an automatic dispenser may be provided as an option.

After incubation, separation in an automatic washer and addition of the signal reagent, enhanced luminescence measurements are possible within more than ten minutes :
measurements are achieved in an automated luminometer within less than 2 minutes for a microplate of 96 wells. The detector is fixed in a high precision XY system which moves above the wells. For each assay, the signal is integrated only during 0.2 seconds.

The light does not cross any optical wall before the reach the detector. This avoids any interference by the optical wall. This concept is used in many recent immunoassay systems like the Stratus, IMX and Cyberfluor.

The method is based on the fact that the slow decreasing of light is proportional for the differents levels of concentration of the calibration solutions and for the specimens.So the validation of the calibration curve is the critical step of the method, helped by several parameters given whitch the calibration curve : the light index, i.e. a limit for the light produced by the highest point of the calibration curve as light intensity, is difficult to fix with precision as long as the time between the addition of the signal reagent and the measurement is not fixed and that the signal is decreasing with time.
The curve fit factor is a precious parameter to appreciate the quality of the curve and to check an eventual discrepant result.

Our proposal should be to go further in control of operations by the microprocessor :

- Fix the time between signal reagent addition and measurements of light production, maybe by an automated process.

- Enhance also the capabilities of the computer to have a good survey of light index, curve fit factor and quality control, related to each test with a statistic and visual representation.

The MAGIC LITE uses competition and extraction-saturation methods, requires a separation step (magnetic) and uses a luminescent label. Here again, molecules of a large range of size and concentration may be measured by this system. (table 3).

Table 3. Magic Lite : available parameters

TOTAL T_4, FREE T_4
TOTAL T_3, T UPTAKE
CORTISOL, H.C.G.
FERRITINE, CK MB
DIGOXINE

Batches are prepared manually in racks containing polystyrene tubes, and solid phase consist of coated magnetic particles.
After washing and separation steps, tubes are introuced in the luminometer manually or automatically (option).
Two reagents are injected by automated pumps in less than 0.2 seconds in the polystyrene tubes. Mixing is achieved by forceable injection.

The luminometer includes a detector chamber with a small light-tight chamber in which the light-emitting occurs in a cuvette placed directly in front of the detector. The walls of the chamber are mirrored to optimize the collection of the photons at the photocathode. Photons are counted and the peak is integrated by the microprocessor.

The light emission last less than two seconds and it is evident that it is the critical step of the assay.
About the integration of the peak for the Magic Lite, the work of Pr Pazzagli (ref 1) about the computer analysis of the kinetics of chemiluminescent reactions should be applied with sucess : automatic study of the shape of the peak by the microprocessor to detect an interfering substance. Usually, the result is related to the total counts during a fixed time interval but a "shape" index should be measured to reveal modifications of the kinetics pattern and then disturbances in the light production efficiency of the chemiluminescent reaction.
Pazzagli proposed the 5/10 ratio to identify changes in the shift of the count distribution and also the Tmax, time where the light production is maximum.

A first improvement of the Magic Lite system should be to recommand before to start measurements on a batch to do a preprogrammed test with a fixed amount of signal reagent and to edit the result for control.
Actually it is difficult to fix the limits in counts because the incubation is at "room temperature" and that the light production is related to temperature. We recommand to fix the incubation temperature in an incubator with thermal stabilisation.

An original feature of the MAGIC LITE is the use of a "MASTER CURVE" introduced in the memory of the luminometer for each lot of a given reagent. The master curve is corrected for each batch by the two points of calibration : we suggest an automatic control of the two calibration points by the calculation of the ratio between the two points with a fixed limit.

LEVEL OF AUTOMATION

The level of automation of the luminescence immunoassay systems is poor, compared with the systems using fluorescence. But we assume that the complete automation is not an absolute target as long as there is a risk of lost of flexibility for testing batches of different sizes on different parameters. Furthermore the concept of profile, or random acess is not transposable to immunoassays because, except for thyroîd tests, profiles are very limited on a single specimen.

We prefer to emphasize the necessity of process control which allows the various operating parameters to be monitored and if necessary automatically adjusted. Priority for automation of an analytical step or self checking of an operating parameter should be defined by their possible interference on the control of measurements by the microprocessor.

QUALITATIVE AND SEMIQUANTITATIVE IMMUNOASSAYS BY PHOTOGRAPHIC DETECTION

An interesting alternative to light measurements by photomultiplier tubes or silicon photodiode, is the combination of luminescence with a photographic films, developed by Larry Kricka and Gary Thorpe, at the Wolfson Laboratories. (ref 2).
The system is composed of a light-tight box located on top of a polaroīd film holder separated by a slidable shutter :

- The MAST chemiluminescent assay system for total IgE and allergen-specific IgE (MAST Immunosystems Inc, Mountain View, CA) is currently the only commercially available assay system which combines chemiluminescence and photography.

- The Camera Luminometer consists of a film-holder, a cover with a timer, and the holder, made in the form of an array of holes to separate the light emission from individual wells.

After the luminescent reaction, the exposed polaroīd film shows positive (white), negative (flash), and weekly positive assays i.e. qualitative results. Semiquantitative results can be obtained by interposing neutral density filters between the glowing reaction vessels and film. Photographic immunoassays based on enhanced luminescence were developed for cytomegalovirus IgG, Factor VIII antigen, Ferritin, IgE, Malaria IgG an rubella specific IgG.
So, multiple assays can be performed simultaneously using low cost, portable instrumentation which requires no power source and a permanent visual record is obtained.

DISCUSSION

Recent luminescence immunoassays, presented as complete systems to the user, allow determinations of a large panel of parameters by competitive or extraction-saturation methods. The main target of automation should be the control of the critical steps of the process. Photographic detection is an ideal tool for screeing methods with qualitative or semi-quantitative results.

CONCLUSION

Chemiluminescence immunoassay systems are a good alternative to radioimmunoassays.

REFERENCES

1. M. Pazzagli, and M. Serio, (1986). On line Computer Analysis of the Kinetics of luminescent reactions : application to luminescent immunoassays. In Bioluminescence and Chemiluminescence, Part B. Methods in Enzymology (DeLuca, M.A. and McElroy, W.D., Eds.) Academic Press, Inc., Florida, 133, pp.
2. M.J. Kricka, and G.H.G. Thorpe, (1986) Photographic detection of chemiluminescent and bioluminescent reactions. In Bioluminescence and Chemiluminescence, Part B. Methods in Enzymology (DeLuca, M.A. and McElroy, W.D., Eds.) Academic Press, Inc., Florida, 133, pp 404-420.

Cell surface analysis with flow cytometry: a comparison of a single color anlaysis with a two color method and a proposal of a flow chart to diagnose hematological disorders

Kazuhiko Nakahara [1], Tetsuya Nakamura [2] and Akiko Yoneyama [2]

Department of Laboratory Medicine [1], The First Department of Internal Medicine [2], Faculty of Medicine, University of Tokyo, Tokyo, Japan

Abstract — Some hematological disorders were analysed with a two color immunofluorescence technique and the results from single color and two color methods were compared. It has been found that adult T cell leukemia cells, which are positive for CD4 (helper/inducer T lymphocytes) in a single color analysis, are derived from suppressor inducer T cells ($CD4^+ - Leu8^+$) in a two color analysis. The increased lymphocytes in infectious mononucleosis have been recognized to be activated cytotoxic T cells ($CD8^+ - CD11^-$ and $CD8^+ - HLA \cdot DR^+$) in a two color analysis. The increased cells in thymoma have also been identified to be positive for both CD4 and CD8 simultaneously ($CD4^+ - CD8^+$). We conclude that a two color analysis is a very useful tool to study more detail and precise cell surface markers. A flow chart to diagnose hematological disorders with cell surface markers is also proposed in this article.

INTRODUCTION

It is quite recognized that the cell surface analysis with a single color technique is a very useful tool to diagnose diseases, especially hematological disorders such as leukemia and lymphoma. Particularly owing to the recent spread of flow cytometry and development of monoclonal antibodies, a single color analysis has become to be used as routine clinical service at many institutions. Recently a two color analysis with fluorescein isothiocyanate (FITC) and phycoerythrin (PE) has become to be easily applied to a cell surface staining and a more detail analysis has become to be available in studying cell surface antigens. It was reported that cytotoxic T lymphocytes (Tc) are positive for CD8 but negative for CD11 ($CD8^+ - CD11^-$) (ref.1) and suppressor T lymphocytes (Ts) express antigens reacted to both CD8 and CD11 ($CD8^+ - CD11^+$) (ref.2,3). Similarly suppressor inducer T lymphocytes (Tsi) and helper T lymphocytes (Th) were reported to be $CD4^+ - Leu8^+$ (ref.4) and $CD4^+ - Leu8^-$ (ref.5) respectively. It has also been published that activated T lymphocytes possess HLA · DR antigens on thier cell surfaces ($CD3^+ - HLA \cdot DR^+$) (ref.6,7). We analysed some hematological disorders with a two color immunofluorescence technique and compared the results from single color and two color methods. We conclude that a two color analysis is a very useful tool to study more detail and precise cell surface markers. A flow chart to diagnose hematological disorders with cell surface markers is also proposed in this article.

A COMPARISON OF A SINGLE COLOR ANALYSIS WITH A TWO COLOR METHOD

Although a single color analysis is a very useful method on the cell surface marker examination, one disadvantage exists. Namely, since CD8 reacts to not only Ts but also Tc, these two subpopulations cannot be distinguished in a single color analysis. It is reported that, by using a two color analysis with both CD8 and CD11, Ts and Tc can be clearly distinguished and identified as mentioned above. Similarly Th and inducer T cells (Ti) cannot be distinguished with a single color analysis using only CD4, but it is published that a two color staining with CD4 and anti—Leu 8 is able to distinguish Th and Tsi. The actual clinical data and the potential application of a two color analysis are presented in the following.

1) Adult T cell leukemia (ATL)

ATL is characterized by oncet in adulthood, a subacute or chronic clinical course with a rapidly progressive terminal course, pleomorphic ATL cells with deeply indented or lobulated nuclei, frequent occurrence of skin lesions and geographic distribution of the patients birthplaces. The discovery that the cause of ATL is human T-lymphocyte tropic virus type I(HTLV-I) attracted many scientists' attention to ATL as the model of leukemogenesis. It was already reported that ATL cells possessed specific surface markers, that is, positive for CD4 and negative for CD8 (ref.8). However, only with a single color analysis, we cannot identify whether the origin of ATL cells is Th or Ti. By using a two color analysis with CD4 and anti-Leu 8, it can be recognized that ATL cells express both CD4 and Leu 8 on a single cell ($CD4^+ - Leu\ 8^+$), namely, the origin of ATL is not Th but Tsi. Table 1 shows a summary of single and two color analyses of ATL. All cases except the case 11 are positive for both CD4 and anti—Leu 8.

2) Infectious mononucleosis (IM)

IM is the disease caused by infection of Epstein—Barr viruses and many atypical lymphocytes appear in peripheral blood. In a single color analysis the number of CD8 positive cells, Ts/c, increases in the peripheral blood of IM patients. However, we cannot identify which subpopulations of Ts or Tc increase in number. A two color analysis clarifies this question. The increased peripheral blood lymphocytes of IM are positive for CD8 and negative for CD11 ($CD8^+ - CD11^-$), which indicates those lymphocytes are not Ts but Tc in a two color analysis. By using a two color method with CD8 and an anti—HLA · DR antibody, those cells also express HLA · DR on the cell surface. It can be suggested that the peripheral blood lymphocytes from IM are activated cytotoxic T lymphocytes. Table 2 shows the results of a two color analysis of IM.

TABLE 1. Single and two color analysis of ATL

case	region	CD 8	CD 4	CD 3	CD 4$^+$– Leu 8$^-$	CD 4$^+$– Leu 8$^+$
1	PBL	6.5%	76.9%	81.1%	ND	ND
2	PBL	9.8	82.9	89.8	15.1%	64.6%
3	PBL	2.8	93.6	96.4	ND	ND
4	PBL	9.6	70.2	77.8	2.8	63.7
	LN	6.0	65.6	71.3	11.7	54.6
5	PBL	7.9	83.1	97.3	4.8	73.8
6	PBL	1.1	93.5	ND	ND	ND
	PBL	2.5	96.5	ND	9.1	74.2
	PBL	0.8	98.4	98.4	7.2	89.1
	PBL	6.0	96.5	98.6	8.9	86.3
7	PBL	10.2	84.7	91.9	9.8	71.2
	PBL	7.7	77.1	ND	ND	ND
8	PBL	9.8	81.1	81.4	5.4	68.7
	BM	7.5	34.6	32.3	4.7	15.5
	PBL	9.0	83.2	70.6	5.0	74.2
	PBL	2.3	90.9	74.6	4.7	87.2
9	PBL	5.7	93.3	95.7	3.2	89.4
	PBL	4.7	91.4	94.1	ND	ND
10	PBL	2.3	85.2	79.4	5.2	77.5
11	PBL	14.6	96.4	97.4	71.7	26.8
	PBL	20.2	91.3	92.7	62.7	27.2
	PBL	14.7	88.3	95.9	54.6	35.4
Normal PBL		34.7±7.4	42.4±8.1	71.8±6.4	7.9±4.9	31.2±9.0

PBL : peripheral blood lymphocytes BM : bone marrow
LN : lymphnode ND : not done

TABLE 2. Two color analysis of IM

		Normal n=16	non IM n=8	IM n=7
CD8$^+$–CD11$^+$	%	8.2±3.2	5.3±4.0	12.5±7.5
	/mm³	(171±80)	(116±64)	(711±510)*
CD8$^+$–CD11$^-$	%	22.1±5.4	22.0±8.1	52.0±14.1**
	/mm³	(478±226)	(600±423)	(3,181±2,637)**
CD4$^+$–Leu8$^+$	%	33.0±7.1	27.3±7.8	11.6±5.8**
	/mm³	(682±248)	(715±522)	(534±166)
CD4$^+$–Leu8$^-$	%	7.6±2.5	8.0±2.1	(4.3±2.9*
	/mm³	(170±108)	(195±79)	(198±143)
CD8$^+$–HLA-DR$^+$	%	1.6±0.5	3.9±3.3	40.0±26.1**
	/mm³	(33±14)	(111±138)	(2,958±3,275)**
CD4$^+$–HLA-DR$^+$	%	1.8±0.8	2.0±1.2	3.2±1.4
	/mm³	(40±23)	(50±39)	(178±91)**
CD3$^+$–HLA-DR$^+$	%	2.7±0.9	6.0±5.3	42.5±22.4**
	/mm³	(59±33)	(181±226)	(2,868±2,854)**

( ) : absolute number IM : infectious mononucleosis
* $P<0.05$ ** $P<0.01$

3) Thymoma

Although it has been recognized that the increased cells in thymoma are positive for CD4 and CD8, it has not been known in a single color analysis whether these antigens reacted to those monoclonal antibodies exist on the same single cell. A two color analysis has clearly indicated that almost all increased cells in thymoma express both antigens reacted to CD4 and CD8 on a single cell simultaneously ($CD4^{+} - CD8^{+}$).

It has been found that ATL cells, which are positive for CD4 (Th/i) in a single color analysis, are derived from Tsi ($CD4^{+} - Leu8^{+}$) in a two color analysis. The increased lymphohcytes in IM have been recognized to be activated cytotoxic T cells ($CD8^{+} - CD11^{-}$ and $CD8^{+} - HLA \cdot DR^{+}$) in a two color analysis. The increased cells in thymoma have also been identified to be positive for both CD4 and CD8 simultaneously ($CD4^{+} - CD8^{+}$). It can be concluded that the two color analysis is a very useful tool to study more detail and precise cell surface markers.

A PROPOSAL OF A FLOW CHART TO DIAGNOSE HEMATOLOGICAL DISORDERS

Recently a tremendous number of monoclonal antibodies have been developed and are available commercially, which is convenient for the study of elucidation of the immune system, etc. However, in the actual clinical fields, since the prompt and accurate diagnosis is really required, it is necessary to diagnose hematological disorders with the minimal number of antibodies. Nevertheless the definite and standard chart for diagnosis of hematological malignancies such as leukemia and lymphoma is not established, and the types and the number of monoclonal antibodies in diagnosing those disorders are different among each institution, which wastes valuable time, money and labor. Fig.1 is our new flow chart to diagnose hematological disorders with cell surface markers and Table 3 shows monoclonal antibodies used for our flow chart.

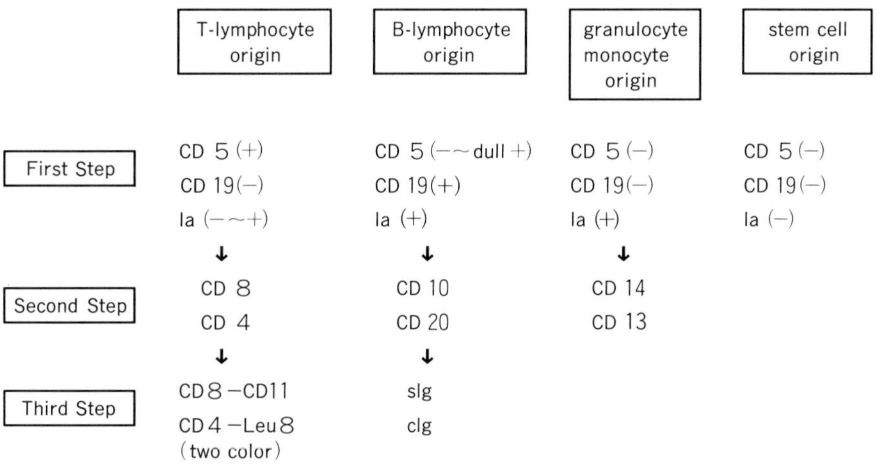

Fig. 1. A flow chart to diagnose hematological disorders using cell surface markers

TABLE 3. Monoclonal antibodies used for our flow chart

CD number	monoclonal antibody	antigen or antigen distribution
CD 5	anti-Leu 1	pan-T
CD 19	anti-Leu 12, B4	pan-B
——	anti-HLA-DR	Ia
CD 8	anti-Leu 2a	suppressor/cytotoxic T
CD 4	anti-Leu 3a	helper/inducer T
CD 10	anti-CALLA	CALLA
CD 20	B 1	mature B
CD 14	MY 4	monocyte
CD 13	MY 7	monocyte, granulocyte

CALLA : common ALL antigen

TABLE 4. Hematological disorders of T−cell origin

case	diagnosis	First step			Second step	
		CD5	CD19	anti-Ia	CD8	CD4
1	T-ALL	+	−	−	−	−
2		+	−	−	−	−
3	T-CLL	+	−	−	−	+
4		−	−	dull+	−	−
5		+	−	−	−	+
6	ATL	+	−	±	−	+
7		+	−	+	−	+
8		+	−	±	−	+
9		+	−	NT	−	+
10		+	−	±	−	+
11		+	−	+	−	+
12		+	−	+	−	+
13		+	−	+	−	+
14	LGL	+	−	+	+	+
15		+	−	−	+	+
16		+	−	−	+	−
17	T-NHL	+	−	+	−	+
18		+	−	+	+	−
19		+	−	±	−	+
20		+	−	±	−	+
21		+	−	±	−	+
22	Thymoma	+	−	−	+	+
23		+	−	−	+	+
24		+	−	−	+	+
25		+	−	−	+	+

ALL : acute lymphocytic leukemia
CLL : chronic lymphocytic leukemia
ATL : adult T-cell leukemia
LGL : large granular lymphocyte leukemia
NHL : non-Hodgkin lymphoma
NT : not tested

TABLE 5. Hematological disorders of B−cell origin

case	diagnosis	First step			Second step	
		CD5	CD19	anti-Ia	CD10	CD20
1	non-T ALL	−	+	+	+	NT
2		−	+	+	+	dull+
3		NT	+	+	+	+
4		−	+	+	+	+
5		dull+	−	±	+	±
6	B-CLL	dull+	+	+	−	NT
7		dull+	+	+	+	NT
8		dull+	+	+	−	NT
9		dull+	+	+	−	NT
10		dull+	+	+	−	NT
11		dull+	+	+	−	NT
12		dull+	+	+	−	+
13		dull+	+	+	−	+
14	B-CLSCL	dull+	+	+	−	NT
15	HCL	−	+	+	NT	NT
16		−	+	+	NT	NT
17		dull+	+	+	NT	NT
18	B-NHL	dull+	+	+	NT	NT
19		−	+	+	NT	NT
20		dull+	+	+	+	NT
21		dull+	+	+	+	NT
22		dull+	+	+	±	NT
23		dull+	+	±	−	NT
24		dull+	+	+	−	NT
25		dull+	+	+	±	NT
26	Hodgkin	−	dull+	+	+	+
27	BC of CML	−	+	+	+	NT

ALL : acute lymphocytic leukemia
CLL : chronic lymphocytic leukemia
CLSCL : chronic lymphosarcoma cell leukemia
HCL : hairy cell leukemia
NHL : non-Hodgkin lymphoma
BC of CML : blastic crisis of chronic myelocytic leukemia
NT : not tested

Our chart is separated into three steps. The major purpose of the first step is to determine the cell origin of the hematological malignancies and it is composed of only three kinds of monoclonal antibodies, that is, CD5, CD19 and anti−Ia. As shown in Fig.1 cells with CD5 (+) , CD19 (−) and Ia (−∼+) are estimated to be T−lymphocyte origin; CD5 (−∼dull +) , CD19 (+) and Ia (+) are B−lymphocyte origin; CD5 (−) , CD19 (−) and Ia (+) are granulocyte or monocyte origin; and CD5 (−) , CD19 (−) and Ia (−) are stem cell origin. Accordingly we can determine the cell origin of the hematological disorders at the first step using only three monoclonal antibodies. If a more detail analysis is needed, we can go forward to the second step. In T−lymphocyte orign more detail subpopulation analysis, Ts/c or Th/i, and the differentiation stage of the hematological disorders are able to be evaluated by using CD8 and CD4. In B−lymphocyte origin the differentiation stage is estimated with CD10 and CD20, and in granulocyte−monocyte origin CD14 and CD13 are used for more detail analysis. Then in case of necessity we advance to the third step and a two color analysis with CD8−CD11 and CD4−anti−Leu8 and a surface or a cytoplasmic immunoglobulin analysis can be examined in T−lymphocyte origin and B−lymphocyte origin, respectively.

In order to evaluate propriety of our flow chart, we investigated it by comparing with the result of 69 cases which were actually examined at our laboratory for these three years. Table 4, Table 5 and Table 6 show the results of T−lymphocyte origin, B−lymphocyte origin and granulocyte−monocyte origin, respectivety.

TABLE 6. Hematological disorders of granulocyte−monocyte origin

case	diagnosis	First step			Second step	
		CD5	CD19	anti-Ia	CD14	CD13
1	AML	−	−	+	NT	NT
2		NT	−	+	−	+
3		NT	−	+	−	+
4		−	−	+	−	+
5	AMMoL	−*	−*	+	NT	NT
6		−*	−*	+	NT	NT
7		−*	−*	+	+	+
8		−	−	+	+	+
9		−*	−*	+	+	+
10	AMoL	−	−	+	NT	NT
11		−	−	+	+	+
12		−*	−*	+	+	+
13	BC of CML	−	−	+	NT	NT
14		−	−	+	NT	NT
15		−	−	+	+	+
16	CML	−	−	+	NT	NT
17	AMgKL	−	−	+	−	−

−* non-specific false positive
AML : acute myelocytic leukemia
AMMoL : acute myelomonocytic leukemia
AMoL acute monocytic leukemia
BC of CML : blastic crisis of chronic myelocytic leukemia
AMgKL : acute megakaryocytic leukemia
NT : not tested

As shown in Table 4 all cases of T−lymphocyte origin except the case 4 were consistent with our chart. As the case 4 was CD5 negative but positive for CD3 which reacts to pan T lymphocytes, we decided the case T−lymphocyte origin. Those CD5 negative and CD3 positive cases are very rare and exceptional. In B−lymphocyte origin all cases except the case 5 were compatible with our chart (Table 5) . Although the case 5 was CD19 negative, we determined the case was B−lymphocyte origin because of CD10 positive and CD20 weakly positive. Those cases negative for CD19 and positive for CD10 and CD20 are also uncommon. As shown in Table 6 all granulocyte−monocyte origin cases except the case 17 were consistent with our chart. Since the case 17 was CD5 (−) , CD19 (−) and Ia (+) , this case must be diagnosed as granulocyte−monocyte origin based on our flow chart. However, this case was platelet peroxidase positive and we diagnosed the case as acute megakaryocytic leukemia. Incidentally when the second step monoclonal antibodies, CD14 and CD13, were examined, we could find it was strange for granulocyte−monocyte origin because of negative for both CD14 and CD13.

All cases except only three out of 69 were consistent with our flow chart. As those three cases were rare or uncommon, we can conclude that our flow chart is useful to diagnose hematological disorders in actual clinical fields.

REFERENCES

1. L. T. Clement, M. K. Dagg and A. Landay, J. Clin. Immunol. 4, 395−402 (1984) .
2. A. Landy, G. L. Gartland and L. T. Clement, J. Immunol. 131, 2757−2761 (1983) .
3. L. T. Clement, C. E. Grossi and G. L. Gartland, J. Immunol. 133, 2461−2468 (1984) .
4. N. K. Damle, N. Mohagheghpour and E. G. Engleman, J. Immunol. 132, 644−650 (1984) .
5. P. A. Gatenby, G. S. Kansas, C. Y. Xian, R. L. Evans and E. G. Engleman, J. Immunol. 129, 1997−2000 (1982) .
6. R. L. Evans, T. J. Faldetta, R. E. Humphreys, D. M. Pratt, E. J. Yunis and S. T. Schlossman, J. Exp. Med. 148, 1440−1445 (1978) .
7. D. T. Y. Yu, R. J. Winchester, S. M. Fu, A. Gibofsky, H. S. Ko and H. G. Kunkel, J. Exp. Med. 151, 91−100 (1980) .
8. K. Nakahara, T. Ōhashi, M. Ichimaru, T. Amagasaki, M. Shimoyama, H. Nakauchi and K. Okumura, Clin. Immunol. Immunopathol.25, 43−52 (1982) .

Flow cytometric analysis of DNA aneuploidy as a tumor marker

Shigeru Takamoto

Department of Blood Transfusion,
Tokyo Metropolitan Komagome Hospital,
3-18-22, Hon-Komagome, Bunkyo-ku, Tokyo, 113, Japan

Abstract - DNA aneuploidy(DA) was examined in 185 adult cases with various types of leukemia using flow cytometry. DA was detected in 50 out of 185 cases (27.0%). Among the subtypes of leukemia, the frequency of DA in adult T-cell leukemia(ATL) was significantly higher(55.3%) when compared with other subtypes, which suggested a special entity of this disease. The DNA index ranged between 0.913 and 2.042, and the average was 1.144, which corresponded to 42, 94 and 53, respectively, for the value for the average size of the chromosomes. Among fifty cases with DA, only two cases showed more than two DA clones, which indicated a less heterogeneous population in leukemic clones than is currently reported. Also, only two cases showed hypodiploidy. In a few cases which we were able to follow up, DA was very useful as a tumor marker for monitoring the clinical course. Furthermore, DA was found to be a good prognostic factor which indicates a poor prognosis in cases with acute non-lymphocytic leukemia(ANLL) and chronic myelocytic leukemia in blastic crisis(CML-BC).

INTRODUCTION

Recently many tumor markers, for example, α 1-fetoprotein, carcinoembryonic antigen, CA-19-9, common ALL antigen(CALLA) and others, have become available in clinical oncology. However, most of these markers are not tumor specific markers, but are oncofetal antigens, differentiation antigens or tumor associated antigens.

It is a well known fact that tumor cells are often associated with chromosomal abnormalities, while normal cells are not. Also chromosomal abnormalities are found in a few congenital diseases, like Down's or Klinefelter's syndromes, where whole cells of individual patients show chromosomal abnormalities. So, with the exception of these rare congenital diseases, chromosomal abnormality could be regarded as a real tumor specific marker by itself.

However, current methods of chromosomal analysis are time-consuming, laborious, not highly quantitative and necessitate skill. Furthermore, the existence of mitotic cells is essential, and that often makes analysis more difficult. These limitations have hindered the use of chromosomal abnormality as a tumor marker.

Since the development of flow cytometry, it has become quite easy to determine relative DNA content per cell. Simply by staining cells with DNA specific fluorescent dye the relative DNA content per cell can be determined fairly quickly, objectively, quantitatively and furthermore, no mitotic cells are necessary. Although qualitative chromosomal abnormalities like translocation are not detectable by this new method, aneuploidy, a quantitative chromosomal abnormality, can easily be detected. In addition, flow cytometric analysis of DNA content per cell could make aneuploidy an actual tumor marker.

Figure 1. shows one example of flow cytometric analysis of DNA aneuploidy(DA). The sample was obtained from a patient with acute myeloblastic leukemia, whose leukemic cells were found to have aneuploidy by current chromosomal analysis methods. On the left is a sample from peripheral blood and the right from bone marrow. On each histogram, the X axis indicates fluorescent intensity, namely relative DNA content per cell, while the Y axis stands for the cell number. In each histogram, two clearly separate peaks are observed. The one on the left is a normal DNA clone from normal hematopoietic cells and the other is an abnormal DNA clone from leukemic cells. For each sample, more than 10,000 cells were determined, which took only a few minutes. Thus, DA was rapidly and easily detected by using flow cytometry.

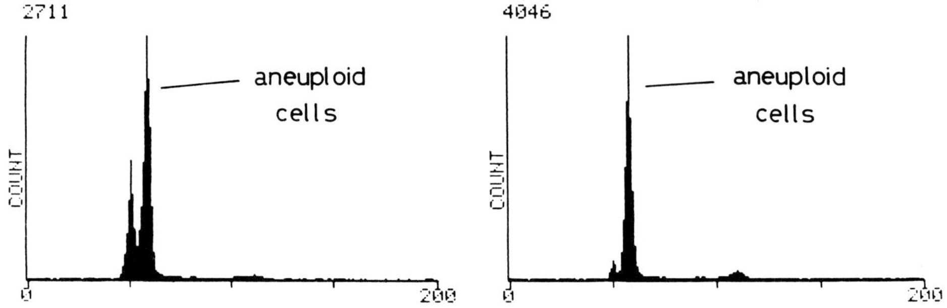

Fig. 1. The DNA histograms of peripheral blood(left) and bone marrow(right) from a case with acute myeloblastic leukemia. The left peak represents normal diploid cells and the right leukemic aneuploid cells.

In this paper, 185 adult cases with various types of leukemia were subjected to analysis of DA using flow cytometry and the clinical implications of DA as a tumor marker are described.
Concerning the terminology, to differentiate the results by flow cytometric analysis from those by current chromosomal analysis, the term "DNA aneuploidy" was used instead of "aneuploidy".

MATERIALS AND METHODS

Peripheral blood or bone marrow was obtained from patients by using a heparinized syringe and was processed by Ficoll-Hypaque density separation. Separated mononuclear cells were divided into two samples. One was mixed with rainbow trout red blood cells(TRBC) as an internal standard and the other was mixed with two standards, namely, normal human diploid cells and TRBC. Then the samples were stained with propidium iodide solution (propidium iodide 50µg/ml in 0.1% sodium citrate with 0.1% Nonidet P-40 and 1mg/ml of ribonuclease A). Samples were kept in a refrigerator and were determined by flow cytometry within 24 hours.
The flow cytometer used in this study was a Cytofluorograf 50-H (Ortho Diagnostic Systems Inc., Westwood, Mass., U.S.A.). Samples were excited at the wavelength of 488nm by 200mW and the emitted fluorescence was determined through a long-pass filter of 600nm. When determining samples, conditions for excitement were properly adjusted so that the small peak of TRBC would appear at a pre-determined channel. For each sample, twenty thousand cells were determined to give a DNA histogram.
Samples with apparently separate peaks from the internal diploid standard were evaluated to have DA. DNA index was calculated based on the internal diploid standard. In practical terms, the peak channel number of the DA clone was divided by that of the internal diploid standard and the value thus calculated represented the DNA index.
Using TRBC as an internal standard, human diploid cells were examined more than one hundred times. As a result, the normal diploid range was defined to be the average value 1.0 ± 0.042. This value corresponded to 2 chromosomes of average size. Thus, by adapting TRBC as an internal standard, we felt it was possible to detect by flow cytometry abnormalities which involved 2 or more chromosomes of average size.
Moreover, the correlation between current chromosomal and flow cytometric analysis was examined. At first two indices were determined. One was karyotype index which was calculated by dividing the chromosomal number of the sample by the normal chromosomal number, 46. The other was the DNA index as described previously. For example, DNA indices of diploid and tetraploid clones are 1.0 and 2.0 respectively. As a result, the indices correlated well (r=0.873). When calculating the karyotype index, the size of abnormal chromosomes were not taken into account. So taking this into consideration, the correlation factor, r, value of 0.873 indicated fairly good correlation between the two analyses, and these results, at the same

time, supported the feasibility of flow cytometric analysis.
Cases analyzed in this study were 185 adult patients with various types of leukemias. With regard to subtypes, there were 38 cases with adult T-cell leukemia(ATL), 35 cases with acute lymphocytic leukemia(ALL), 71 cases with acute non-lymphocytic leukemia(ANLL), 25 cases with chronic myelocytic leukemia in blastic crisis(CML-BC) and 16 cases with chronic lymphocytic leukemia(CLL). The cases included 92 male and 93 female patients.

RESULTS

Patterns of the DNA histograms

When samples with TRBC alone were determined, the patterns of the DNA histograms were basically divided into two groups. One group showed only one peak, while the other showed more than two peaks in addition to the small peak due to TRBC. Among the former group, three types were observed. The first type included samples with peaks at the diploid channel and the second type had a peak at a channel other than the diploid channel. The third type showed a very asymmetric peak. With the exception of the first type, the other two types showed 2 separate peaks when samples with two internal standards, namely TRBC and diploid standard, were determined; these samples were thought to have DA. Samples with more than two peaks were also considered to have DA.

Frequency of DNA aneuploidy

Out of the 185 cases examined, 50 cases showed DA, as shown in Table 1, and that made the over-all frequency 27%. This value was similar to those currently reported by other researchers. No differences were observed between the sexes. With regard to subtypes of leukemia, 21 cases out of 38 cases(55.3%) showed DA in ATL, similarly 9/35 cases(25.7%) in ALL, 12/71 cases(16.9%) in ANLL, 7/25 cases(28.0%) in CML-BC and 1/16 cases(6.3%) showed DA. Frequency in ATL was significantly higher when compared with those in other subtypes ($p<0.01$). A low frequency was recognized in CLL, however it was not statistically significant. To examine if the high frequency in ATL could be attributed to the cell surface phenotype, namely T-cell origin, phenotypes of lymphocytic leukemic cells were examined. However no relationship was found between phenotypes and frequency of DA in other subtypes of leukemia. ATL is characterized among subtypes of leukemia by being more prevalent in Southwest Japan and also by having special relevance to human T-cell leukemia virus I. Therefore, the high frequency of DA in ATL is possibly attributable to the specific entity of this disease.

TABLE 1. Frequency of DNA aneuploidy in subtypes of leukemia

Subtype	ATL	ALL	ANLL	CML-BC	CLL	Total
Cases	21/38	9/35	12/71	7/25	1/16	50/185
Percentage	55.3*	25.7	16.9	28.0	6.3	27.0

*$p<0.01$ Male:28/92(30.4%), Female:22/93(23.7%)

DNA index

DNA indices of 50 cases with DA ranged between 0.913 and 2.042, with the average being 1.144. These values corresponded to 42, 94 and 53, respectively for the value for the average size of the chromosomes. There was a tendency for high DNA indices to be observed in ATL and ALL, however no significant differences were found in the average values of DNA indices among subtypes of leukemia. Among 50 cases, only two cases showed two leukemic DNA clones, while the rest, 48 cases, showed only one leukemic DNA clone. This suggested that leukemic cells have much less heterogeneity than expected by current chromosomal analysis from the point of view of DNA content. Also, only two cases showed DNA indices lower than 1.0, which indicated hypodiploidy.

DNA aneuploidy and laboratory data

Correlations between DA and laboratory data, for example, the percentage of leukemic cells, absolute leukemic cell number, red blood cell number, LDH value and others, were analyzed, however, no significant correlations were observed. Neither symptoms or physical signs showed relationship with DA.

Monitoring the clinical course by DNA aneuploidy

In this study, follow-up of the clinical course was only possible in a few cases. Nevertheless in two cases DA was found to be useful as a tumor marker for monitoring the clinical course. One case had DA that was nearly tetraploid. After induction chemotherapy, the patient achieved complete remission and it lasted for several months. During complete remission, a bone marrow specimen showed a normal DNA histogram shown in the left of Fig. 2. At a later date, bone marrow specimen revealed a DNA histogram slightly different from the normal one, it had a small sharp peak at tetraploid position, as shown in the middle of Fig. 2, that suggested "relapse". However, morphological examination of a bone marrow smear at this point resulted in a diagnosis of remission, although a few leukemic cells were observed. A week later, morphological examination revealed a relapse and a bone marrow specimen gave the DNA histogram shown in the right of Fig. 2. Thus, DA was very useful as a tumor marker for the early detection of relapse in this case.

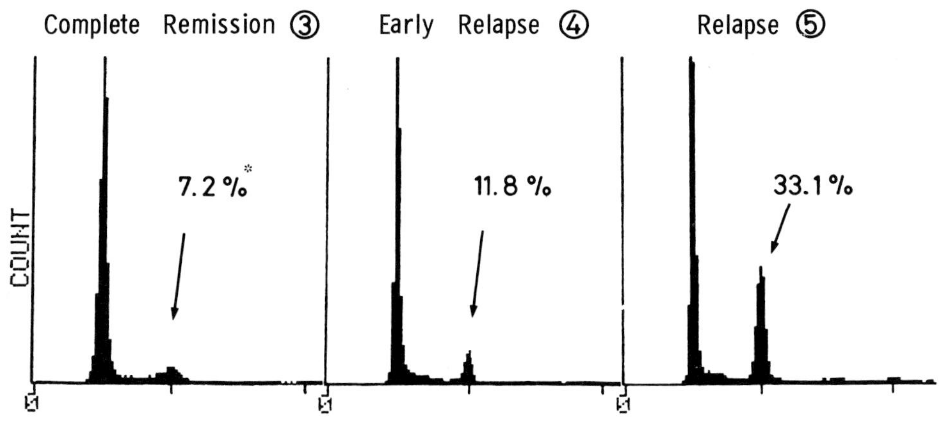

Fig. 2. Early detection of relapse by DNA aneuploidy as a tumor marker. An ALL case with DNA aneuploidy of nearly tetraploid clone. Percentages of the second peak represent G2+M fractions of normal diploid cells and G0+G1 fractions of leukemic cells.

The other case with ALL showed a single apparent DA clone at the onset. This case relapsed twice during the clinical course, through which times no changes of leukemic cells were observed by morphological examinations. However, flow cytometric analyses clearly showed changes in the leukemic DNA clone, namely from one to two leukemic clones at the first relapse and then back to the same one leukemic clone at the second relapse.
These were good examples of the usefulness of DA as a tumor marker for monitoring the clinical course of patient.

DNA aneuploidy as a prognostic factor

Finally, correlation between DA and survival time of patient was analyzed. Since the treatment of the leukemia varied depending on subtype, analysis was performed for each subtype of leukemia. As shown in Fig. 3, in ANLL, cases with DA, expressed by open squares, apparently showed shorter survival compared with cases without DA, expressed by closed squares ($p<0.01$). The same result was obtained in CML-BC ($p<0.05$). For other subtypes, no significant differences were obtained between cases with and without DA. These results indicated the usefulness of DA as a prognostic factor, its appearance suggesting a poor prognosis in cases with ANLL and CML-BC.

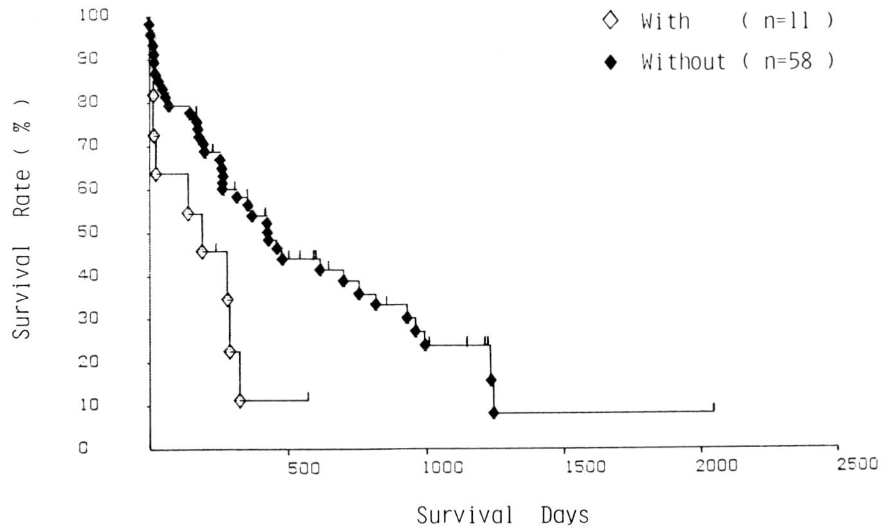

Fig. 3. Cumulative survival curve of cases with (◇) and without (◆) DNA aneuploidy. Acute non-lymphocytic leukemia. ($p<0.01$)

Recent advance on analysis of anti-platelet antibody—special reference to application of flow cytometry

Shosaku Nomura and Terutoshi Kokawa

The First Department of Internal Medicine, Kansai Medical University, Fumizono-cho, Moriguchi, Osaka 570 Japan

Abstract - Idiopathic thrombocytopenic purpura (ITP) is a syndrome caused by circulating antibodies reactive with the platelet membrane. We characterized new monoclonal antibodies that react with a determinant specific to the GPIb and GPIIb/IIIa complex, and used flow cytometry to investigate platelets from patients with ITP to elucidate the antigenic determinants to which their autoantibodies are directed. Platelets from forty cases with ITP were analyzed using the platelet suspension immunofluorescence test. The monoclonal antibodies used were: 5 against the GPIIb/IIIa complex and 2 against GPIb. The reactivity of the monoclonal antibodies was inhibited by the presence of autoantibody on the platelets of some ITP patients. Direct method (using ITP platelets) showed a decrease in the binding rate of monoclonal anti-GPIIb/IIIa complex antibodies for platelets from 11 of 40 patients, and indirect method (using ITP plasma) demonstrated monoclonal anti-GPIIb/IIIa complex antibodies in 4 of 40 patients and monoclonal anti-GPIb antibodies from 1 of 40 patients. Differences in inhibition were found not only among monoclonal antibodies but also among cases. These results suggest that some ITP patients have circulating antibodies to GPIb or GPIIb/IIIa, and that heterogeneous antibodies are present on platelets. Moreover, the presence of these autoantibodies may aggravate or initiate a bleeding diathesis.

INTRODUCTION

Flow cytometry has become available for research into cell surface antigens since Herzenberg et al. (ref. 1) introduced what is called FACS (fluorescence activated cell sorter). The distribution (histogram) of cell surface antigen can be grasped by flow cytometry, unlike previous serum assay methods (ref. 2). Therefore, the antigenic change of cell surface (antigenic modulation (ref. 3)) can be analyzed progressively and quantitatively.

On the other hand, idiopathic thrombocytopenic purpura (ITP) occurs at all ages, in acute and chronic forms, and is a syndrome caused by a circulating antibody reactive with the platelet membrane (ref. 4,5). Both forms are now thought to be due to an anti-platelet antibody, usually of platelet-associated IgG (PAIgG), which coats autologous platelets and leads to their phagocytosis and destruction by the reticuloendothelial system (ref. 5). However, at present the antigenic specificity of these antibodies is unknown. Autoantibodies against GPIb or GPIIb/IIIa were recently found in patients with chronic ITP (ref. 6,7).

In this study we characterized new monoclonal antibodies that react with a determinant specific to the GPIb or GPIIb/IIIa complex, and used flow cytometry to investigate platelets from patients with ITP to elucidate the antigenic determinants to which the autoantibodies are directed.

MATERIALS AND METHODS

1. Monoclonal antibodies

Monoclonal antibodies against human platelet membrane glycoproteins were produced by immunizing BALB/c mice with intraperitoneal injections of washed platelet suspensions, without Freund's adjuvant. BALB/c mice were injected three times with 10^9 washed platelets at 2-wk intervals. Three days after the last injection, the spleen cells were fused with a myeloma cell line (NS-1) using standard technology (ref. 8). Positive hybridomas producing anti-platelet antibodies were selected by enzyme-linked immunosorbent assay (ELISA)(ref. 9). Positive hybridomas were subcloned twice by limiting cell dilution (ref. 10). The molecular weight (MW) of the antigen corresponding to anti-GPIIb/IIIa complex antibodies was determined by immunoprecipitation using platelets surface-labeled with ^{125}I. The MW of the antigen corresponding to anti-GPIb antibodies was determined by SDS-polyacrylamide gel electrophoresis and Avidin-Biothin Peroxidase Complex (ABC) method.

2. Aggregation studies
Platelet rich plasma (PRP) or a washed platelet suspension was incubated with 10 μg/ml of monoclonal antibody for 5 min at 37°C before the addition of a platelet-aggregating agent. Final concentrations of platelet agonists were as follows: ADP was used at 8 μM, epinephrine at 2 μM, collagen at 4 μg/ml, thrombin at 0.5 U/ml, and ristocetin at 1.5 mg/ml.

3. Preparation of washed human platelets
Whole blood anticoagulated with 3.8% sodium citrate (9 vol blood to 1 vol Na citrate) was centrifuged at 200 g for 10 min at room temperature. After centrifugation, the supernatant consisting of diluted PRP was collected without disturbing the other fractions. PRP was transferred to a second plastic tube and centrifuged at 1,400 g for 10 min at room temperature. The platelet-poor supernatant was discarded and the pellet resuspended in 6.0 ml of washing buffer (9 mM Na_2EDTA, 26.4 mM Na_2HPO_4 $2H_2O$, 140 mM NaCl, pH 7.2) and centrifuged again at 1,400 g for 10 min at room temperature. The resuspension and centrifugation was repeated three more times.

4. Preparation of paraformaldehyde-treated platelets
The platelets were resuspended in 1% paraformaldehyde solution (PFA), dispersed by gentle pipetting, and incubated at room temperature for 5 min. They were then pelleted and resuspended in washing buffer two more times under the same conditions. After the final centrifugation, the platelets were resuspended in stock solution (9 mM Na_2EDTA, 26.4 mM Na_2HPO_4 $2H_2O$, 140 mM NaCl, 0.1% NaN_3, 2% Foetal Bovine Serum, pH 7.2) and stored at 4°C until analysis.

5. Fluorescence flow cytometry
PFA-treated platelets were washed 3 times in washing buffer and diluted to 2×10^6 platelets per 100 ul. They were then incubated with monoclonal antibody (suspended in the same buffer) for 30 min at room temperature, again washed 3 times by centrifugation (1,400 g for 10 min at room temperature), and resuspended in the same buffer. The treated platelets were incubated with fluorescein-labeled goat anti-mouse antibody for 30 min at room temperature, and washed 3 times by centrifugation. After the final wash, the platelets were resuspended in 500 ul of EDTA-PBS(-), transferred to a plastic tube (Falcon 2052 tube), and stored on ice until analysis, which was done within 24 hours.

6. Operating conditions for the FACS Analyzer
The labeled platelets were analyzed on a Becton Dickinson FACS Research Analyzer. The assay was performed using the 50-micron orifice. Instrument settings were as follows: volume, current 0.35 unit, log mode, threshold minimum; fluorescence, PMT 550, log mode, threshold off. The variable gain of the FL1 channel was adjusted using 2.0-micron diameter beads. Volume gates were set at channel 10 and channel 255. This excludes debris below the normal platelet size distribution. A flow rate of 500 to 800 events per second was maintained. For the one-parameter mode analysis, FL1 markers were set at channel 0 and 255. The negative control (autofluorescence) was set at 0 and 50. The rate of positive fluorescence was calculated from the total platelet counts above channel 51. To quantify fluorescence, SIGMA was defined as

$$\text{SIGMA} = [\text{ Mean channel of positive region} \times \text{total platelet counts of positive region }] / 10^3$$

10,000 events were analyzed in the one-parameter mode.
For the two-parameter mode analysis, volume was set at Gate 1 and FL1 was Gate 2. 3,000 events were analyzed in the two-parameter mode (Fig. 1).

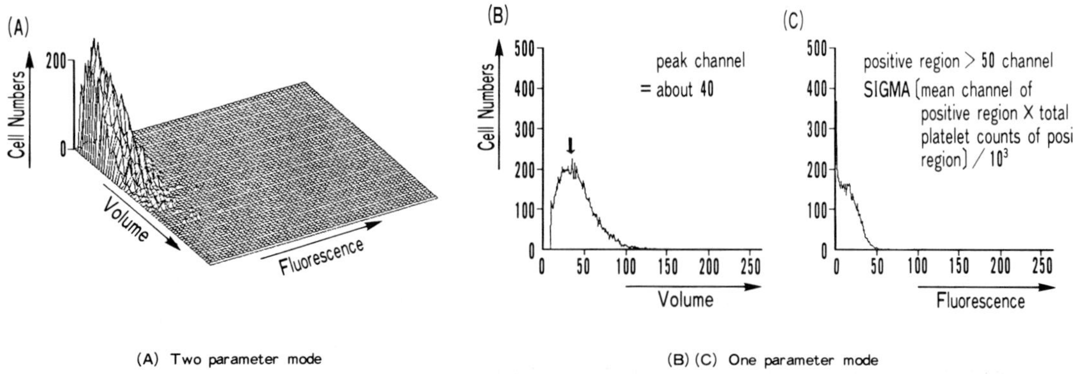

Fig. 1 Flow cytometric histogram of unstained healthy control platelets

7. Investigation of pdrtelet size
For small platelets, the volume gates were set at channel 10 and the volume peak channel (about 40); for large platelets, the volume gates were set at the volume peak channel and channel 255.

8. Assay protocol
Samples (platelet and plasma) were obtained from 40 patients with chronic ITP. All patients with chronic ITP satisfied the usual clinical criteria and had not received transfusions. Measurements were performed by the platelet suspension immunofluorescence test (PSIFT) as described by von dem Borne et al. (ref. 11). Fig. 2 outlines the assay procedure. The change in the binding percentage of monoclonal antibodies was assessed by SIGMA and peak channel. In the case which SIGMA and peak channel were less than or equal to 3SD under the mean of the normal control, which was provided as significant decline. Platelet-associated IgG (PAIgG) and platelet-binding IgG (PBIgG) were measured by PSIFT using flow cytometry. PBIgG was measured by indirect immunofluorescence applying a platelet panel from selected group O blood donors.

3.8% Sodium Citrate : Blood (from patients or healthy O type donor)
= 1 : 9
↓
Centrifugation
↓
Washed 3 times with EDTA-PBS(-)
↓
Fixation 1% paraformaldehyde (PFA)
↓
Washed twice with EDTA-PBS(-)
↓

Direct method	Indirect method
	↓ Incubation with patients plasma 100 µl
	↓ Washed 3 times with EDTA-PBS(-)

↓
Incubation with monoclonal antibody 100 µl
↓
Washed 3 times with EDTA-PBS(-)
↓
Staining with FITC conjugated anti-mouse IgG 100 µl
↓
Washed twice with EDTA-PBS 0.1% NaN_3, 2% FBS
↓
Resuspended in EDTA-PBS 0.1% NaN_3, 2% FBS
↓
Flow Cytometry

Fig. 2 Assay procedure

RESULTS

1. Characteristics of monoclonal antibodies
The monoclonal antibodies used were 5 against GPIIb/IIIa complex (NNKY1-32, NNKY2-5, NNKY2-6, NNKY2-11, NNKY2-18) and 2 against GPIb (NNKY5-4, NNKY5-5). Table 1 shows their characteristics. The MW of the platelet-membrane antigens recognized by monoclonal antibodies were determined to be respectively 130 kDa (kilo daltons) and 110 kDa under reducing conditions and 140 kDa and 95 kDa under non-reducing conditions for NNKY1-32, NNKY2-5, NNKY2-6, NNKY2-11 and NNKY2-18, and 150 kDa under reducing conditions for NNKY5-4 and NNKY5-5. The binding of NNKY1-32, NNKY2-5, NNKY2-6, NNKY2-11 and NNKY2-18 to platelets reduced remarkably by incubation with EDTA at 37°C, and these monoclonal antibodies hardly bound to platelets of Glanzmann's thrombasthenia (Type I)(ref. 12). On the other hand, NNKY5-4 and NNKY5-5 hardly to platelets of Bernard Soulier syndrome. NNKY1-32, NNKY2-5 and NNKY2-6 completely inhibited aggregation induced by ADP, epinephrine, collagen and thrombin, but NNKY2-11 and NNKY2-18 showed partial inhibition. It is speculated that the epitopes recognized by NNKY1-32, NNKY 2-5 or NNKY2-6 are located near the fibrinogen receptor on the GPIIb/IIIa complex. Neither NNKY5-4 and NNKY5-5 significantly influenced the aggregation induced by ADP, epinephrine, collagen, or thrombin, nor did NNKY5-4 affect ristocetin-induced agglutination. NNKY5-5 however, inhibited ristocetin-induced agglutination almost completely. It is speculated

that epitope recognized by NNKY5-5 is located near the von Willebrand factor receptor but far from the thrombin receptor on GPIb, while the epitope recognized by NNKY5-4 is far from both receptors.

TABLE 1. Characteristics of monoclonal antibodies

Antibody Designation	Subclass	Epitope	Inhibition of platelet aggregation				
			ADP	Epinephrine	Collagen	Thrombin	Ristocetin
NNKY1-32	IgG2b	GPIIb/IIIa	++	++	++	++	+
NNKY2-5	IgG3	GPIIb/IIIa	++	++	++	++	+
NNKY2-6	IgG1	GPIIb/IIIa	++	++	++	++	+
NNKY2-11	IgG2a	GPIIb/IIIa	+	+	+	+	-
NNKY2-18	IgG1	GPIIb/IIIa	+	+	+	+	-
NNKY5-4	IgG1	GPIb	-	-	-	-	-
NNKY5-5	IgG2b	GPIb	-	-	-	-	++

++: complete inhibition, +: partial inhibition, -: no inhibition

2. Analysis of platelet surface antigens using FACS

Fig. 3 shows the fluorescence histogram patterns, percent positivity, peak channel and SIGMA of the monoclonal antibodies for healthy O-type platelets. The percent positivity, peak channel and SIGMA are shown as the mean+SD of 30 normal subjects. The correlation between peak channel and SIGMA was analyzed (Fig. 4). A statistically significant correlation was found for both NNKY1-32 and NNKY5-5. However, no correlation was found percent positivity and peak channel (data not shown). The SIGMA of large platelets was higher than that of small platelets (Fig. 5). The incubation of intact platelets with EDTA at 37°C is said to cause progressive dissociation of the GPIIb/IIIa complex (ref. 12,13). As Fig. 6 shows, the binding of monoclonal antibodies decreased with the dissociation of GPIIb/IIIa complex on the platelet surface. In this case, both SIGMA and peak channel dicreased similarly. On the other hand, in mixing experiment with GPIIb/IIIa complex deficient and normal platelets, SIGMA showed a decrease with the increase in the proportion of Glanzmann's thrombasthenia platelets (Fig. 7). In this case, however, the peak channel shows little change.

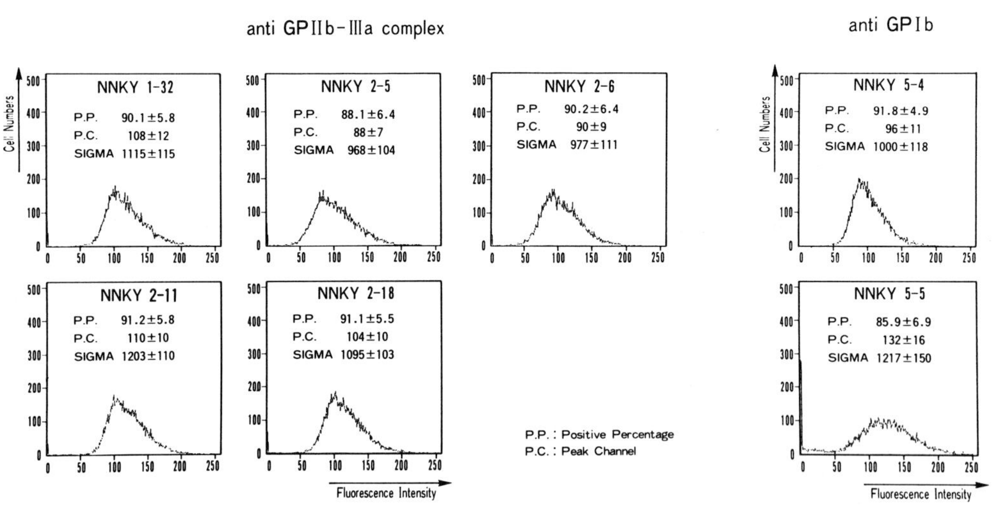

Fig. 3 Fluorescence histogram of monoclonal antibodies for healthy O-type platelets

3. ITP patient characteristics

Forty cases of ITP (11 men, 29 women) were studied. The age range of the patients was 19 to 85 years. Sixteen patients had been treated, and 24 were untreated. In 20 patients, platelet counts were less than or equal to 50,000 /mm^3. The mean±SD of the platelet counts (/mm^3), PAIgG (%) and PBIgG (%) was 68,600±55,900, 20.0±10.5 and 43.5±12.3, respectively. There was a definite negative correlation between the platelet counts and PAIgG (r=-0.59, P=0.0002).

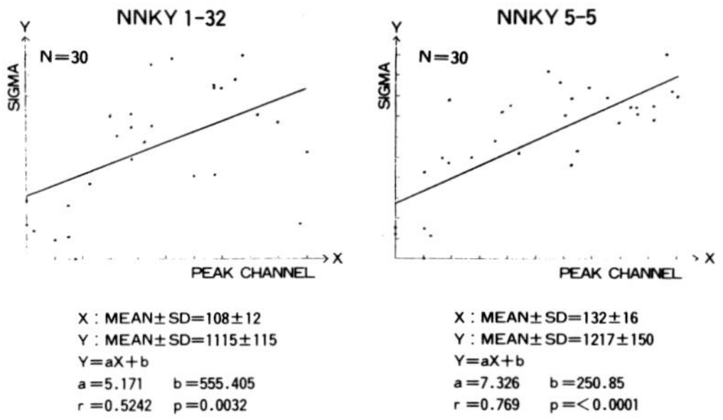

Fig. 4 Correlation between peak channel and SIGMA

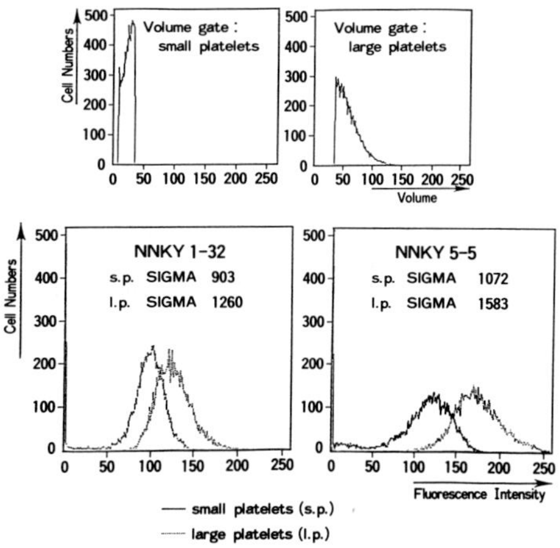

Fig. 5 Investigation of platelet size

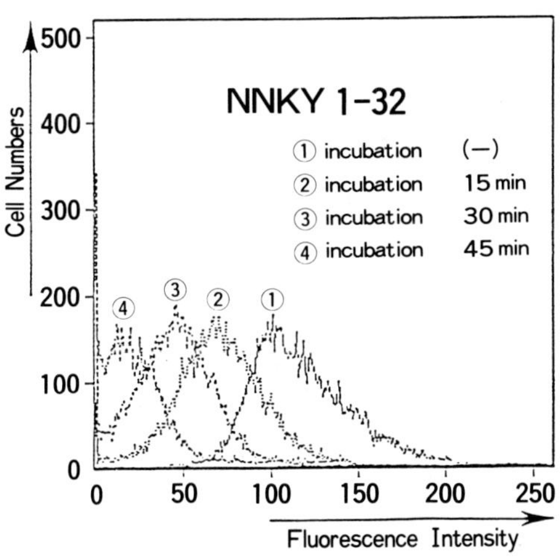

Fig. 6 Effect of EDTA on fluorescence histogram

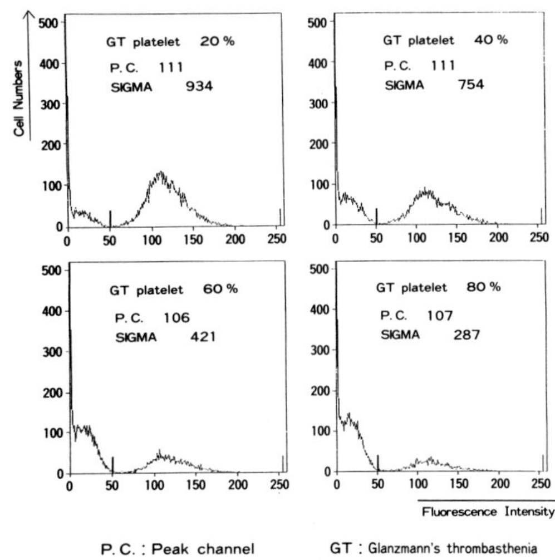

Fig. 7 Change of monoclonal anti-GPIIb/IIIa complex antibody binding to mixtures of PFA-treated platelets of Glanzmann's thrombasthenia and normal subjects

4. Analysis of platelet antigen for anti-platelet antibodies in ITP

Fig. 8 shows the principle of measurement. Monoclonal antibodies bind closely to the specific antigens on the surface of normal platelets, but in ITP the presence of autoantibodies inhibits this binding. The homologous antigen for the anti-platelet antibody was analyzed from the inhibition rate of this monoclonal antibody binding.

[Direct method]

The monoclonal anti-GPIIb/IIIa complex antibodies showed decreased reactivity for platelets from 11 of 40 patients with ITP. Differences in inhibition were found not only among monoclonal antibodies but also among cases (Table 2). The number of cases showing dominant inhibition by each type of antibody were as follows: NNKY1-32, 4 cases; NNKY2-5, 9 cases; NNKY2-6, 9 cases; NNKY2-11, none; NNKY2-18, 2 cases. Fig. 9 shows the two-parameter mode analysis of monoclonal anti-GPIIb/IIIa complex antibodies for platelets from Case 9. The reactivity of NNKY1-32 and NNKY2-6 for the patient's platelets was significantly decreased.

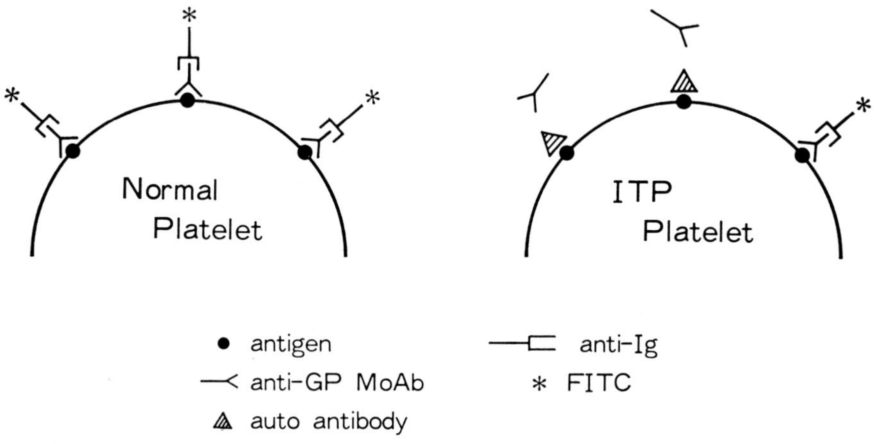

Fig. 8 Principle of measurement

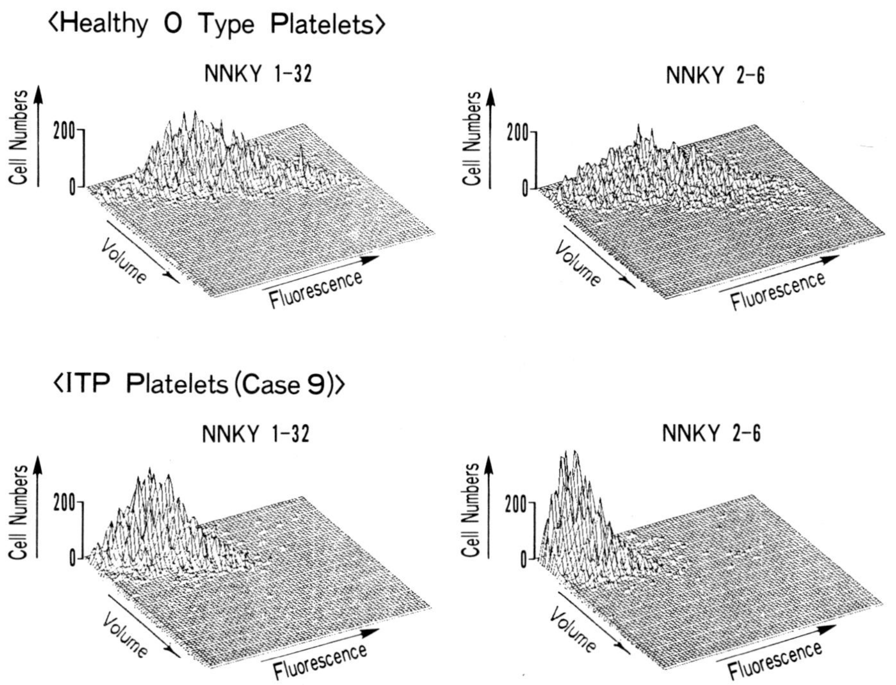

Fig. 9 The two-parameter mode histogram of ITP platelets using monoclonal anti-GPIIb/IIIa complex antibodies

[Indirect method]
Plasma from 4 of the 40 patients with ITP inhibited the reactivity for healthy type O platelet of monoclonal anti-GPIIb/IIIa complex antibodies, and the plasma from 1 of the 40 patients inhibited the reactivity of monoclonal anti-GPIb antibodies. Differences in inhibition as well as direct method were found not only among monoclonal antibodies but also among

cases (Table 2). The number of cases showing dominant inhibition by each type of antibody were as follows: NNKY1-32, none; NNKY2-5, 4 cases; NNKY2-6, 1 case; NNKY2-11, none; NNKY2-18, none; NNKY5-4, none; NNKY5-5, 1 case.

The reactivity of monoclonal antibodies was much lower when measured by the direct method than by the indirect method. On the other hand, there was no definite correlation between the monoclonal antibodies and PAIgG or PBIgG which used a platelet panel from selected group O blood donors.

TABLE 2. The reactivity of monoclonal antibody and ITP platelet or serum using flow cytometry

Patients	Sex	Age	% S.R. of monoclonal antibody (NNKY)					platelet count (/mm^3)	Therapy	PAIgG (%)	PBIgG (%)
			1-32	2-5	2-6	2-18	5-5				
Case 2	F	23	32/87	14/105	16/116	106/112	105/67	191000	S.N.	14.0	45.2
Case 6	F	33	63/100	46/104	40/109	78/111	100/76	244000	AP	8.6	58.4
Case 9	M	57	63/83	62/49	30/111	69/69	94/121	40000	(-)	16.2	35.2
Case 10	F	60	62/83	52/57	50/67	67/83	98/78	32000	PSL	29.8	37.4
Case 11	M	68	84/65	83/57	88/73	92/70	111/66	53000	PSL	40.7	42.6
Case 14	F	37	26/91	22/104	41/111	127/99	111/73	39000	(-)	22.0	48.8
Case 15	F	29	31/97	29/84	24/86	49/91	97/96	64000	(-)	14.7	20.2
Case 20	F	19	75/54	66/42	78/44	87/60	70/45	63000	(-)	12.0	62.4
Case 23	F	20	64/83	50/67	48/61	75/81	84/67	15000	(-)	37.1	37.8
Case 24	F	30	85/72	55/52	83/61	85/84	66/72	47000	(-)	16.2	44.3
Case 25	F	61	54/101	39/67	47/93	60/88	100/45	65000	PZ	25.7	45.3
Case 32	F	70	110/95	107/98	62/55	109/96	92/107	40000	PSL	26.8	37.8
Case 39	F	85	74/104	61/91	59/100	74/89	43/91	20000	(-)	20.3	25.4

S.N.: splenectomy, AP: azathioprine, PSL: prednisolone, PZ: parameson
% S.R. = SIGMA of Patients / SIGMA of Control x 100
D/I D: direct method, I: indirect method
— : significant decline
Each box contains the D/I results of each patient.

DISCUSSION

Flow cytometry allows measurement of low fluorescence levels with the improvement of apparatus. Using flow cytometry and monoclonal antibodies, we investigated platelets from patients with ITP to elucidate the antigenic determinants to which their autoantibodies are directed. The results obtained from this fundamental study using flow cytometry indicated the followings.

(1) In fluorescence histogram of monoclonal antibodies for healthy platelet, there existed a definite correlation between peak channel and SIGMA.
(2) SIGMA of large platelets was higher than that of small platelets.
(3) The incubation of intact platelets with EDTA at 37°C caused the progressive dissociation of GPIIb-IIIa complexes, and this effect was observed as the decrease of both SIGMA and peak channel.
(4) In mixing experiment with GPIIb-IIIa complex deficient and normal platelets, SIGMA only showed a decrease with the increase in the proportion of Glanzmann's thrombasthenia platelets.

From these results, it appears to be best to observe both peak channel and SIGMA in order to investigate the antigen on the platelet surface using flow cytometry.

It is clear from works already reported that ITP is a clinical syndrome characterized by the destruction of platelets due to an anti-platelet antibody (ref. 4). Considerable information has been accumlated with respect to the nature of the antibody and its presence on platelets (ref. 14). However, little is known regarding the platelet antigen to which the autoantibodies are directed. Recently, Woods and co-workers (ref. 6,7) have demonstrated directly the presence of anti-GPIb and anti-GPIIb/IIIa autoantibodies in the serum of patients with chronic ITP. These results suggest that some ITP patients have circulating antibodies to GPIb or GPIIb/IIIa. However, there are still many points to be clarified as to the nature and extent of the influence of anti-platelet antibodies upon the mechanisms of ITP.

In the present investigation, direct method(using ITP platelets) showed a decrease in the binding rate of monoclonal anti-GPIIb/IIIa complex antibodies for platelets from 11 of 40 patients, and indirect method (using ITP plasma) demonstrated monoclonal anti-GPIIb/IIIa complex antibodies in 4 of 40 patients and monoclonal anti-GPIb antibodies from 1 of 40 patients. When comparing the direct and indirect method with regard to the degree of inhibition seen in the binding of monoclonal antibodies to the patients' platelets, the indirect method showed less inhibition of binding (Table 2). That is to say, the direct method may be more specific than the indirect method. However, in case 20, the indirect method showed strong inhibition, so the best technique is to use both methods (Table 2).

Generally, it is said that the epitope which monoclonal antibody recognizes is composed of a few amino acids (under 10-15). Therefore, even if a monoclonal antibody recognizes both GPIb and GPIIb/IIIa, the binding site differs a little. In this study, differences in inhibition were found not only among monoclonal antibodies but also among cases. These findings provide support for the concept that heterogeneous antigens are present on platelets.

In a previous communication, a significant inverse correlation between platelet counts and PAIgG was observed (ref. 15). Our present study using flow cytometry confirms this inverse correlation between platelet counts and PAIgG.

It is said that platelet GPIIb and GPIIIa are major constituents of platelet membrane and are critically involved in the formation of the cell surface fibrinogen receptor on activated platelets (ref. 16). And recently, a case was reported which was interpreted as an example of acquired thrombasthenia due to an anti-GPIIb/IIIa autoantibody (ref. 17). As all 5 monoclonal antibodies against GPIIb/IIIa complex which were used in the present study influenced platelet function, it was supposed that the cited case may represent a platelet function disorder in which the binding of monoclonal antibody inhibited normal platelet function. It was suggested that the closer the autoantibodies are to fibrinogen binding sites, the more likely it is for a bleeding problem to develop and the presence of anti-GPIIb/IIIa autoantibodies may aggravate or initiate a bleeding diathesis.

REFERENCES

1. L.A. Herzenberg and R.G. Sweet, Sci. Am., 234, 108-117 (1976).
2. B. Adelman, A.D. Michelson, R.I. Handin and K.A. Ault, Blood, 66, 423-427 (1985).
3. J. Ritz and S.F. Schlossman, Blood, 59, 1-11 (1982).
4. R. McMillan, N. Engl. J. Med., 304, 1135-1147 (1981).
5. T.R. Burns and A. Saleen, Am. J. Med., 75, 1001-1007 (1983).
6. V.L. Woods, E.H. Oh, D. Mason and R. McMillan, Blood, 63, 368-375 (1984).
7. V.L. Woods, Y. Kurata, R.P. Montgomery, P. Tani, D. Mason, E.H. Oh and R. McMillan, Blood, 64, 156-160 (1984).
8. B.S. Coller, E.I. Peerschke, L.E. Scudder and C.A. Sulliran, J. Clin. Invest., 72, 325-338 (1983).
9. J.R. Clamp, K.W. Hughes and J.C. McPherson, Immunochemistry, 8, 871-879 (1971).
10. H.A. Coller and B.S. Coller, Hybridoma, 2, 91-96 (1983).
11. A.E.G.Kr. von dem Borne, F.W.A. Verheugt, F. Oosterhof, E. von Riese, A. Brutel de la Riviere and C.P. Englefriet, Br. J. Haematol., 39, 195-207 (1978).
12. S. Nomura, H. Nagata, K. Oda, T. Kokawa and K. Yasunaga, Thromb. Res., 47, 47-58 (1987).
13. L.A. Fitzgerald and D.R. Phillips, J. Biol. Chem., 260, 11366-11374 (1985).
14. S. Karpatkin, Blood, 56, 329-343 (1980).
15. S. Panzer, S. Szamait, R-H. Bodeker, O.A. Hoas, A. Haubenstock and C. Mueller-Eckhardt, Am. J. Haematol., 23, 89-99 (1986).
16. J.S. Bennett, J.A. Hoxie, S.F. Leitman, G. Vilaire and D.B. Cines, Proc. Natl. Acad. Sci., USA 80, 2417-2421 (1983).
17. H. Niessner, K.J. Clemetson, S. Panzer, C. Mueller-Eckhardt, S. Santoso and P. Bettelheim, Blood, 68, 571-576 (1986).

Introduction to new techniques in hematology

Kazuo Niitani[1] and Noriyuki Tatsumi[2]

1: Kanto Teishin Hospital, Shinagawa-Ku, Tokyo, 141, Japan
2: Osaka City University Medical School, Abeno-Ku, Osaka, 545, Japan

Abstract - Recent advances in medical engineering are prominent and the results have been rapidly introduced into the hematology laboratory. The main effect has been in reducing manpower, but it is obvious that new technology provides information never obtained by traditional methodologies. Volumetric analysis and pattern recognition of blood cells show remarkable development and give fresh impact to laboratory medicine.

VOLUMETRIC ANALYSIS

Volumetric analysis has been used in mean corpuscular volume (MCV) or hematocrit determination in blood cell counters. But in the early stages, it was not practical and only theoretical. So the cause of discrepancies between Price-Jones curves and particle size distribution curves (PSDC) had to be resolved before using PSDC in medical practice (ref. 1). Sheath flow (ref. 2) or back sweep mechanisms have been introduced. So it is not now a problem in practice, and volumetric analyses are used in red blood cell (RBC), white blood cell (WBC), and platelet (PLT) determinations, providing new information about these cells.

The differential (hemogram) is a time-consuming and labor-intensive task in the hematology laboratory. Using volumetric techniques in the WBC channel of the blood cell counter, distribution curves of WBC shows three peaks. From small to large volume, it shows lymphocyte-, mixed cell-, and granulocyte-peaks respectively. This is the 3 part differential and shows an advantage in reproducibility but also a disadvantage in the uncertainty of the constituents of the mixed cell peak, compared with the ordinary differential. Cytochemical flow systems have provided 5 part differentials (ref. 3). Recently in electric detection systems, the 5 part differential is also available in Coulter's VCS or Sysmex's NE-series. In 3 part differentials, it was difficult to get a consensus of clinicians but it has a great future as an effective screening test.

Volumetric analysis is also effective in reticulocyte counting combined with fluorometry using auramine O stain. Fluorocytes are separated by automatic gating from mature RBC and throughput reaches sixty samples per hour. The relationship between reticulocytes and fluorocytes is an interesting subject in clinical hematology.

PATTERN RECOGNITION

Pattern recognition is one of main fields of computer technology. But its application had been restricted within use for research works. Now according to the development of technology many pattern recognition machines have been installed into routine laboratories and perform many differentials and reticulocyte counts. Set ordinary stained blood smears under an automatic focusing microscope, then information about blood cells coming through a television camera or flying spot scanner are processed and compared with stored differential criteria. This method is easily accepted by clinical doctors.

This is in typical use in clinical laboratories, but the main contribution of pattern recognition is the fact that it provides quantitative morphology against ordinary quantitative ones. There are many applications in hematology, for example a study of fine nuclear changes of blast in leukemia therapy, karyotyping, and other quantitative changes of blood cells.

REFERENCES

1. C.F.T. Mattern, F.S. Brackett and B.j. Olson, J. Appl. Physiol., 10, 56-70 (1957)
2. R. Thom, A. Hampe and G. Sauerbrey, Z.ges.exp.Med., 151, 331-349 (1969)
3. A. Simons, P. Leaverlon and G. Elbert, J. Clin. Pathol., 27, 55-58 (1974)

Fully automated blood cell differential system and its application

Akihide Hashizume Jun Motoike Ryouhei Yabe[1]

Central Research Lab., Hitachi, Ltd.
Kokubunji, Tokyo 185, Japan

[1]Naka Works, Hitachi, Ltd.
Katsuta, Ibaraki 312, Japan

Abstract - There are two kinds of blood cell differential counters. One is a system using the pattern recognition technique, and the other is a flow system using cytochemical reaction. This paper describes a fully automated blood cell differential, called the Hitachi 8200 system. It classifies blood cells using the pattern recognition technique. What is important for any kind of blood cell differential counter is high classification accuracy as well as a reduction in the time and labor required for examination, including a review of the samples. The new system achieves high classification accuracy through improvement of the pattern recognition technique and through automatic slide preparation to make the processing conditions constant. Moreover, the system enables an effective review of samples by technologists in comparison with the flow system.

INTRODUCTION

More than ten years have passed since automated blood cell differential counters (ref. 1 and 2) were put on the market. At present, there are two kinds of blood cell differential counters. One is a system that classifies blood cells according to the criterion for conventional morphological classification using the pattern recognition technique. The other is a flow system that utilizes the cytochemical reactions of blood cells.

There are many problems with automated blood cell differential counters, such as classification accuracy, processing capacity, cost and the ability to reduce examination time and labor. What are most important from the viewpoint of screening are high classification accuracy and a reduction in examination time and labor. In this paper, a system is described that can handle samples completely automatically from slide preparation to classification and thereby resolve these two problems.

This system, the Hitachi 8200, has four classification functions : white blood cell (WBC) differential counting, the detection of morphological and chromatic abnormalities of red blood cells (RBC), indirect platelet counting and reticulocyte counting. Slides that have received May-Giemsa staining are used for the former three functions, while those stained by new methyleneblue are used for the last one. This paper focuses on the WBC differential counting.

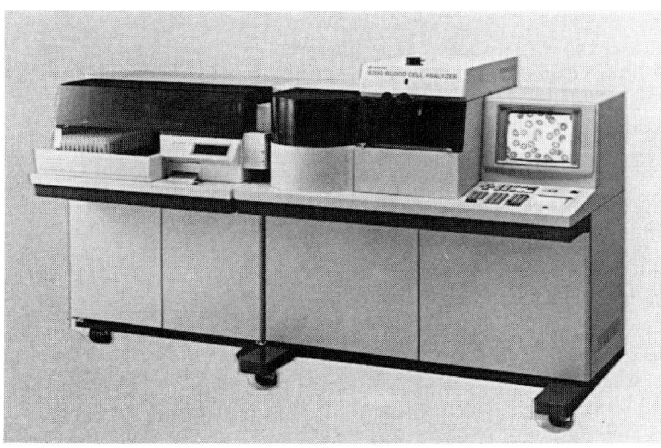

Fig. 1. Entire system

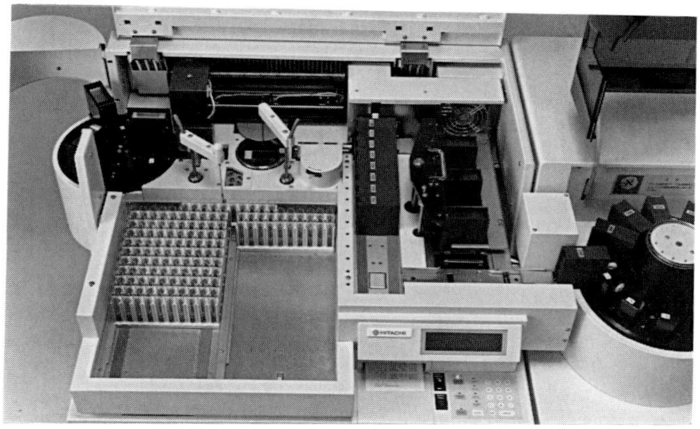

Fig. 2. Automatic slide preparation unit of system

WHOLE SETUP

The whole system is shown in Fig. 1. On the left is the automatic slide preparation unit. It contains the sampler, spinner, dryer and stainer shown in Fig. 2. On the right in Fig. 1 is the automatic classification unit.

The maximum capacity of the test tube rack area in the automatic slide preparation unit shown on the left in Fig. 2 is 150 samples (10 samples x 15 racks). That of both the automatic slide preparation area and automatic classification area is 300 samples (25 samples x 12 cassettes). All together, 300 samples can be reviewed. The processing capacity for the automatic slide preparation is 150 samples/hour and that for the automatic classification is 120 samples/hour.

The only thing technologists have to do is put a rack with the samples in the automatic slide preparation area and review the cells classified as "other" after automatic classification. Up to 300 samples can be reviewed together using the system's optical unit, which can magnify an object to 1,000 times its original size.

CLASSIFICATION ACCURACY

To achieve high classification accuracy, it is important to make data deviation as small as possible. It is also important to develop an adaptive pattern recognition system based on blood cell properties.

Fully automatic slide preparation

Fully automatic slide preparation, which is the complete integration of functions such as sampling blood from a test tube, spinning, drying and staining, results in small data deviation, especially regarding cell size, in comparison with discrete automatic slide preparation and manual slide preparation.

Pattern recognition improvement

Pattern recognition improvement is the main factor in obtaining high classification accuracy. For this improvement, it is first necessary to choose an optical system that makes it possible to obtain an image with high resolution and good color information on the blood cells. Next, .it is necessary to develop reliable feature extraction techniques (ref. 3). Finally, classification logic matching the properties of blood cells is required.

Image input. This system has an oil emersion objective lens with magnification of 100. The sampling pitch of an image is 0.23 μm, which makes it possible to capture the image with high resolution.

The spectrum characteristics of blood cells that received May-Giemsa staining are shown in Fig. 3. The x axis is for the wavelength and the y axis is for the absorbance. Based on these characteristics, three optical filters were chosen for attachment to a color TV camera. One is blue and has a principle wavelength of 415nm. This means it can separate RBC from WBC. The other two are green and red, with principle wavelengths of 525nm and 590nm, respectively. These two are suitable for emphasizing the color difference between redish and bluish cytoplasm.

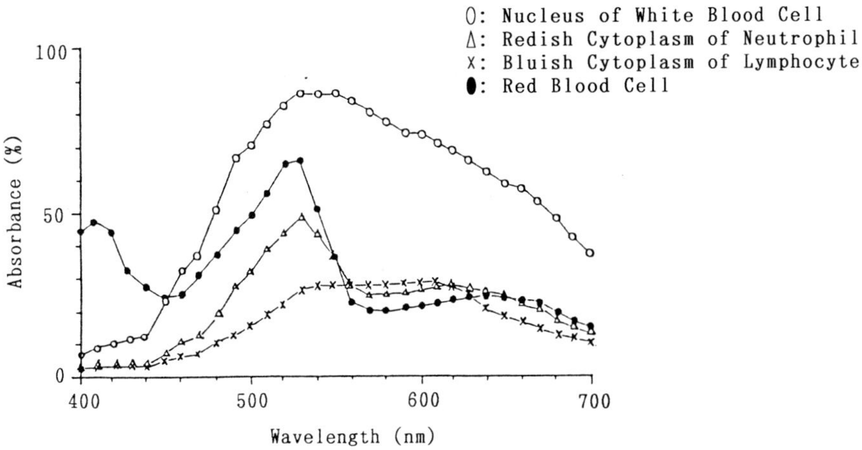

Fig. 3. Spectrum characteristics of blood cells that received May-Giemsa staining

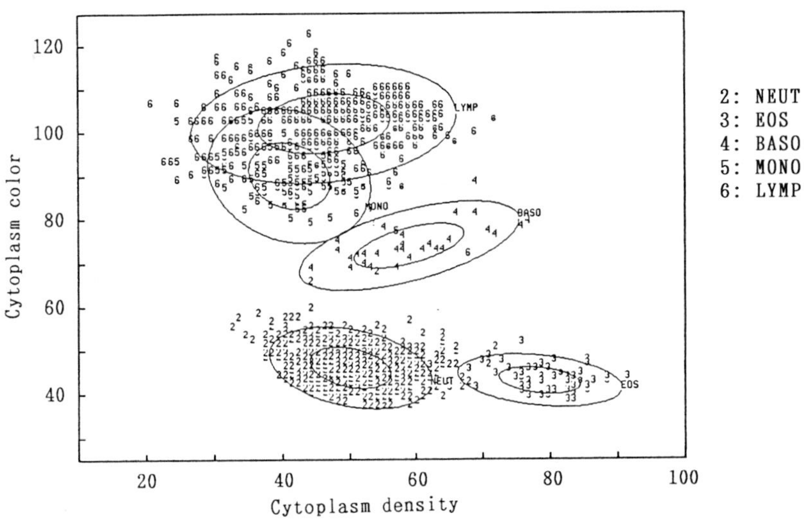

Fig. 4. Distribution of feature parameters

Feature parameters. An example of the feature parameter distribution is presented in Fig. 4. The x axis is for cytoplasm density, which is the ratio of the average cytoplasm density to the average nucleus density in a green image. The y axis is for cytoplasm color, which is the ratio of the average cytoplasm density in a red image to that in a green one. The ellipses in Fig. 4 show one and two times the standard deviation of each distribution.

Neutrophil and eosinophil, both having redish cytoplasm and the latter having redish granules in the cytoplasm, are the two distributions at the bottom of this figure. Monocyte and lymphocyte, which have bluish cytoplasm, are at the top, while basophil is in the middle. The monocyte and lymphocyte distributions overlap and thus need to be viewed as one grouping in this plane. About ninety feature parameters are utilized in classification logic. Nevertheless, normal WBCs can be roughly classified into four categories using only the two feature parameters of cytoplasm density and color.

Multistage classifier. A conceptual flow of the system's multistage classifier and conceptual charts of the classified results are shown in Fig. 5 and Fig. 6, respectively. At the first stage, a WBC is classified into one of five normal categories or as an abnormal. It should be noted that a nontypical immature cell is put in one of the normal categories at this stage. At the second stage, WBCs classified as normal at the first stage are checked again (in each category) using feature parameters different from those used in the first stage. Finally, at the third stage, WBCs classified as abnormal at the first or second stage are put into one of the four abnormal categories (ref. 3).

The reasons this multistage classifier was developed are as follows. First, the differential distribution of immature cells in peripheral blood is much smaller than that of mature ones. Second, the deviation of the feature parameters of immature cells is much larger than that of mature ones. Therefore, it is difficult to generate discriminant functions if abnormal categories are treated the same as normal ones.

Classification results

Classification accuracy (cell-by-cell comparison). Classification accuracy in the case of cell-by-cell comparison is shown in Table 1. This shows the results after a technologist input the IDs of cells, which are automatically put in the visual field of the photomicroscope, one by one after the system analyzed 87 samples, including abnormal ones. The horizontal column at the top shows the IDs given by the system, while the vertical one at the left has the IDs from the technologist. The rate for classifying as the five categories in true negative is 98.8% and is based on the figures in the central part of Table 1 surrounded by the dark line. False positive is 3.2%, and true positive (the detection rate of immature cells) is 95.0%.

Classification accuracy (sample-by-sample comparison). Classification accuracy in the case of sample-by-sample comparison is shown in Fig. 7. It shows correlations on differential counting of neutrophil and lymphocyte by the technologist and the system. Using the same slides, the system and the technologist analyzed 100 WBCs per sample independently. This shows good correlation, the correlation coefficient being 0.882 and 0.841 for neutrophil and lymphocyte, respectively.

Abnormal sample detection capability. The capability of the system to detect abnormal samples is shown in Fig. 8. Using 254 samples, the technologist analyzed 100 WBCs per sample while the system analyzed 100 WBCs plus "other" cells per sample. The technologist only reviewed the "other" cells. With this method, the technologist was able to detect 105 abnormal samples out of the 254 samples, while the system found 110 abnormal ones. The number of abnormal samples detected by both the technologist and system was 80, which includes all of the blast dominant samples. The system's true positive for detecting the abnormal samples was 81.4%, which is comparable to the ability of technologists.

EFFECTIVE SAMPLE REVIEW

What is necessary to achieve effective sample review are a reduction in the number of cells or samples to be reviewed by high classification accuracy and a decrease in the work related to reviewing.

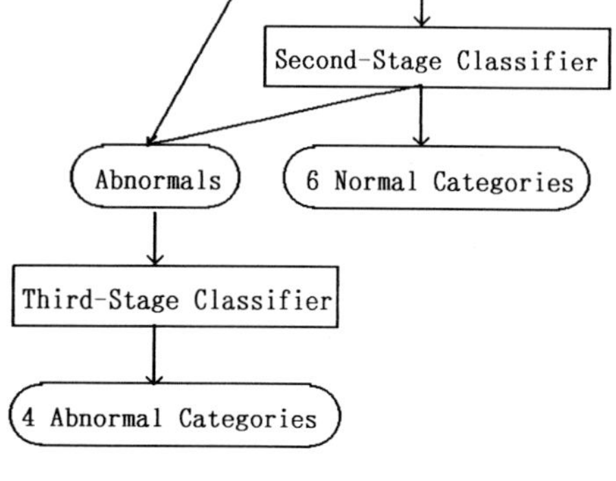

Fig. 5. Multistage classifier

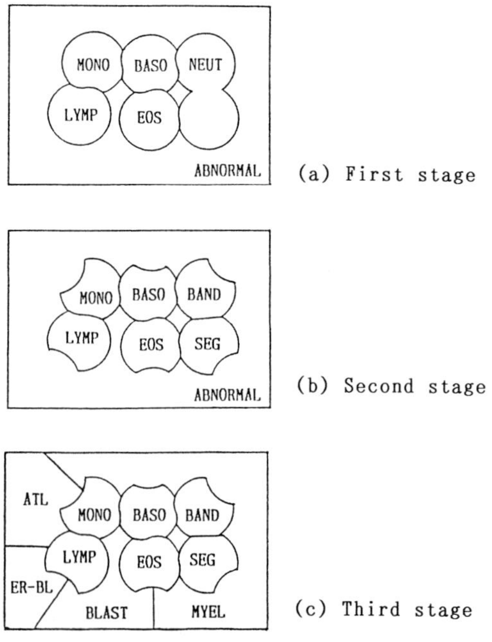

Fig. 6. Conceptual charts of classified results

TABLE 1. Classification accuracy (cell-by-cell comparison)

		SYSTEM									
		BAND	SEG	EOS	BASO	MONO	LYMP	OTH	Σ	Coincidence Rate (%)	Detection Rate (%)
	BLAST							14	14		100.0
T	PROMYELO.				2			5	7		71.4
E	MYELOCYTE		1		1			16	18		88.9
C	METAMYELO.		1		1			21	23		91.3
H	BAND NEUT.	116	170		1		2	28	317	99.7	
N	SEG. NEUT.	128	3656	3	3		2	75	3867		
O	EOSINOPHIL		24	157	1			7	189	86.8	
L	BASOPHIL				39	4	1	13	57	91.2	
O	MONOCYTE					649	17	38	704	97.6	
G	LYMPHOCYTE					38	3203	83	3324	98.9	
I	ATYP. LYMP.					3		95	98		96.9
S	PLASMA CELL								0		
T	OTHER		1		3	3	3	37	47		
	ERY. BLAST							19	19		100.0
	Σ	244	3853	160	50	698	3228	451	8684		
	Coincidence Rate (%)	99.3		98.1	78.0	93.0	99.2				

n = 87

Classification (Five Categories) in True Negative: 98.8 %
False Positive: 3.2 %
True Positive: 95.0 %

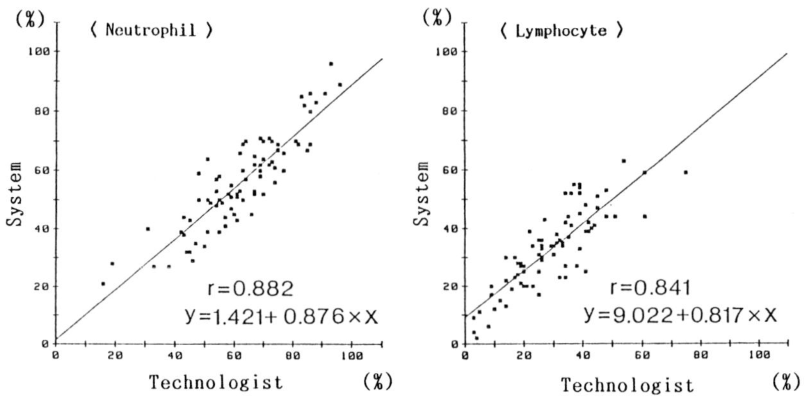

Fig. 7. Classification accuracy (sample-by-sample comparison)
100-cell counting

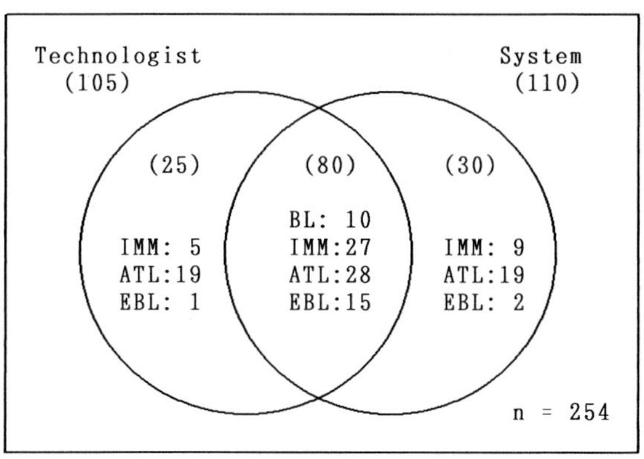

Method:
Technologist: 100-cell counting
System: 100-cell counting & "others"
Only reviewed cells classified as "other"

BL: Blast dominant sample
IMM: Juvenile dominant sample
ATL: Atypical lymphocyte dominant sample
EBL: Erythroblast dominant sample

(i): Number of detected samples

Fig. 8. Abnormal sample detection capability

As mentioned in the previous section, the system can detect cells with high accuracy for review by a technologist, that is, the false positive is 3.2% and the true positive is 95.0%.

To decrease the work related to reviewing, the environment needs to be the same as that which technologists normally use. The new system can locate the "other" cells in the visual field of the photomicroscope with an accuracy of ±5 μm. Therefore, the technologist only has to observe the WBCs in the center of the visual field, even when there are more than two WBCs in the field. As the slide is dryed by a gentle cool breeze and undergoes May-Giemsa double staining in the system, the technologist can review the cells precisely without any preparation. In addition, the optical system has a total magnification power of 1,000 with an oil emersion objective lens that magnifies 100 times. These are the same environment as that technologists presently utilize to precisely observe samples. Moreover, the technologist can review up to 300 samples all together. These are advantages of the system that enable effective sample review.

TABLE 2. Pattern recognition system versus flow system (WBC differential)

		Pattern	Flow
Classification accuracy	Statistically	△	○
	Screening	○	△[1]
Time & labor for review		○	×
Processing capacity		○	△~○
Speed of processing a sample		△	○
Ease of use		○	○

○: good, △: fair, ×: bad 1: (ref. 4)

CONCLUSION (PATTERN versus FLOW)

A comparison between the pattern recognition system and the flow system in terms of WBC differential counting is shown in Table 2. The flow system has a statistical classification accuracy advantage because the pattern recognition system can only analyze 200 WBCs per sample at most in a reasonable amount of time, while the flow system can do from 5,000 to 10,000 WBCs per sample. As for the screening rate, however, the pattern recognition system is better than the flow system at least at present.

Another advantage of the pattern recognition system is that it is much more effective for reviewing than the flow system. However, the flow system can analyze a sample within two minutes, including the sample preparation, versus the pattern recognition system's twenty minutes.

Each system has advantages as well as disadvantages. However, if the purpose of automation is to reduce the time and labor required for total examination, the pattern recognition system is better than the flow system at present.

FUTURE APPLICATION

A new application under research is automatic classification of bone marrow samples. To achieve this, the classification logic must be improved and the method to separate cells from each other by slide preparation or image processing (segmentation) must be developed.

At this time, research is being conducted on the automatic classification of the bone marrow specimens of experimental animals. This is because the number of samples examined by the phamaceutical industry is large and human bone marrow specimens are difficult to obtain in large quantities.

ACKNOWLEDGEMENT

The authors greatly appreciate the advice and comments of Mr. Shigeaki Naito of the Instrument Division, Hitachi, Ltd., during the cource of this work.

REFERENCES

1. G.K. Megla, Acta Cytologica, 17, 3 - 14 (1973)
2. M.N. Miller, 2nd International Conference on Pattern Recognition, 517 (1974)
3. R. Suzuki, A. Hashizume, H. Matsushita and R. Yabe, IECON '84 (International Conference on Industrial Electronics, Control and Instrument), 1152 - 1157 (1984)
4. T. Morii, Y. Ashida, H. Shibata and T. Chishio, JSCLA '86 (Japan Society of Clinical Laboratory Automation), 31 (1986) (in Japanese)

The usefulness of cytochemical leukocyte differentials using the technicon H6000 system

Takayuki Takubo

Department of Clinical Pathology, Osaka Medical College, 2-7 Daigaku-machi, Takatsuki, Osaka, Japan

Abstract - The Technicon H6000 System automatically differentiates leukocytes on the basis of their cytochemical and optical properties. Leukocyte differentials are obtained by processing leukocyte cytograms using the H6000. The clinical utility of thus derived differentials in acute leukemia cases - M1, M2, M3, L1, and L2 according to FAB classification - were studied and the results were as follows. In M1 and M2 acute myeloblastic leukemias, the cell population distributed in four main regions, that is, in the monocyte, neutrophil, eosinophil, and High Peroxidase Activity Cells (HPX) regions of the cytograms. In acute promyelocytic leukemia (M3) the cell population distributed in the regions defined to represent neutrophils and eosinophils, the acute lymphoblastic leukemia (L1, L2) cell populations fell into two regions - those of Large Unstained Cells (LUC) and Lymphocytes, and in cases of chronic myelocytic leukemia, the cells fell into two regions consisting of neutrophils and HPX. It was concluded from this study that the differentials were useful in FAB classification of leukemias and clinical diagnosis of chronic myelocytic leukemia. In addition, two unusual types of cases were revealed - cases in which the neutrophil population had shifted into the regions of monocytes and LUCs, and cases in which the eosinophils shifted into the monocyte region. These kinds of results indicated how we might detect neutrophil or eosinophil populations with low peroxidase activity. Using the conventional eye count method these cases were undetectable, with the H6000 they were easily detectable.

INTRODUCTION

The Technicon H6000 System (Technicon Instrument Corporation, Tarrytown, N.Y., U.S.A.) automatically differentiates leukocytes using both cytochemical and optical methods. A leukocyte differential can be obtained by processing the leukocyte cytogram using the H6000. As the differential of leukocytes can be quite useful in the diagnosis and classification of a variety of leukemias, we studied the clinical utility of the H6000 in the analysis of blood samples from a wide range of leukemic cases. In addition, to study the ability of the H6000 to reveal peroxidase activity abnormalities in non-leukemic cases, we also screened many cases with a variety of non-leukemic diagnoses.

MATERIALS AND METHODS

The leukocyte cytograms and differentials generated in this study were produced as follows. Peripheral blood was collected, and after hemolysis (approximately 2 to 3 hours after collection), the leukocytes were stained for peroxidase activity using H_2O_2/4-chloro-1-naphthol as the chromogen. The cell size, based on forward light scatter, and peroxidase activity, based on absorbance photometry were determined for each cell in a sample by flow cytometry. Each of approximately 10,000 cells in each sample were determined in this way and were plotted by computer onto a two-dimensional graph where cell size is on the ordinate and peroxidase activity is on the abcissa (Fig. 1). The plotted leukocytes distributed into one of 6 predetermined regions which represent neutrophils, lymphocytes, monocytes, eosinophils, basophils, LUC, and HPX. The differential was then generated simply by counting all of the points in each of the 6 regions. This counting is performed by the H6000, which then produces a differential or rather, gives the percentage of cells found in each region. Wright-Giemsa stains were also done on blood smears from these patients, and the conventional eye count was also performed. The results from these two methods - H6000 differential and eye count - were compared.

Basophils distribute in the same region as the monocytes, and so they have to be stained with Alcian blue to be differentiated from the monocytes. Eosinophils, with the highest peroxidase activity, distribute in the region labelled 'EOS' in Fig. 1, whereas the 'LUC'

LEUKOCYTE CYTOGRAMS USING H6000

region contains large, peroxidase negative cells. Large, peroxidase positive cells distribute in the HPX region. Normally, only 0 to 1% of the cells will be found in the LUC and HPX regions.

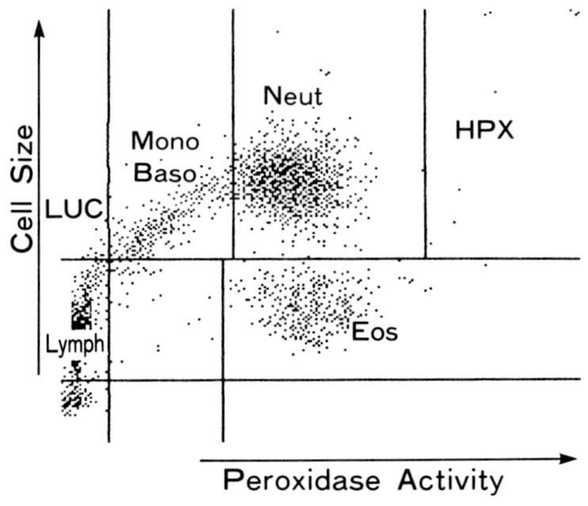

Fig. 1. Normal leukocyte cytogram using the H6000.

Neut; Neutrophils, Lymph; Lymphocytes, Mono; Monocytes, Eos; Eosinophils, Baso; Basophils, LUC; Large Unstained Cells, HPX; High Peroxidase Active Cells.

Differentials from a wide variety of both leukemic and non-leukemic clinical cases were studied. The leukemic cases included M1 and M2 acute myeloblastic leukemias, M3 acute promyelocytic leukemia, L1 and L2 acute lymphoblastic leukemias, and chronic myelocytic leukemia (CML). The non-leukemic cases studied included myelitis, aortitis syndrome, uterine cancer, gastric ulcer, lung cancer, Hashimoto's disease, pregnancy, diabetes mellitus, allergic purpura, traumatic injury, urticaria, iron-deficient anemia, and three cases of unknown diagnosis.

In addition to leukocyte cell population analysis, further studies were performed on blood smears from the patients, including Sudan black B stain for phospholipids, Neutrophil Alkaline Phosphatase Activity (NAP) measurement, the phospholipid reaction test, and the peroxidase histochemical stain.

RESULTS

Acute myeloblastic leukemia (M1).

The leukemia cells in M1 acute myeloblastic leukemia (ref. 1) are peroxidase positive and therefore distributed in the neutrophil and HPX regions on the cytogram. By the eye count, 89% of the cells in the leukemic cell population are myeloblasts. The H6000 leukocyte differential indicated that 86.3% of the cells were neutrophils and 14.1% were HPX (Fig. 2).

Acute myeloblastic leukemia (M2).

In the eye count, the cell population of M2 FAB-classified acute myeloblastic leukemia consisted of 58.0% myeloblasts, 2.0% promyelocytes, and 0.5% myelocytes. The cell population distributed widely in the cytogram throughout 4 regions - those of the neutrophils, monocytes, eosinophils, and HPX cells (Fig. 3). These cells are peroxidase positive. The H6000 differential also supports this as it revealed that 44.6% of the cells were neutrophils, 12.0% were monocytes, and 8.3% were HPX cells.

Acute promyelocytic leukemia (M3).

For M3 acute promyelocytic leukemia, the eye count indicated that 77% of the cells were promyelocytes, and in the cytogram the cells fell into the regions of neutrophils and eosinophils (Fig. 4) as these cells, like those in M2 acute myeloblastic leukemia, are peroxidase positive. The H6000 differential showed values for neutrophils and eosinophils of 50.7% and 36.3% respectively. The distinguishing characteristic of M3 acute promyelocytic leukemia, as compared to M1 and M2 acute myeloblastic leukemia, is the large number of cells which distribute in the eosinophil region of the cytogram. This is due to the even greater peroxidase activity of leukemic cells in M3 cases, as compared to M1 or M2 - a level of activity the same as that of eosinophils.

	Leukocyte Cytogram	Wright-Giemsa
	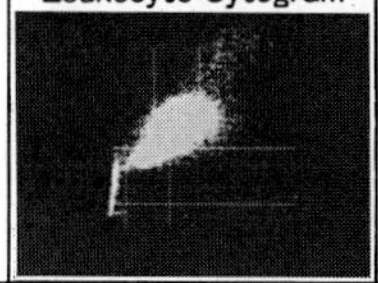	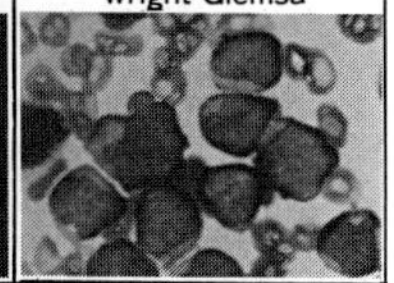
Differential	H6000(%)	Eye Count(%)
Neut	86.3	2.0
Lymph	7.4	4.5
Mono	4.8	3.5
Eos	1.3	0
Baso	0	0
LUC	0.1	—
HPX	14.1	—
Blast	—	89.0
Promyelo	—	1.0

Fig. 2. Acute myeloblastic leukemia (M1) according to the FAB classification.

(Leukocyte cytogram, Wright-Giemsa stain and the Leukocyte differential using the H6000 and the eye count are shown in Fig. 2 to Fig. 7.)

	Leukocyte Cytogram	Wright-Giemsa
	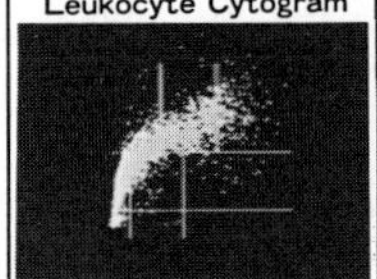	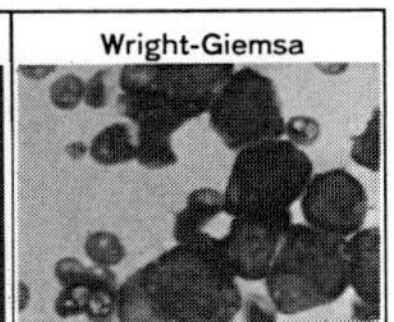
Differential	H6000(%)	Eye Count(%)
Neut	44.6	3.5
Lymph	41.4	35.0
Mono	12.0	0
Eos	0.8	0.5
Baso	0.1	0
LUC	1.1	—
HPX	8.3	—
Blast	—	58.0
Promyelo	—	2.0
Myelo	—	0.5

Fig. 3. Acute myeloblastic leukemia (M2).

Acute lymphoblastic leukemia (L1).

The L1 acute lymphoblastic leukemia cell population, when counted by eye, consisted of 62.5% lymphoblasts. These cells distribute in the lymphocyte and LUC regions in the cytogram (Fig. 5) because these cells are peroxidase negative. The H6000 differential reflects these results by indicating that 91.2% of the cells are lymphocytes and 6.5% are LUC.

Acute lymphoblastic leukemia (L2).

In the L2 acute lymphoblastic cell population there were 68.0% lymphoblasts according to the eye count. In the cytogram the cells distribute in the lymphocyte and LUC regions (Fig. 6) as these cells are peroxidase negative. Lymphocytes account for 74.3% of the cells in the H6000 differential, and LUC 5.8%.

LEUKOCYTE CYTOGRAMS USING H6000

Leukocyte Cytogram | Wright-Giemsa

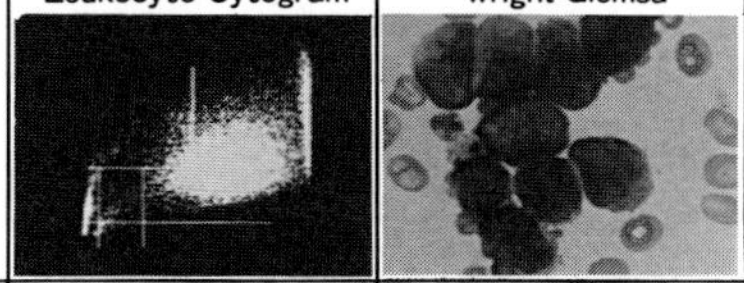

Differential	H6000 (%)	Eye Count (%)
Neut	50.7	2.0
Lymph	9.3	10.0
Mono	3.2	0
Eos	36.2	0
Baso	0.5	0
LUC	0.1	—
HPX	2.1	—
Blast	—	2.5
Promyelo	—	77.0
Myelo	—	8.5

Fig. 4. Acute promyelocytic leukemia (M3).

Leukocyte Cytogram | Wright-Giemsa

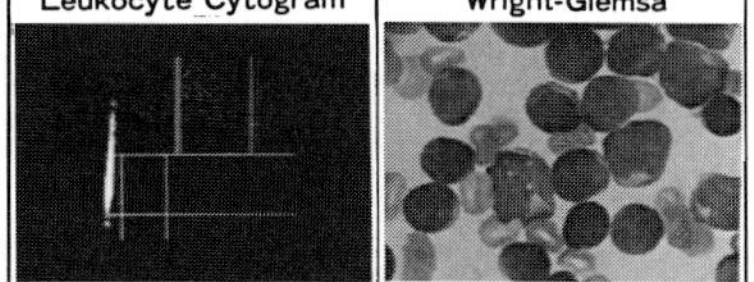

Differential	H6000 (%)	Eye Count (%)
Neut	1.7	0.5
Lymph	91.2	35.0
Mono	0.2	0.5
Eos	0.2	0
Baso	0.1	0
LUC	6.5	—
HPX	0.1	—
Blast	—	62.5
Aty-Lymph	—	1.5

Fig. 5. Acute lymphoblastic leukemia (L1).

Leukocyte Cytogram | Wright-Giemsa

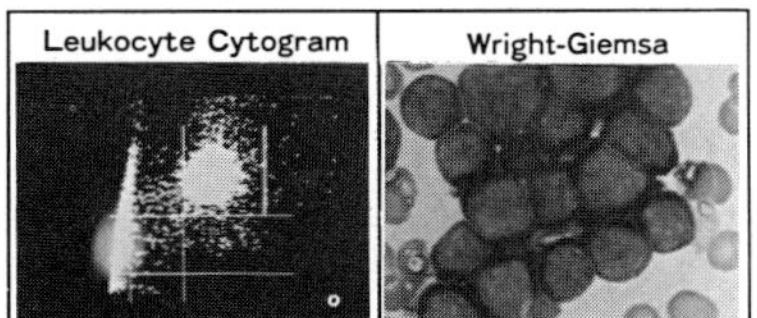

Differential	H6000 (%)	Eye Count (%)
Neut	17.7	20.5
Lymph	74.3	11.0
Mono	1.8	0
Eos	0.4	0
Baso	0	0
LUC	5.8	—
HPX	0.2	—
Blast	—	68.0

Fig. 6. Acute lymphoblastic leukemia (L2).

LEUKOCYTE CYTOGRAMS USING H6000

Chronic myelocytic leukemia (CML).

The chronic myelocytic leukemia cell population consisted of 7.3% myeloblasts, 8.0% promyelocytes, 6.0% myelocytes, and 4.0% metamyelocytes when counted by eye. This cell population distributed into two regions, that of the neutrophils and that of the HPX cells, as seen in Fig. 7. On the H6000 differential there are 80.7% neutrophils and 27% HPX cells. It is the large number of cells distributing in the HPX region which distinguishes this leukemia from the others. This distribution is due to the large number of myeloblasts, promyelocytes, myelocytes and metamyelocytes, all of which have greater peroxidase activity than neutrophils.

	Leukocyte Cytogram	Wright-Giemsa
	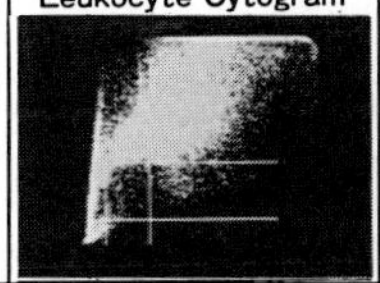	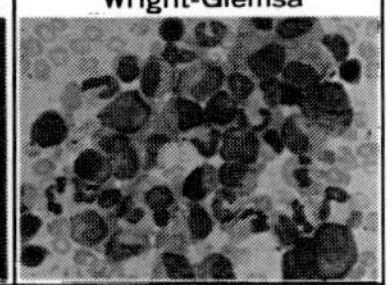
Differential	H6000 (%)	Eye Count(%)
Neut	80.7	58.3
Lymph	10.4	5.7
Mono	1.5	2.3
Eos	0.6	2.3
Baso	4.3	6.0
LUC	2.5	—
HPX	27.0	—
Blast	—	7.3
Promyelo	—	8.0
Myelo	—	6.0
Meta	—	4.0

Fig. 7. Chronic myelocytic leukemia.

Neutrophils with lowered peroxidase activity.

Six of the non-leukemic cases studied showed evidence of having neutrophils with lowered peroxidase activity. The results in these cases all looked like Fig. 8 - where the neutrophil population had apparently shifted over to the LUC and monocyte regions (indicated by the arrow) on the cytogram. This suggests that peroxidase activity of the neutrophils is decreased. The H6000 differential indicates the percentage of LUC to be 15.8%, and this is also seen in the cytogram itself (Table 1).

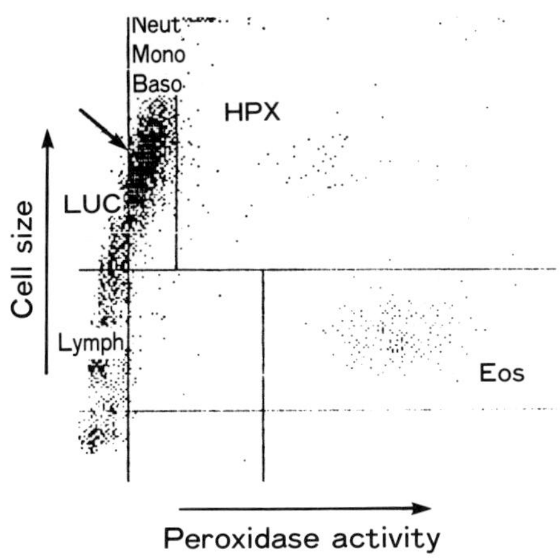

Fig. 8. Leukocyte cytogram of lowered neutrophil peroxidase activity using the H6000.

LEUKOCYTE CYTOGRAMS USING H6000

TABLE 1. Leukocyte differential of patient's peripheral blood of lowered neutrophil peroxidase activity using the H6000 and the eye count.

Differential	H6000(%)	Eye Count(%)
Neut	70.6	76.0
Lymph	11.7	13.0
Mono	–	9.0
Eos	1.9	2.0
Baso	0.3	0
HPX	2.1	–
LUC	15.8	–

In Fig. 9, when cells were stained for peroxidase activity using H_2O_2/Diaminobenzidine as a chromogen, the neutrophils were negative for the peroxidase reaction, as indicated by the arrow. This result reemphasizes that peroxidase activity of the neutrophils was decreased.

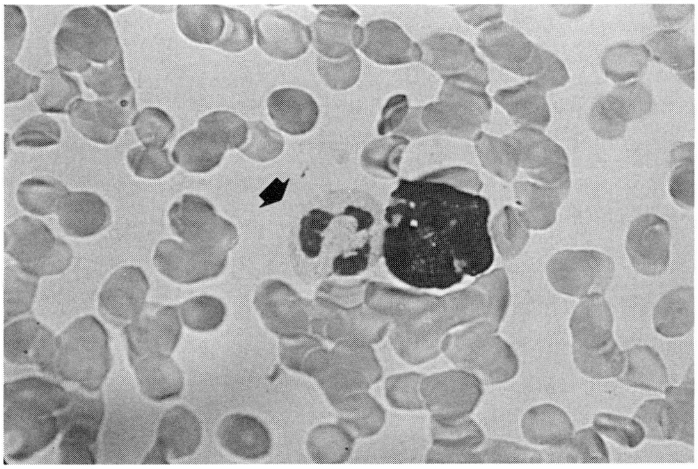

Fig. 9. Negative peroxidase stain of neutrophil (an arrow) and positive peroxidase stain of eosinophil of patient's peripheral blood using H_2O_2/Diaminobenzidine as a chromogen.

Upon analysis of their cytograms, six cases were found in which the neutrophils had lowered peroxidase activities. Four of these patients were female and two were male. At the time the cytogram was generated from their blood specimens, the diagnoses of these patients included one case of myelitis, one aortitis syndrome, one uterine cancer, one gastric ulcer, and two were unknown (Table 2).

Summarizing the results of morphological and cytochemical analyses of neutrophils from these cases, neutrophils in all of these cases were peroxidase negative and the phospholipid reaction was either negative or only weakly positive, and Neutrophil Alkaline Phosphatase (NAP) activity was low in one case, normal in four cases, and was not tested in one case. There were no other morphological abnormalities, such as in nuclear segmentation or cytoplasmic granulation (Table 3).

LEUKOCYTE CYTOGRAMS USING H6000

TABLE 2. Patients with lowered neutrophil peroxidase activity found using the H6000.

No	Name	Sex	Age	Clinical Diagnosis
1	F.N.	F.	54	Myelitis
2	M.M.	F.	16	Aortitis syndrome
3	K.M.	F.	43	(?)
4	Y.N.	F.	60	Uterine cancer
5	N.H.	M.	37	(?)
6	Y.Y.	M.	24	Gastric ulcer

TABLE 3. Morphological and cytochemical characteristics of neutrophils with lowered peroxidase activity.

*N; Normal, NAP; Neutrophil Alkaline Phosphatase, N.T.; Not Tested.

Case No.	Neutrophils (%)	LUC* (%)	Percentage of lobulation No. of lobes					Evaluation*	NAP*		Phospholipid Reaction
			stab	II	III	IV	V		Rate (%)	Score	
1	65.5	7.2	4	36	28	32		N	59	147	N.T.
2	49.5	2.5	4	24	48	20	4	N	72	134	±
3	54.0	13.3	2	44	48	6		N	78	223	−
4	88.5	N.T.	5	46	42	7		N	91	292	±
5	65.0	2.3	2	32	46	18	2	N	45	88	±
6	76.0	15.8	18	46	24	11	1	N	N.T.	N.T.	−

Eosinophils with lowered peroxidase activity.

In cases with eosinophils with lowered peroxidase activity, the eosinophil population was observed in the monocyte region in the cytogram (Fig. 10), as indicated by the arrow. From this, it was concluded that eosinophil peroxidase activity must have been low. According to the leukocyte differential using the H6000, and as seen in the cytogram itself, the monocytes were 20.7%, and eosinophils were as low as 0.2%, but in the leukocyte differential using the eye count, 13% of the leukocytes were eosinophils (Table 4). In Fig. 11, one can see that the peroxidase reaction was negative for eosinophils, as indicated by the arrow, and was positive for the neutrophils. From these results it is evident that eosinophil phospholipid reaction was negative and the neutrophil phospholipid reaction was positive when using the Sudan black B phospholipid stain.

LEUKOCYTE CYTOGRAMS USING H6000

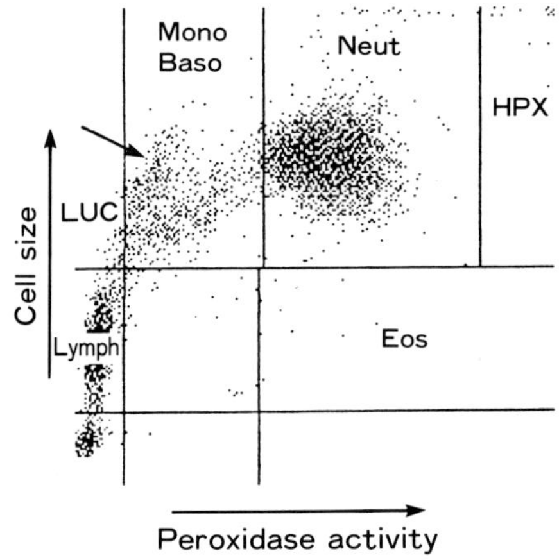

Fig. 10. Leukocyte cytogram of lowered eosinophil peroxidase activity using the H6000.

TABLE 4. Leukocyte differential of patient's peripheral blood of lowered eosinophil peroxidase activity using the H6000 and eye count.

Differential	H6000(%)	Eye Count(%)
Neut	50.7	44.0
Lymph	26.5	27.5
Mono	20.7	12.5
Eos	0.2	13.0
Baso	1.3	1.5
HPX	0.6	–
LUC	0.1	–

Nine cases with low peroxidase activity eosinophils were found using the cytogram and differential. Four males and five females showed these kinds of results. At the time the H6000 differential was generated the diagnoses for these cases were one case of lung cancer, one of Hashimoto's disease, one case of pregnancy, one of diabetes mellitus, one allergic purpura, one traumatic injury, one urticaria, one iron-deficient anemia, and one unknown (Table 5 & 6).

As seen in the Wright-Giemsa stained blood smears from these patients, some morphological abnormalities were found in the eosinophils (Fig. 12). Abnormal nuclear morphology (B and H) and a reduction in cytoplasmic granulation (B and D to J) can be seen in these smears. Eosinophils in all of these cases were peroxidase negative and phospholipid reaction negative, one case showed a tendency toward hypersegmentation in the nuclei of the eosinophils and the other eight cases showed normal segmentation. Furthermore, eosinophils in two other cases showed abnormal nuclear morphology and eight cases showed a reduction in granulation.

LEUKOCYTE CYTOGRAMS USING H6000

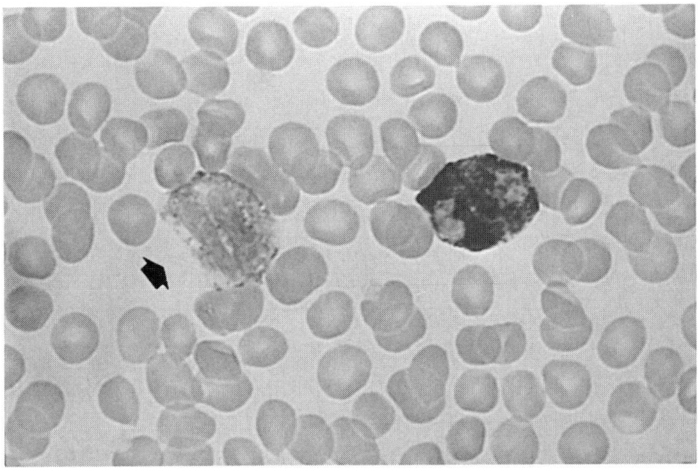

Fig. 11. Negative peroxidase stain of eosinophil (an arrow) and positive peroxidase stain of neutrophil of patient's peripheral blood using H_2O_2/Diaminobenzidine as a chromogen.

TABLE 5. Patients with lowered eosinophil peroxidase activity found using the H6000.

No	Name	Sex	Age	Clinical Diagnosis
1	M.M.	M.	45	Lung cancer
2	T.S.	F.	41	Hashimoto's disease
3	S.O.	F.	33	Pregnancy
4	Y.H.	M.	66	Diabetes Mellitus,Gallstone
5	T.H.	M.	4	(Allergic) purpura
6	K.W.	F.	29	(?)
7	M.O.	F.	54	Traumatic injury
8	H.S.	M.	31	Urticaria
9	N.I.	F.	43	Iron deficiency anemia

DISCUSSION

The results of this study indicate that the leukemic cell population in acute and chronic leukemias distributes characteristically on the flow cytometric cytogram into regions corresponding to predetermined levels of peroxidase activity and cell size and that this distribution is reflected in the H6000 differential generated from analysis of the cytogram. This has been seen in other studies as well (ref. 2). The cytogram and H6000 differential are therefore thought to be useful in supporting the FAB classification of acute leukemias and the clinical diagnosis of chronic myelocytic leukemia (ref. 2 & 3). Furthermore, it is thought that cases in which either neutrophil or eosinophil peroxidase activity is low can be more easily identified in routine examinations by using the leukocyte cytograms and by processing the cytograms using the H6000 to generate a differential (ref. 4, 5, 6, 7, 8, 9, & 10).

LEUKOCYTE CYTOGRAMS USING H6000

TABLE 6. Morphological and cytochemical characteristics of eosinophils with lowered peroxidase activity.

*N; Normal, HS; Hypersegmentation, SG; Scarce Granulation, DG; Decreased Granulation.

Case No.	Eosinophils (%)	Percentage of lobulation					Evaluation*	Phospholipid and Peroxidase Reactions*	Granulation*
		No. of lobes							
		meta	I	II	III	IV			
1	13.0		16	82	2		N	–	N
2	2.0		20	50	30		N	–	SG
3	4.5	+	10	83	7		N	–	DG ~ N
4	0.5		27	60	13		N	–	DG ~ SG
5	1.5		10	80	10		N	–	SG
6	2.5		10	83	7		N	–	DG ~ SG
7	1.0	+	44	52	4		N	–	SG
8	4.0		2	54	44		HS ?	–	N ~ DG
9	3.0		10	56	34		N	–	DG

Fig. 12. Wright-Giemsa stain of eosinophils of normal and patient's peripheral blood.

A; Normal, B to J; Patients.

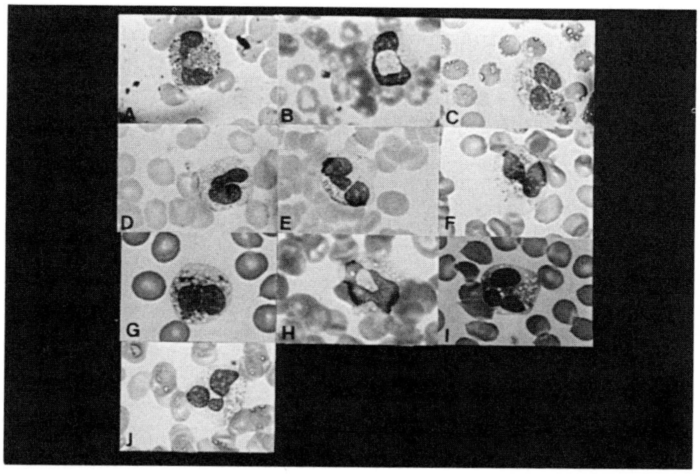

REFERENCES

1. J.M. Bennet, D. Catovsky, M.T. Daniel, G. Flandrin, D.A.G. Galton, H.R. Granlnick and C. Salton, Brit.J.Haemat. 33, 451-458 (1976).
2. B. Drewinko, P. Bollinger, C. Brailas, S. Moyle, J. Wyatt, E. Simson, D. Johnston and J.M. Trujillo, Brit.J.Haemat. 65, 27-36 (1987).
3. B. Drewinko, P. Bollinger, C. Brailas, J. Wyatt, E. Simson and J.M. Trujillo, Brit.J.Haemat. 67 157-165 (1987).
4. F. Lanza, A. Fietta, S. Spisani, G.L. Castoldi and S. Traniello, J.Clin.Lab.Immunol., 22, 175-180 (1987).
5. L. Pasini, G. Briani, P. Boccato, and U. Lippi, Haematologica 70, 83-85 (1985).
6. J.J.M.L. Hoffmann and A.G.W.M. Tielens, Blut, 54, 165-169 (1987).

LEUKOCYTE CYTOGRAMS USING H6000

7. P. Lepelly, M. Zandecki, S. Paquet, B. Lerche, M.H. Estienne, P. Fenax, G. Torpier and A. Cosson, Eur.J.Haematol. 39, 77-81 (1987).
8. M.D. Valdes and M.A. Calero, Acta haemat. 78, 265 (1987).
9. F. Lanza, G.I. Castoldi and M. Masotti, Blut 56, 143-144 (1988).
10. T. Takubo, T. Kikuchi, H. Harunari, A. Takeuchi and S. Inai, Clin.Lab.Haemat. 9, 289-296 (1987).

The reticulocyte counter sysmex R-1000

Keiji Fujimoto

R&D Department, TOA Medical Electronics Co.,Ltd. POBOX 1002

KOBE,JAPAN.

Abstract - The SYSMEX R-1000 is a fully automated instrument which measures absolute number and percentage of reticulocytes in whole blood specimen by means of a gas laser and a dye. The instrument requires 100 μl whole blood for measurement. 60 samples can be measured in one hour. The reproducibility and the precision were good for routine and investigation purposes with time saving.

INTRODUCTION

Recent development of fully automated instruments in clinical laboratories can help medical technologists to reduce their time for measurements a lot of kind of patients parameters. In the hematology laboratories, since about ten years ago, fully automated blood cell counters have been introduced.
Using those instruments, counting data of white blood cells(WBC),red blood cells(RBC),platelets(PLT) and hemoglobin concentration (HGB),which are the most basic clinical data of patients, can be obtained with high reliability in a minute. Reticulocyte counts are also one of the basic parameters which tells the red cell production ability of bone marrow (ref.1,ref.2).
The measurement process by manual, however, is very time-consuming and low-reliable (ref.3,ref.4).
Recently, the SYSMEX fully automated reticulocyte counter R-1000 (TOA Medical Electronics,Kobe,Japan) was introduced in the market. In this paper, the basic evaluation of this instrument is described.

GENERAL EXPLANATION OF THE INSTRUMENT

The instrument aspirates 100 μl anticoagulated whole blood. After 90 seconds, on a CRT which is assembled in the instrument, reticulocyte percentage(RET%) ,reticulocyte absolute number(RET#) and RBC absolute number(RBC#) are displayed with a scattergram of analyzed cells. The scattergram shows signal intensity of fluorescence by each counting cell excited by argon-ion laser belong to the horizontal axis and signal height of forward scattered by each counting cell belong to the vertical axis. The fluorescence intensity indicates the concentration of DNA and RNA in a analyzed cell. The intensity of forward scatter indicates the cell size. Fig.1 shows one example of the scattergram.

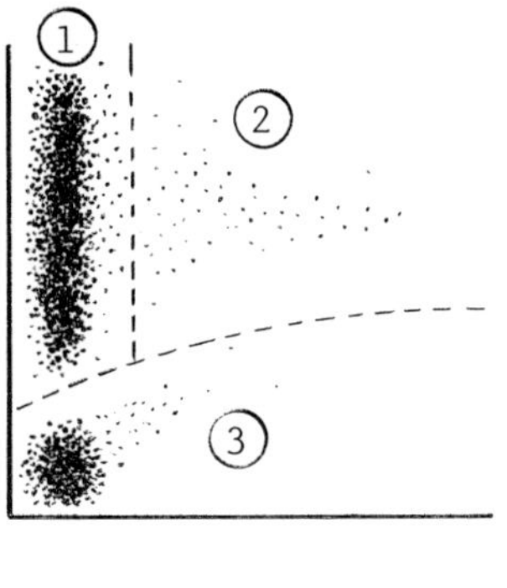

Fig.1. An example of the scattergram
The horizontal axis shows intensity of fluorescence and the vertical axis shows intensity of forward scatter.
Matured red cells are in 1 area.
Platelets are in 3 area.
Reticulocytes are in 2 area.
Two dotted lines are the moving discriminators between 1,2 and 3 area.

Assembled computer algorism automatically separates reticulocytes area from maturated erythrocytes(MRBC) and platelets area. A fixed dişcriminator also separates reticulocytes from large stained cell like WBCs,erythroblasts and nuclear RBCs(NRBC).
500 counting data can be stored in the memory. The scattergrams can be printouted on time with counting data.
The lapped sequence program for fluid circuits accomplished 60 samples measurement per one hour.
Optionally, a fully automated sampler,on which 100 samples can be set, is available(ref.5).

MATERIAL AND METHOD

Samples - EDTA-2K anticoagulated whole blood samples were used in this evaluation. Except special purpose, samples were from healthy donors.
For the confirmation of signal positions of WBCs and erythloblasts in the scattergram, a ALL(acute lymphocytic leukemia) and a bone marrow specimens were used.

Stain for manual method - For the comparison of the counting results by the instrument and by manual eye count, new methylene blue(NMB) was used by Brecher's method (ref.6,ref.7).

RESULTS

Reproducibility - Using three samples which had different concentration of reticulocytes (i.e. low, normal and high reticulocytes specimens), the reproducibility of the instrument was examined. Table.1 shows the result.

Table 1. The reproducibility of RET%,RET# and RBC# for Low-,Normal- and High-RET specimens.

	RET %		RET #		RBC #	
	X (%)	C.V.	X ($x10^3/\mu l$)	C.V.	X ($x10^6/\mu l$)	C.V.
LOW	0.24	12.1%	9.8	11.8%	4.12	0.9%
NORMAL	0.78	6.8%	35.9	7.1%	4.60	0.5%
HIGH	5.43	3.3%	165.2	3.8%	3.04	0.9%

(Each specimen was measured 10 times)

Comparability of R-1000 and Manual method - Using 135 samples, the comparability of R-1000 and manual method was examined. The reproducibility of manual eye count(i.e. 1000 or 2000 RBC count) is poor (ref.3,ref.4). Then in this evaluation, 6000 RBC eye count was done for each 135 samples. That is each of three technologists counted 2000 RBCs (i.e. 3 persons x 2000 RBCs). Fig.2 shows the comparability of R-1000 and manual method.

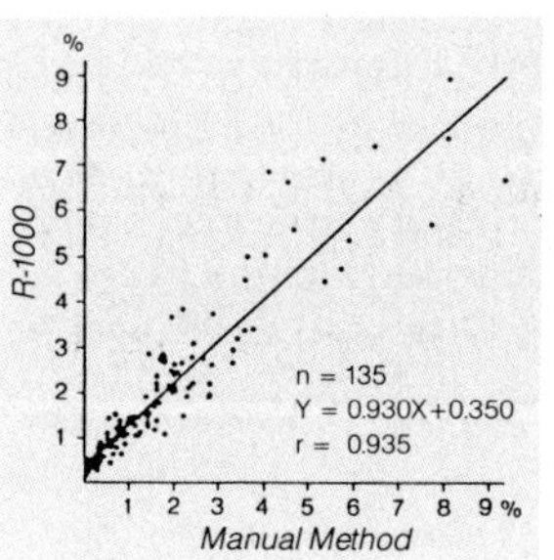

Fig.2. Correlation with results of manual method.
6000 RBCs were counted for each specimen.

Data stability - Data stability was examined for 5 samples which were normal samples. Each specimen was divided into two aliquots and one of each aliquot was storaged at room temperature and another was storaged at 4°c.
Each aliquot was measured by R-1000 on just after taking specimen from donors ,after 2 hours,4 hours,8 hours,24 hours and 48 hours.
Fig.3 is the profile of data stability. Using t-test , data differences between 4°c and room temperature storaged samples were examined.
Until 8 hours in all 5 specimens, there was no significant difference. After 24 and 48 hours, data of samples storaged at room temperature showed much lower than samples' storaged at 4°c depend on the time.

Fig.3. Time dependence of reticulocyte counts storaged at 4°c and room temperature.
(Only two of five samples data were shown. Other samples had the same tendency)

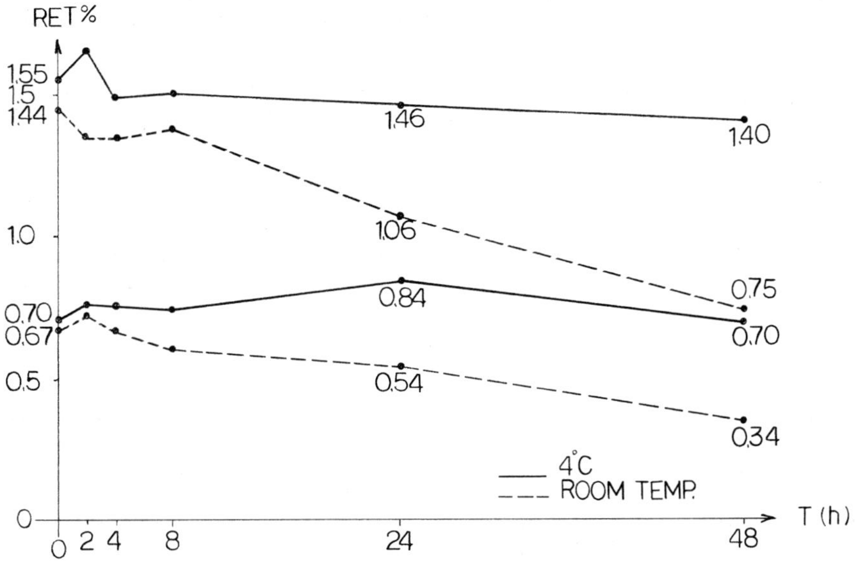

Discrimination of large stained cells - Auramine-O is the stain of R-1000 which can stain not only RNA but also DNA. Then the discrimination of reticulocytes and large stained cells is important.(ref.8)
Using a bone marrow specimen and a ALL specimen, the signal positions of WBCs and erythroblasts in scattergrams were confirmed.
The reticulocytes area in scattergrams are between the lower moving discriminator and the 254th channel. The area of WBCs was over the 600th channel which was not displayed on CRT. The area of erythroblasts were between the 300th channel and around the 500th channel. Those positions of WBCs and erythroblasts were far from the positions of reticulocytes.

Linearlity - Data linearlity was examined using purified matured red cells and purified reticulocyte. Some different mixing ratio of red cells and reticulocytes were measured by R-1000 and by manual. Manual data were calibrated by those hemoglobin concentrations. Between 0.1% and 15% of reticulocyte concentration, the linearlity of data was exellent. Over 15%, however, data had the tendency to be saturated a little.

DISCUSSION

R-1000 analyzes about 30,000 cells in one measurement. In normal samples, the concentration ratio of WBC:RBC:PLT:RET is 1:1000:30:10. Then around 300 reticulocytes are analyzed in one measurement.
The theoretical reproducibility in C.V.(Coefficient of variation) is

$$C.V. = \frac{100}{(N)^{\frac{1}{2}}} \%$$

where N is the total counted number of reticulocyte

Then in this case

$$C.V. = \frac{100}{(300)^{\frac{1}{2}}} \% = 5.8\%$$

Actual C.V. in normal specimen was 6.8% (Table.1.),which was nearly the same of theoretical value.
In current method(i.e. manual eye count), about 20 reticulocytes were counted by 2000 red cell count in normal specimens. Then the C.V. of manual method is

$$C.V. = \frac{100}{(20)^{\frac{1}{2}}} = 22.4\%$$

Those calculations indicate the R-1000 has much better reproducibility than manual eye count.
The definition of reticulocyte has been discussed(ref.1). In routine,even if the definition is concluded, there is a lot of kind of cells which require careful observation to technologists for avoiding mis-read as reticulocytes. The R-1000 avoids those mis-separations by means of two moving discriminators and a fixed discriminator (ref.5).
The stability data were interesting for the issue of reticulocyte maturation in vitro. Because of poor reproducibility of manual method, the conclusion of reticulocyte maturation in vitro has not been gotten.
The R-1000 counted decreased reticulocytes after 24 and 48 hours for room temperature storaged samples. This phenomenon suggests the maturation of reticulocytes in vitro. In the opposite side, this may suggest the interaction of Auramine-O and the membrane of stainable cells.
The linearlity of R-1000 was acceptable. Generally, the most important range of reticulocyte count is so-called low abnormal samples. In such low range, R-1000 can get reliable data which is useful for monitoring bone marrow activity after bone marrow transplant or during treatment of amemia.

REFERENCES

1. J.F.Koepke,J.A.Koepke, Clin.Lab.Haemat.,8,169-179 (1986)
2. E.W.Friedman, Diagnostic Medicine, July,29-33 (1984)
3. R.A.Savage,D.P.Skoog,A.Rabinovitch, Blood Cells, 11,97-112 (1985)
4. E.R.Greenberg, J.R.Beck, Arch.Pathol.Lab.Med., 108, 396-398 (1984)
5. T.Takami et.al.,Sysmex Journal, 2, 18-26 (1988)
6. C.A.Finch, P.N.Marshall, G.Brecher, F.E.Trobaugh, O.W.van Assendelft, NCCLS Proposed standard, H16P,225-233 (1985)
7. G.Brecher, Am.J.Clin.Pathol., 19, 895-896 (1949)
8. L.Brand, J.R.Gohlke, Ann.Rev.Biochem., 41,843-864 (1972)